Community Health Nursing–II

for GNM Nursing Students

(As per the New Syllabus of INC for GNM)

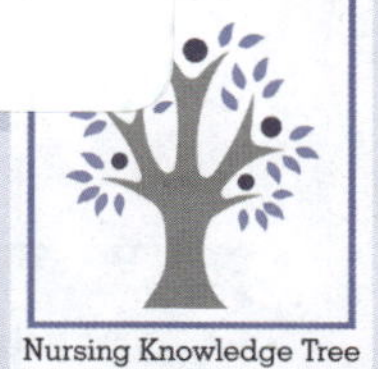

—— **Second Edition** ——

Lt. Col. KK GILL RN, RM, DNE, BSc (N) PB, MSc (CHN)

Former Principal
State Institute of Nursing and Paramedical Sciences, Badal, Punjab
and
Amar Professional College of Nursing, Mohali, Punjab

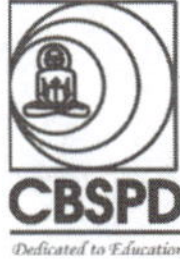

CBS Publishers & Distributors Pvt Ltd

• New Delhi • Bengaluru • Chennai • Kochi • Kolkata • Lucknow • Mumbai
• Hyderabad • Jharkhand • Nagpur • Patna • Pune • Uttarakhand

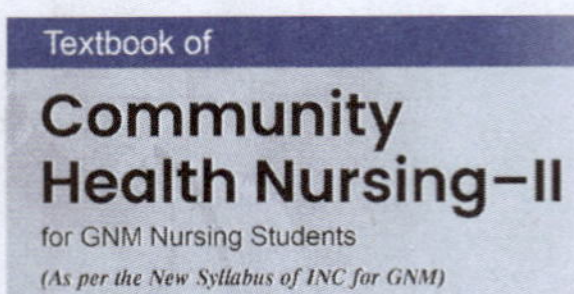

ISBN: 978-81-977500-2-1

Copyright © Publishers

Reprint: 2026

Second Edition: 2025

First Edition: 2020

Published by **Satish Kumar Jain** and produced by **Varun Jain** for

CBS Publishers and Distributors Pvt Ltd

4819/XI Prahlad Street, 24 Ansari Road, Daryaganj, New Delhi 110 002, India.
Ph: +91-11-23289259, 23266861, 23266867   Website: www.cbspd.com
Fax: 011-23243014
e-mail: delhi@cbspd.com; cbspubs@airtelmail.in.

Corporate Office: 204 FIE, Industrial Area, Patparganj, Delhi 110 092
Ph: +91-11-4934 4934   Fax: 4934 4935
e-mail: feedback@cbspd.com

Branches

- **Bengaluru:** Seema House 2975, 17th Cross, K.R. Road, Banashankari 2nd Stage, Bengaluru-560 070, Karnataka
  Ph: +91-80-26771678/79   Fax: +91-80-26771680   e-mail: bangalore@cbspd.com

- **Chennai:** 7, Subbaraya Street, Shenoy Nagar, Chennai-600 030, Tamil Nadu
  Ph: +91-44-26680620, 26681266   Fax: +91-44-42032115   e-mail: chennai@cbspd.com

- **Kochi:** 68/1534, 35, 36-Power House Road, Opp. KSEB, Cochin-682018, Kochi, Kerala
  Ph: +91-484-4059061-65   Fax: +91-484-4059065   e-mail: kochi@cbspd.com

- **Kolkata:** Hind Ceramics Compound, 1st Floor, 147, Nilganj Road, Belghoria, Kolkata-700056, West Bengal
  Ph: +91-033-2563-3055/56   e-mail: kolkata@cbspd.com

- **Lucknow:** Basement, Khushnuma Complex, 7-Meerabai Marg (Behind Jawahar Bhawan), Lucknow-226001, Uttar Pradesh
  Ph: +0522-4000032   e-mail: tiwari.lucknow@cbspd.com

- **Mumbai:** PWD Shed, Gala No. 25/26, Ramchandra Bhatt Marg, Next to J.J. Hospital Gate No. 2, Opp. Union Bank of India, Noor Baug, Mumbai-400009, Maharashtra
  Ph: +91-22-66661880/89   Fax: +91-22-24902342   e-mail: mumbai@cbspd.com

Representatives

• **Hyderabad**	+91-9885175004		• **Jharkhand**	+91-9811541605
• **Nagpur**	+91-9421945513		• **Patna**	+91-9334159340
• **Pune**	+91-9623451994		• **Uttarakhand**	+91-9716462459

Printed at : Goyal Offset Works Pvt. Ltd. Haryana

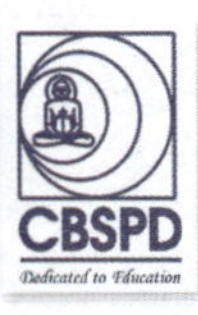

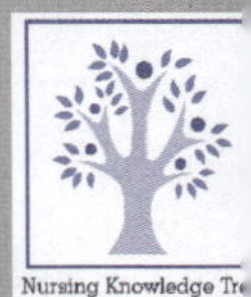

CBS Nursing Knowledge Tree

Extends its Tribute to

Florence Nightingale

For glorifying the role of women as nurses,
For holding the title of " The Lady with the Lamp,"
For working tirelessly for humanity—
Florence Nightingale will always be
remembered for her
selfless and memorable services to the
human race.

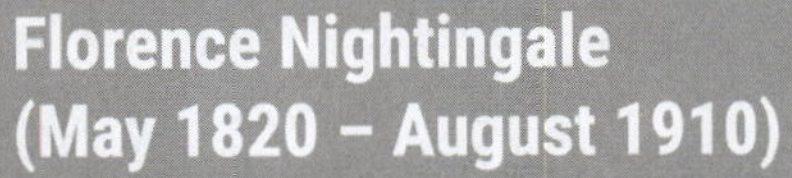

Florence Nightingale
(May 1820 – August 1910)

Dedicated to

My family for their unconventional
support and constant encouragement
throughout the venture.

Preface to the Second Edition

Community Health Nursing is a rapidly growing field. According to Global Commitment of Health for All and to achieve **Millennium Development Goals** (MDGs), the Comprehensive Primary Health Care (CPHC) has been implemented through health and wellness centers (HWCs) by transforming existing Sub Centers (SCs), and Primary Health Centers (PHCs) into the basic pillars of Ayushman Bharat as a foundation of India's Health System.

The role of Accredited Social Health Activist (ASHA) has expanded. ASHA's roles now include educating and promoting health, facilitating access to health services, providing first aid, keeping records and improving sanitation. A Community Health Officer (CHO) is appointed to coordinate and accelerate the services of community health nursing team at HWC-SC and HWC-PHC.

COVID-19 has been added under the epidemiology of communicable diseases. The book is updated according to the changes made in the delivery of comprehensive primary healthcare. I hope that this edition will be useful for nursing students, teachers and other healthcare professionals to meet their requirements.

Lt. Col. KK Gill (Retd.)

Preface to the First Edition

Nurses are the frontline fighters in the battle for health and wellness of society. They are the backbone of the healthcare delivery system at all levels, be it rural or urban community, hospitals, clinics or industries. Community Health Nursing is a multidisciplinary, rapidly growing subject. The primary objective of community health nursing is to help people attain an optimal level of health through healthy lifestyle. Sound basic knowledge of community health nursing will help nursing students to assess health problems of community and take appropriate action at grass root level.

The community health nurse needs to know about the community, its social and cultural patterns, principles of community health nursing, community diagnosis, community development, expanded health programs and roles and responsibilities of community health nurse in shaping the health-seeking behavior of the community.

It gives me immense pleasure to present this book titled *Textbook of Community Health Nursing–II for GNM Nursing Students*. This book is not only useful for students but also for the educators.

It is written in simple language according to new syllabus of GNM prescribed by the Indian Nursing Council for Community Health Nursing-II.

This book will meet the requirements of the students and will help in strengthening their basic knowledge of the subject so that they can become better equipped to provide primary health care to the community, thus keeping the commitment of the country to achieve "Health for All".

I invite constructive comments and suggestions from students, teachers and experts for the improvement of this book in future editions.

Lt. Col. KK Gill (Retd.)

Acknowledgments

First of all, I must bow my head before the Almighty God for bestowing upon me the strength, courage and wisdom to sustain myself through this endeavor. Writing a book is like undertaking a long journey of ardor and self-discovery, and without a guiding light that constantly shows the way, an author is bound to get lost in the vast sea of knowledge.

I extend my deep sense of gratitude to my children, **Dr Navneet Gill** and **Er. Kamalpreet Singh Gill.** Without their constant presence by my side, the completion of this herculean endeavor would not have been possible.

I would like to thank **Mr Satish Kumar Jain** (Chairman) and **Mr Varun Jain** (Managing Director), M/s CBS Publishers and Distributors Pvt Ltd for providing me the platform in bringing out the book. I have no words to describe the role, efforts, inputs and initiatives undertaken by **Mr Bhupesh Aarora** [Sr. Vice President – Publishing and Marketing (Health Sciences Division)] for helping and motivating me.

I sincerely thank the entire CBS team for bringing out the book with utmost care and attractive presentation. I would like to thank Ms Nitasha Arora (Assistant General Manager – Publishing) and Dr Anju Dhir (Sr. Product Manager cum Commissioning Editor) for their publishing support. I would also like to extend my thanks to Ms Surbhi Gupta (Sr. Editor cum Team Lead), Mr Ashutosh Pathak (Assistant Production Manager cum TL) and all the production team members for devoting laborious hours in editing, designing and typesetting the book.

Reviewers

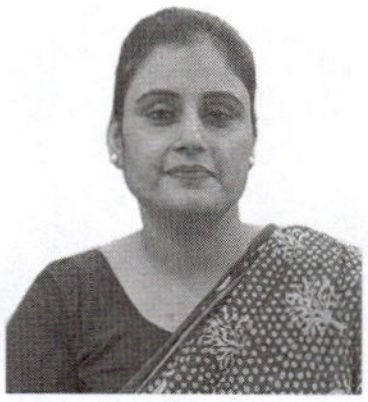

Amritpal Kaur
PhD (N), MSc (Community Health Nursing)
Professor cum Vice Principal
SGL Nursing College
Jalandhar, Punjab

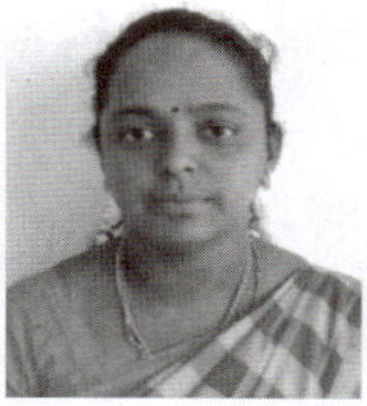

Anbumalar J
MSc (Community Health Nursing)
Vice Principal
White Memorial College of Nursing
Attoor, Veeyanoor, Tamil Nadu

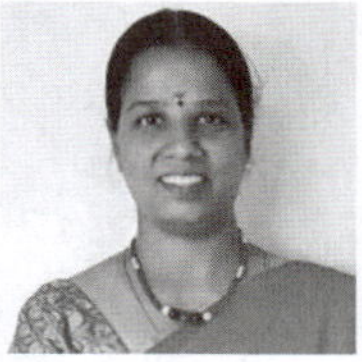

Arulmozhi Baskaran P M
PhD (N), MSc (Community Health Nursing)
Principal
PES University Institute of Nursing
Bengaluru, Karnataka

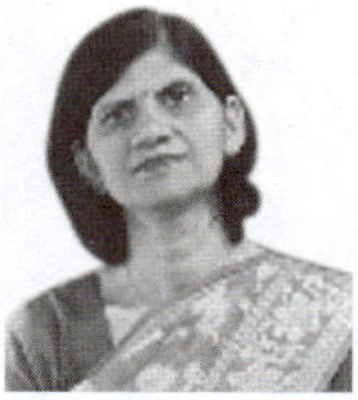

Bandana
PhD (N), MSc (Community Health Nursing)
Principal
Shri Lal Bahadur Shastri Government College of Nursing
Mandi, Himachal Pradesh

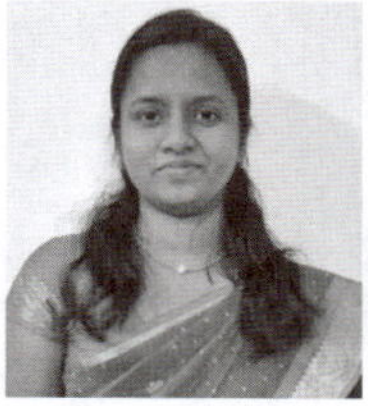

Deva Pon Pushpam
PhD Scholar, MSc (Community Health Nursing)
Professor cum HOD
BEE ENN College of Nursing
Jammu and Kashmir

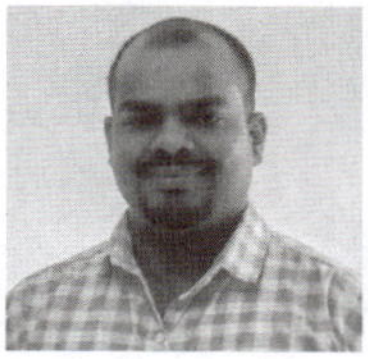

Dinesh Kumar Kachhawa
MSc (Community Health Nursing)
Professor cum Vice Principal
Sunder Devi Nursing College
Bhopal, Madhya Pradesh

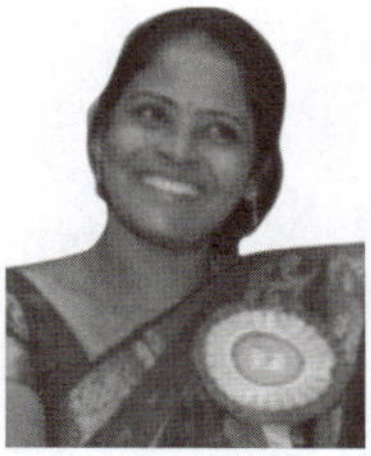

Kalpana Boddu
PhD Scholar, MSc (Community Health Nursing)
Professor
Sree Narayana Nursing College
Nellore, Andhra Pradesh

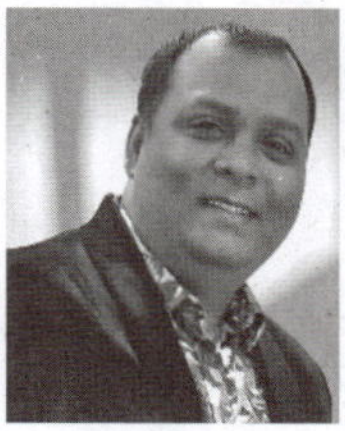

Pratul Prasann Nand
PhD (N), MSc (Community Health Nursing)
Vice Principal
Sanjivani Institute of Technology
Bilaspur, Chhattisgarh

The names of the reviewers are arranged in alphabetical order.

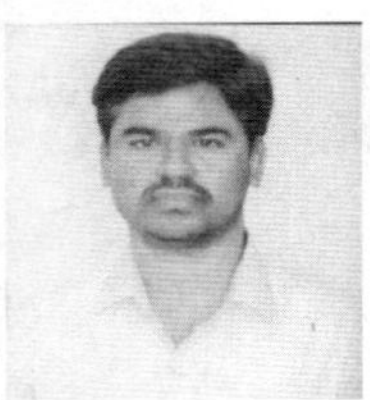

Ramakrishna Degani
MSc (Community Health Nursing)

Professor & HOD
Adesh University
Bathinda, Punjab

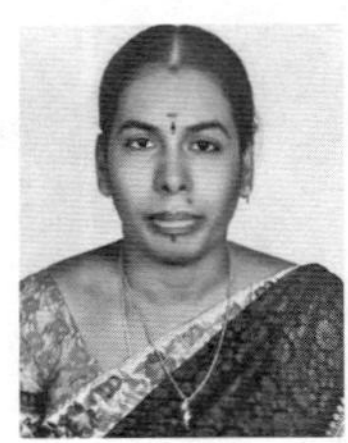

Viruthasarani K
PhD Scholar, MSc (Community Health Nursing)

Professor cum Vice Principal
Vivekanandha Nursing College
Pondicherry

The names of the reviewers are arranged in alphabetical order.

Dear Reader,

Nursing Education has a rich history, often characterized by traditional teaching techniques that have evolved over time. Primarily, teaching took place within classroom settings. Lectures, textbooks, and clinical rotations were the core teaching tools; and students majorly relied on textbooks by local or foreign publishers for quality education. However, today, technology has completely transformed the field of nursing education, making it an integral part of the curriculum. It has evolved to include a range of technological tools that enhance the learning experience and better prepare students for clinical practice.

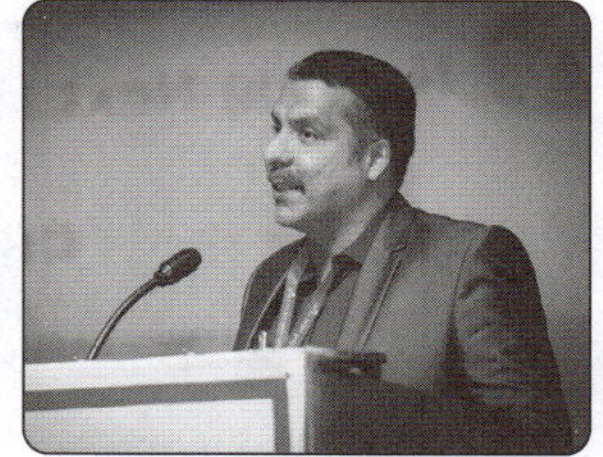

As publishers, we've been contributing to the field of Medical Science, Nursing and Allied Sciences and earned the trust of many. By supporting **Indian authors**, coupled with **nursing webinars and conferences**, we have paved an easier path for aspiring nurses, empowering them to excel in national and state level exams. With this, we're not only enhancing the quality of patient care but also enabling future nurses to adapt to new challenges and innovations in the rapidly evolving world of healthcare. Following the ideology of **Bringing learning to people instead of people going for learning**, so far, we've been doing our part by:

- Developing quality content by qualified and well-versed authors
- Building a strong community of faculty and students
- Introducing a smart approach with Digital/Hybrid Books, and
- Offering simulation Nursing Procedures, etc.

Innovative teaching methodologies, such as modern-age Phygital Books, have sparked the interest of the Next-Gen students in pursuing advanced education. The enhancement of educational standards through **Omnipresent Knowledge Sharing Platforms** has further facilitated learning, bridging the gap between doctors and nurses.

At Nursing Next Live, a sister concern of CBS Publishers & Distributors, we have long recognized the immense potential within the nursing field. Our journey in innovating nursing education has allowed us to make substantial and meaningful contributions. With the vision of strengthening learning at every stage, we have introduced several plans that cater to the specific needs of the students, including but not limited to **Plan UG** for undergraduates, **Plan MSc** for postgraduate aspirants, **Plan FDP** for upskilling faculties, **SDL** for integrated learning and **Plan NP** for bridging the gap between theoretical & practical learning. Additionally, we have successfully completed seven series of our **Target High** Book in a very short period, setting a milestone in the education industry. We have been able to achieve all this just with the sole vision of laying the foundation of diversified knowledge for all. With the rise of a new generation of educated, tech-savvy individuals, we anticipate even more remarkable advancements in the coming years.

We take immense pride in our achievements and eagerly look forward to the future, brimming with new opportunities for innovation, growth and collaborations with experienced minds such as yourself who can contribute to our mission as Authors, Reviewers and/or Faculties. Together, let's foster a generation of nurses who are confident, competent, and prepared to succeed in a technology-driven healthcare system.

Mr Bhupesh Aarora
(Sr Vice President – Publishing & Marketing)
bhupeshaarora@cbspd.com| +91 95553 53330

Special Features of the Book

LEARNING OBJECTIVES

After the completion of the unit, the readers will be able to:
- Explain the health systems in India.
- Identify the areas of responsibility of central government, state government, center and state with regard to healthcare.
- Describe the local self-government in urban areas of districts in India.
- Describe the structure and functions of healthcare organization.

Learning Objectives given in all the units focus on the areas that a student shall gain after completing the unit.

UNIT OUTLINE

- Introduction
- Health
- Community
- Public Health
- Community Health
- Community Health Nursing
- Organization of Health System in India

Every unit starts with a **Unit Outline** that gives the glimpse of the content covered in the unit.

KEY TERMS

- **Community:** A group of people living together in a particular geographical area.
- **Community health:** It is the science and art of preventing disease, prolonging life and promoting health through organized efforts. This includes informed choices of society, organization, public and private sectors, community and individual.

Abbreviations

- **BDO:** Block Development Officer
- **CEO:** Chief Executive Officer
- **CMO:** Chief Medical Officer
- **DGHS:** Directorate General of Health Services
- **WHO:** World Health Organization

Important terms used in the unit are enlisted under **Key Terms**.

TABLE 7.19: Advantages and disadvantages of Cu-T

Advantages	Disadvantages
• An effective contraceptive • Fertility can be restored • Inexpensive and easy to use • Does not require continuous supervision • Can be used up to 10 years • Free from any harmful effects	• Pain and bleeding • Ectopic pregnancy may occur • Spontaneous expulsion may take place • Infection of pelvis • Perforation of uterus

Numerous Tables are used in the text to provide you with necessary data and information to supplement the text.

Several **images and diagrams** have been used at relevant places to simplify the concepts for the students.

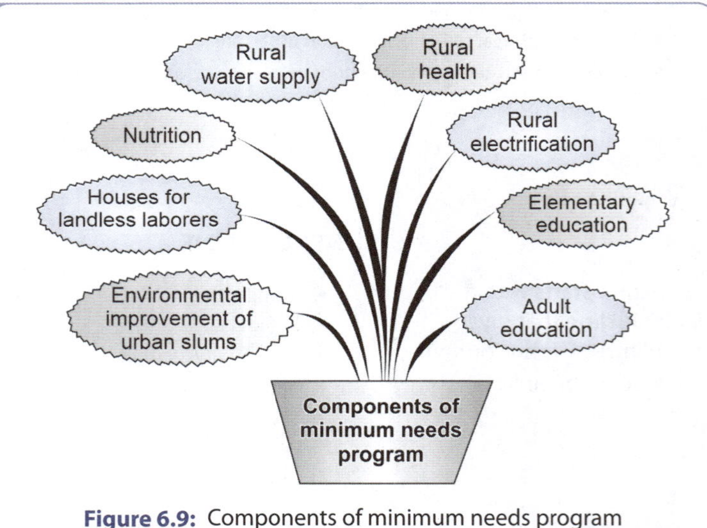

Figure 6.9: Components of minimum needs program

Nursing Considerations

Elements of Case Management

The case management of a sick child brought to the first level health facility includes the following steps:

1. **Outpatient health facility (OPD cases)**
   - Assessment
   - Classification and identification of treatment
   - Referral, treatment or counseling of child's caretaker
   - Follow-up care
2. **Referrals health facility**
   - Emergency triage assessment and treatment
   - Diagnosis, treatment and monitoring the patient's progress

Nursing Consideration boxes are covered throughout the book for implementation of better clinical practices.

Recent Update

Electronic Vaccine Intelligence Network (eVIN)

The Government of India has rolled out an Electronic Vaccine Intelligence Network (eVIN) system that digitizes the entire vaccine stock management, their logistics and temperature tracking at all levels of vaccine storage – from national to the subdistrict. This enables program managers to have real time view of the vaccine stock position and their storage temperature across all the cold chain points providing a detailed overview of the vaccine cold chain logistics system across the entire country. eVIN is to be scaled up to entire country.

Recent Update keeps students aware of all the latest advances and developments in the field.

High Yield Point

The UNICEF is promoting a campaign known as GOBI campaign to encourage four strategies for a "Child Health Revolution".
  G: For growth charts to better monitor child development
  O: For oral rehydration to treat all mild and moderate dehydration
  B: For breastfeeding
  I: For immunization against measles, diphtheria, polio, pertussis, tetanus and tuberculosis

High Yield Points are covered to add extra value to student's knowledge.

Must Know

Branches of Rehabilitation

- Medical rehabilitation—Restoration of function.
- Vocational rehabilitation—Restoration of the capacity to earn a livelihood.
- Social rehabilitation—Restoration of family and social relationship.
- Psychological rehabilitation—Restoration of personal dignity and confidence.

  Nurses play vital role in providing all these services to the individuals, families and community.

Must Know boxes covering valuable facts are strategically placed to highlight critical information, ensuring readers are well-informed of key concepts and important details.

Summary

- Healthcare services are a multitude of services provided to individual, families and community by the healthcare agency for the purpose of promoting, preventing, caring and restoring the health of individuals.
- The concept of the healthcare is to provide universal healthcare at the grassroots level to the underserved rural and urban poor through a primary healthcare approach with full participation of the community to achieve the goal of "health for all" by 2000 AD.
- There are three levels of healthcare: (1) Primary (2) Secondary and (3) Tertiary.
- The Bhore Committee (1946) used the term 'comprehensive healthcare' which means provision of integrated preventive, curative and promotive services from 'womb to tomb' to every individual residing in a defined geographical area.

Each and every unit ends with **Summarized one-liner** for quick revision of the chapter.

Student Assignment in the form of comprehensive exercises in each and every unit will facilitate structured learning and revision of the material provided in the respective units.

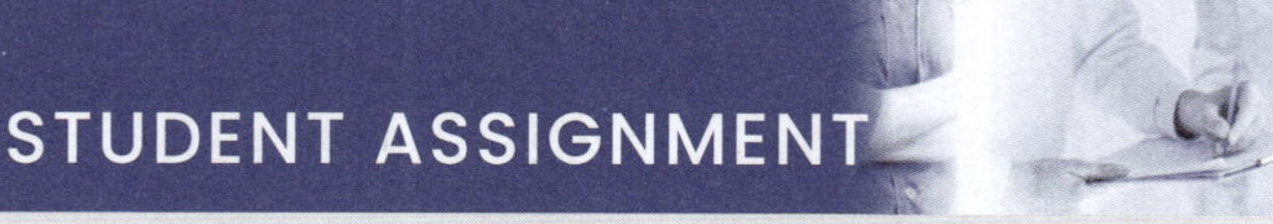

STUDENT ASSIGNMENT

LONG ANSWER TYPE QUESTIONS

1. Explain briefly the major health problems in India.
2. Describe the major communicable disease problems in India.

SHORT ANSWER TYPE QUESTIONS

1. State the causes of poor health services in the rural areas of India.
2. List the communicable diseases causing major health problems in India.

MULTIPLE CHOICE QUESTIONS

1. **Which of the following is not a communicable disease?**
   a. Diabetes mellitus
   b. Tuberculosis
   c. Malaria
   d. AIDS
2. **Which of the following is not a noncommunicable disease?**
   a. Cardiovascular accidents
   b. Mental disorders
   c. Cancer
   d. Filaria

COMMUNITY HEALTH NURSING-II

GNM Nursing

Placement: Third Year (Part – I)   **Total Hours – 90**

Unit	Learning Objectives	Contents	Hours	Teaching Learning Activities	Assessment Methods
I.	Explain the health system in India.	**Heath System in India** Organization and administration of health system in India at • Central level ▪ Union Ministry ▪ Directorate General of Health Services ▪ Central Council of Health • State level ▪ State Health Administration ▪ State Ministry of Health ▪ State Health Directorate • District level ▪ Sub-divisions ▪ Tehsils/Talukas ▪ Villages ▪ Municipalities and Corporation ▪ Panchayats	10	• Lecture cum discussion • Organizational chart of various levels • Visit to Municipality Office, Panchayat office, Health block office, CHC	• Short answer • Objective type • Essay type
II.	Describe the health care services in India and discuss the role of the nurse in these services.	**Health Care Delivery System** • Heath care concept and trends • Health care services—Public sector, rural, urban • Private sector • Public private partnership (PPP) • Other agencies • Indigenous systems of medicine Ayurvedha, Yoga, Unani, Siddha and Homeopathy (AYUSH) • Voluntary health services • National Health Programs • Nurse role in health care services	8	• Lecture cum discussion • Visit to different health care agencies	• Short answer • Objective type • Essay type

Contd...

Unit	Learning Objectives	Contents	Hours	Teaching Learning Activities	Assessment Methods
III.	Describe health planning in India.	**Health Planning in India** • National health planning • Five-year plans • Health committees and reports • National health policy	10	Lecture cum discussion and reports	• Short answer • Essay type
IV.	Describe the different specialized community health services and the nurse's role in these services.	**Specialized Community Health Services and Nurse's Role** • Reproductive and child health care (RCH) • National Health Mission (rural/urban) • Janani Sishu Suraksha Karaykaram (JSSK) • Emergency ambulance services • Government health insurance schemes • School health services • Occupational health nursing (including health care providers) • Geriatric nursing • Care of differently abled—physical and mental • Rehabilitation nursing	18	• Lecture cum discussion • Visit to different agencies of specialized services, factory, old age home, homes for the differently abled	• Short answer • Objective type • Essay type
V.	Describe the major health problems in India.	**National Health Problems** Health problems in India • Communicable diseases • Noncommunicable diseases • Nutritional problems • Environmental sanitation • Population	5	• Lecture cum discussion • Quiz	• Short answer • Objective type
VI.	Describe the national health and family welfare programs in India and the role of the nurse.	**National Health Program** • National ARI program • Revised national tuberculosis control program (RNTCP) • National antimalaria program • National filarial control program • National guinea worm eradication program • National leprosy eradication program • National AIDS control program • STD control program • National program for control of blindness • Iodine deficiency control program	15	• Lecture cum discussion • Government of India program flyers	• Short answer • Objective type

Contd...

Unit	Learning Objectives	Contents	Hours	Teaching Learning Activities	Assessment Methods
		• Expanded program of immunization • National family welfare program • National water supply and sanitation program • Minimum needs program • National diabetes control program • Polio eradication: Pulse polio program • National cancer control program • Yaws eradication program • National nutritional anemia prophylaxis program • 20 point program • ICDS program • Midday meal program • National mental health program • Adolescent health program • Role of nurse in the national health program			
VII.	Explain the meaning of demography and describe the national family welfare programs.	**Demography and Family Welfare** • Demography ▪ Concept ▪ Trends in the world and in India ▪ Concept of fertility and infertility ▪ Small family norm • Family welfare ▪ Concept, importance, aims and objectives ▪ Family planning methods ▪ Family planning counseling ▪ National family welfare policy ▪ National family welfare program ▪ Role of a nurse in the family planning program	18	• Lecture cum discussion • Show and explain family planning devices • Role play • Demonstration	• Short answer • Objective type • Essay type

Contd...

Unit	Learning Objectives	Contents	Hours	Teaching Learning Activities	Assessment Methods

VIII.	Describe the concept and functions of health team and the role of nursing personnel at various levels.	**Health Team**
		• Concept
		  ■ Composition
		  ■ Functions
		• Role of nursing personnel at various levels:
		  ■ District public health nursing officer
		  ■ Block health nurse
		  ■ Public health nurse
		  ■ Lady health visitor/health supervisor
		  ■ Health worker female/ANM
			7	• Lecture cum discussion
				• Interaction with health team members: Job description as per the Indian Public Health Standards (IPHS)
					• Short answer
					• Objective type
					• Essay type

IX.	Explain the concept and uses of health information system.	**Health Information System** • Concepts, components, uses, sources • Vital statistics: ■ Important rates and indicators • Vital health records and their uses • Basic statistical methods • Descriptive statistics	6	• Lecturer cum discussion • Exercises	• Short answer • Objective type • Exercises

X.	Describe the national and international health agencies.	**Health Agencies**
		• International:
		  ■ WHO
		  ■ UNFPA
		  ■ UNDP
		  ■ World Bank
		  ■ FAO
		  ■ UNICEF
		  ■ DANIDA
		  ■ European Commission (EU)
		  ■ Red Cross
		  ■ USAID
		  ■ UNESCO
		  ■ ILO
		  ■ CARE
		• National:
		  ■ Indian Red Cross
		  ■ Indian Council for Child Welfare
		  ■ Family Planning Association of India
		  ■ Other NGOs
			3	• Lecture cum discussion
				• Seminar
					• Short answer
					• Objective type

Contents

Preface to the Second Edition vii
Preface to the First Edition ix
Acknowledgments xi
Reviewers xiii
Special Features of the Book xvii
Syllabus xxi

Unit 1 Health System in India 1–18

Introduction *2*
Health *2*
Community *3*
Public Health *3*

Community Health *4*
Community Health Nursing *5*
Organization of Health System in India *6*

Unit 2 Healthcare Delivery System 19–66

Introduction *20*
Concepts of Healthcare *20*
Healthcare System *21*
Trends in Healthcare or Changing Concepts *23*
Healthcare Model *27*
Primary Healthcare in India *32*
Community Health Centers *47*

Community Development Program *50*
Healthcare Agencies *50*
Public-Private Partnership *52*
Indigenous System of Medicine *53*
Voluntary Health Services *57*
National Health Programs *60*
Nurses' Role in Healthcare Services *60*

Unit 3 Health Planning in India 67–102

Introduction *68*
Planning *68*
Health Planning *69*
National Health Planning *70*
Twenty Point Program *71*
Planning Commission *71*

Health Sector Planning *72*
National Development Council *74*
Five-Year Plans *74*
Health Committees and Reports *88*
National Health Policy *94*

Unit 4 Specialized Community Health Services and Nurses' Role 103–171

Introduction *104*
Specialized Community Health Services *104*
Reproductive and Child Health Program *104*
National Health Mission *117*

Janani Shishu Suraksha Karyakram *122*
Emergency Ambulance Services *124*
Government Health Insurance Schemes *124*
School Health Services *128*

Occupational Health Nursing or
 Industrial Nursing   *135*
Geriatric Nursing   *144*

Physically and Mentally Challenged People   *154*
Rehabilitation Nursing   *163*

Unit 5   National Health Problems 173–184

Introduction   *174*

Health Problems in India   *174*

Unit 6   National Health Programs 185–263

Introduction   *186*
Major Health Problems in India   *186*
National Health Programs   *187*
Acute Respiratory Infection   *187*
Revised National Tuberculosis Control Program   *189*
National Strategic Plan for
 TB Elimination (2017–2025)   *196*
National Antimalaria Program   *198*
National Filaria Control Program   *201*
National Guinea Worm Eradication Program   *204*
National Leprosy Eradication Program   *204*
National AIDS Control Program   *213*
National Strategic Plan for HIV/AIDS
 and STI 2017–2024   *217*
National STD Control Program   *218*
National Program for Control of Blindness   *219*
Iodine Deficiency Disorder Control Program   *222*
Expanded Program on Immunization   *223*
National Family Welfare Program   *231*
National Water Supply and Sanitation Program   *232*
Drinking Water Supply Programs and Policies   *232*
Swajaldhara   *233*
National Sanitation Program   *233*

Nirmal Bharat Abhiyan   *234*
Swachh Bharat Mission   *234*
Minimum Needs Program   *235*
Ayushman Bharat Program   *236*
National Diabetes Control Program   *238*
Polio Eradication—Pulse Polio Program   *239*
National Cancer Control Program   *241*
Yaws Eradication Program   *242*
National Nutritional Anemia Prophylaxis
 Program   *244*
Twenty Point Program   *245*
Integrated Child Development Scheme Program   *246*
Midday Meal Program   *248*
Midday Meal Scheme   *249*
National Mental Health Program   *250*
Mental Health Policy   *250*
Integration of Mental Health with Primary
 Healthcare   *251*
District Mental Health Program   *252*
Adolescent Health Program   *253*
Tribal Health   *255*
Role of a Nurse in National Health Programs   *258*

Unit 7   Demography and Family Welfare 265–337

Demography

Introduction   *266*
Concepts   *266*
Definition   *267*
History of Demographic Studies   *267*
Demographic Cycle   *267*
Demographic Processes   *268*
Sources of Demography   *268*
Demographic Trends in the World   *268*

Demographic Trends in India   *271*
Population Explosion   *282*
National Population Policy, 2000 (NPP 2000)   *284*
New National Population Policy, 2000
 (NNPP 2000)   *284*
Concepts of Fertility and Infertility   *285*
Small Family Norms   *294*

Family Welfare

Concepts of Family Welfare   *298*
Services Included in the Family Welfare Program   *299*
Importance of Family Welfare   *300*
Aspects of Family Welfare   *301*

Aims and Objectives of Family Welfare   *301*
Family Planning   *302*
Method of Family Planning   *304*
Types of Contraceptives   *305*

Elements of Success in Family Planning *320*
Family Planning Counseling *320*
National Family Welfare Policy *322*

National Family Welfare Program *323*
National Family Planning Insurance Scheme *328*
Role of Nurse in Family Welfare Program *330*

Unit 8 Health Team 339–363

Introduction *340*
Concepts of Health Team *340*
Medical and Nonmedical Health Team *340*

Community Health Nursing Team *341*
Role of Nursing Personnel at Various Levels *346*

Unit 9 Health Information System.. 365–397

Introduction *366*
Health Management Information System
  Planners *366*
Sources of Health Information System *369*
Vital Statistics *372*
Important Rates and Indicators *374*
Useful Rates and Indicators *375*

Vital Health Record *380*
Basic Statistical Methods *381*
Statistic Average *387*
Measures of Dispersion or Variability *388*
Descriptive Statistics *391*
Responsibility of Community Health Nurse in
  Vital Statistic *394*

Unit 10 Health Agencies 399–428

International Health Agencies

World Health Organization *400*
United Nations Fund for Population Activities *404*
United Nations Development Program *404*
World Bank *405*
Food and Agriculture Organization *406*
United Nations International Children's
  Emergency Fund *407*
Danish International Development Agency *410*
European Commission *410*

International Red Cross *411*
United States Agency for International
  Development *412*
United Nations Educational, Scientific and
  Cultural Organization *413*
International Labor Organization *415*
Cooperation for Assistance and
  Relief Everywhere *415*

National Voluntary Health Agencies of India

Indian Red Cross Society *417*
Indian Council for Child Welfare *418*
Family Planning Association of India *419*
Tuberculosis Association of India *420*
Hind Kusht Nivaran Sangh *420*

Central Social Welfare Board *421*
All India Women's Conference *422*
All India Blind Relief Society *423*
Bharat Sevak Samaj *424*
Kasturba Memorial Fund *424*

Appendix Management of Biomedical Waste 429–436

Policy on Healthcare Waste Management *429*
Definition of Biomedical Waste *429*
Sources of Healthcare Waste *429*
Health Hazards of Healthcare Waste *430*
Categories of Biomedical Waste and their
  Collection *431*
Segregation of Biomedical Waste *433*

Collection of Biomedical Waste *434*
Storage of Waste *434*
Transportation of Waste within the Hospital *435*
Transportation of Waste for Disposal Outside
  the Hospital *435*
Training in Handling Biomedical Waste *435*
Waste Management in Subcenters *436*

Index 437

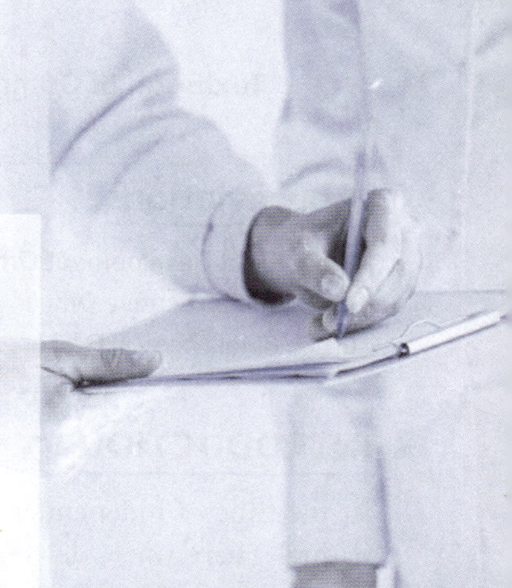

1

Health System in India
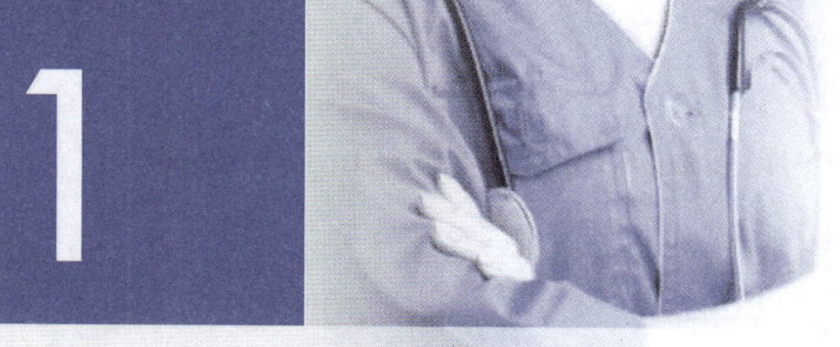

LEARNING OBJECTIVES

After the completion of the unit, the readers will be able to:
- Explain the health systems in India.
- Identify the areas of responsibility of central government, state government, center and state with regard to healthcare.
- Describe the local self-government in urban areas of districts in India.
- Describe the structure and functions of healthcare organization.

UNIT OUTLINE

- Introduction
- Health
- Community
- Public Health

- Community Health
- Community Health Nursing
- Organization of Health System in India

KEY TERMS

Community: A group of people living together in a particular geographical area.

Community health: It is the science and art of preventing disease, prolonging life and promoting health through organized efforts. This includes informed choices of society, organization, public and private sectors, community and individual.

Community health nursing: Nursing services provided to community at homes, schools, industries and various health centers.

Gram Panchayat: It is an executive organ of the Gram Sabha and is responsible for overall planning and development of the village.

Gram Sabha: The assembly of all adults of the village which meet at least twice a year.

Health system: A system that involves planning, organization and management to deliver the health services to the entire community to improve their health through the use of available resources and knowledge.

Nyaya Panchayat: It comprises 5 members from the Panchayat who try to solve the village disputes on mutual consent.

Panchayat Samiti: An agency comprising all village Sarpanches in a block, local MLAs, MPs and representatives of women, SCs, STs and cooperative societies. It is responsible for block development activities under the community development program.

Abbreviations

BDO: Block Development Officer
CEO: Chief Executive Officer
CMO: Chief Medical Officer

DGHS: Directorate General of Health Services
WHO: World Health Organization

INTRODUCTION

At the time of independence, the healthcare services were urban-oriented and mainly curative in nature. There was a dense rural population with high degree of illiteracy; low per capita income and deprived of health services. After independence there has been vast improvement in healthcare services. The organization and infrastructure have undergone extensive changes and expansion in shapes followed by increase in a number of expert committees. At present, there is a wide spread network of healthcare services so that it can reach both the rural and urban areas equally well.

After the Alma-Ata (1978) Declaration of "Health for All" by 2000 AD, rapid advancement has taken place in biomedical science and technology. This was essential as under the changing demographic structures, needs, demands, advancement in health and behavioral sciences, there was also a need to improve the health status of the people throughout the country. Primary healthcare has laid a framework within which the Indian states are developing their healthcare services system, as health is a fundamental human right. Every individual in India has the right of availing health services to protect and promote his health, beyond being personal responsibility; it is also the national and international responsibility. Community has influence on the health of the people and is the basic unit of improving the health status of the people. Every state is responsible for the health of its own people. National government is striving to expand and improve health services.

HEALTH

Health is a general condition of a person in all aspects. It is also a level of functional or metabolic efficiency of a person. Health is highly individualized perception. It is not something that a person achieves suddenly at a specific time. Many factors affect individual's expectation of self, age and sociocultural influences. Therefore, it is an ongoing process.

Definitions

There are many definitions of health but the widely accepted definition of health given by WHO in 1948 is as follows:

"Health is a state of complete physical, mental and social well-being and not merely an absence of disease or infirmity."   **—World Health Organization (1948)**

"The condition of being sound in body, mind or spirit, especially freedom from disease or pain."
                                    —Webster English Dictionary

"Soundness of body and mind, the condition in which its functions are duly and efficiently discharged."   **—Oxford English Dictionary**

"A state of relative equilibrium of body form and functions which result from its dynamic adjustment of forces tending to disturb it. It is not passive interplay between body substance and forces infringing upon it but an active response of the body forces working toward adjustment."
                                                                                                    —**Perkins**

New Philosophy of Health

The new philosophy of health may be stated as under:
* Health is a fundamental human right.
* Health is the essence of productive life and not the result of ever increasing expenditure on medical care.
* Health is intersectoral.
* Health is an integral part of development.
* Health is central to the concept of quality of life.
* Health involves individuals, state and international responsibility.
* Health and its maintenance is a major social investment.
* Health is a worldwide social goal.

COMMUNITY

Community is a group in which organisms interact and share populated environment. The community has been described as the most useful area for improving the health status of people by providing them better healthcare services. The fact is that the social, physical and cultural aspects of community influence the health status of an individual.

Definitions

"A community is a social group characterized by geographical boundaries, common values and interests. Its members know and interact with each other. It functions within a particular social structure and exhibits certain norms, values and social institutions. An individual belongs to the broader society through his family and community."   —**World Health Organization (1947)**

"A group of people who share same type of bond, who interact with each other and who function collectively regarding common concerns."   —**Green and Anderson (1986)**

"A community is defined as a group of people having intimacy, informal relations, common culture and living together in specific geographical boundaries."   —**Paul B Horton (1992)**

PUBLIC HEALTH

Public health is the science and art of preventing disease, prolonging life and promoting health. This is done through organized efforts and informed choices of society, organization, public-private sectors, community and individuals.

Definitions

"Public health nursing is a population focused on community nursing practice with the goal of prevention of a disease and disability by creating the conditions where people can be healthy."
                                                                                                    —**ANA (1999)**

"Public health nursing is the practice of promoting and protecting the health of population using knowledge from nursing, social and public health sciences."

—American Public Health Association (Public Health Nursing Section, 1996)

Distinct Characteristics of Public Health

- The focus of public health intervention is to prevent rather than treat a disease through surveillance of causes and promoting people to adopt healthy behavior.
- "Public health" deals with preventive rather than curative aspect of health.
- It deals with the population level rather than individual level health issues.
- Sometimes during the outbreak of an infectious disease, treatment becomes vital to prevent it.

COMMUNITY HEALTH

Community health is a systematic way of studying the health and disease present in the community. It also involves studying the patterns of delivery of care, both of which influence the amount and nature of disease.

The term community health has replaced the term public health in many countries. It is because of the changing nature of public health which focuses on individual responsibility and community participation.

Definitions

"Community health is referred to as the health status of the members of the community, problems affecting their health and in totality of health provided to community."

—World Health Organization (1979)

"Community (public) health is the science and art of preventing disease, prolonging life and promoting health and efficiency through organized efforts by the sanitation of the environment, the control of infections, the education of the individual in principles of personal hygiene, the organization of medical and nursing service and the early diagnosis and preventive treatment of disease and the development of social machinery which will ensure to every individual a standard of living adequate for maintenance of health. It is the organizing of these benefits in such a fashion as to enable every citizen to realize his birth right of health and longevity."   **—Winslow (1920)**

"The mission of public health is to fulfill society's interests in assuring conditions in which people can be healthy."   **—United States Institute of Medicine**

Public health has often been defined as "a science dealing with the determinants and defense of health at the population level, while clinical medicine deals with multiple maladies and their remedies at the level of an individual patient. Public health aims to understand and influence the social, cultural and economic determinants of health as well as to study and structure health system as efficient channels for health services delivery. Public health is thus a discipline built on the academic tradition of inquiry involving research, teaching and professional practice to prevent disease and promote health in populations".   **—Public Health Foundation of India**

COMMUNITY HEALTH NURSING

Community health nurses are the first-line healthcare providers to the community. Community health nursing has been affected by several new developments that have taken place in the field of medicine, nursing and other scientific discipline. The advancement of new technology in medicine and nursing has brought a tremendous change in the practice of community health nursing. There has been a significant shift from institution-based care to community-based care because of change from curative aspect to preventive aspect. The duration of hospitalization has become shortened. There is a challenge for the community health nurses to provide high quality, cost effective and innovative system of care which is accessible to the population operating within an increasingly complex and changing environment.

Definitions

Community health nursing is defined as "synthesis of nursing and public health practice applied to promoting and preserving the health of populations. It also involves "treating population as a whole." Focus on individual, family, groups, community, utilizing health promotion, health maintenance, health education and management, coordination and continuity of care for meeting population needs."

                                                                      —**ANA (2000)**

Community health nursing is "a collaborative application of nursing and public health measures within the framework of the total community health efforts."   —**Freeman (1970)**

Community health nursing is learned practice disciplines with the ultimate goal of contributing as individuals and in collaboration with others to the promotion of patient's optimum level of functioning through teaching and delivery of care.   —**Margaret J Jacobson**

"Community health nursing, a synthesis of both public health science and nursing science, is theoretically responsive to our prevailing ideas of social justice and the methods of distributing healthcare resources as chosen by the community."   —**Archer S E (1982)**

Community-Based Nursing

"The philosophy of nursing that guides nursing care provided for individuals, families and groups at their homes or workplace, industries and schools."

Population-Based Nursing

The focus of population-based practice is to identify the problems of the population under care, population-based data guide in identifying the problems of the community. The identified problems are approached on priority base.

Population-based nursing is similar to the community-based nursing but the only difference is that the population-based nursing practice refers to the people who are not organized and have no identity as a group or locality; nurses are involved in taking actions and condition to promote, protect and preserve their health.

ORGANIZATION OF HEALTH SYSTEM IN INDIA

India is a democratic country having 28 States and 8 Union Territories. The President of India is the constitutional head. The real executive powers are vested in the council of ministers with prime minister collectively responsible to Lok Sabha. Since health is a fundamental right of every citizen of India and it is also fundamental to the national progress. So, under the Constitution of India, the states are largely independent regarding the delivery of healthcare to the people. Each state has developed its own system of healthcare delivery independent of the central government. The central responsibility is mainly of policy making, planning, guiding, assisting, evaluating and coordinating the work of the state health ministers so that health services cover every part of the country and no state is left for want of these services.

The organization of health system in India (Fig. 1.1) works at three main levels as follows:

1. At the central level
2. At the state level
3. At the district level

Health Organization at the Central Level

The official "organ" of the health system at the national level consists of the following (Fig. 1.2):

- Ministry of Health and Family Welfare
- Directorate General of Health Services (DGHS)
- Central Council of Health and Family Welfare

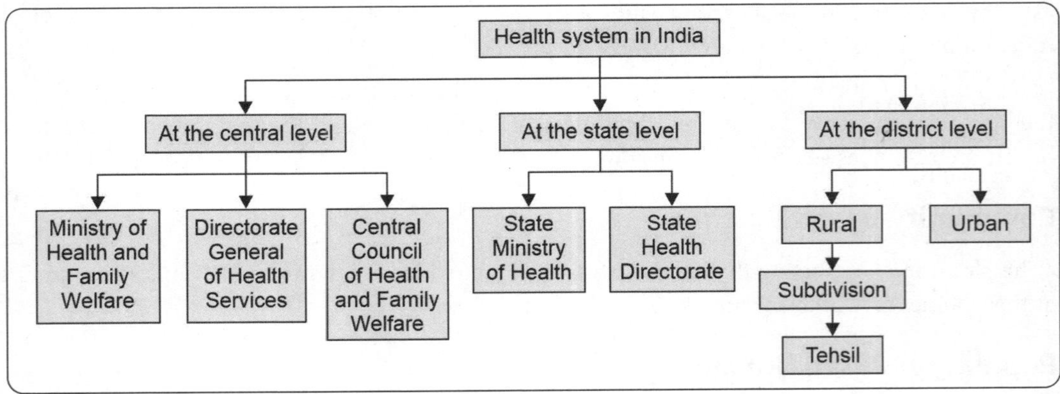

Figure 1.1: Organization of health system in India

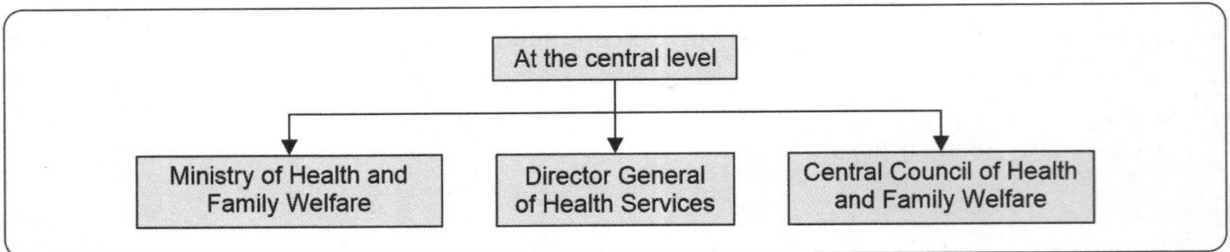

Figure 1.2: Health organization at the central level

Union Ministry of Health and Family Welfare

It is headed (Fig. 1.3) by the following:

- Cabinet Ministers
- Ministers of State
- Deputy Health Minister

Organization

It has got the following departments:

- **Department of Health:** It is headed by secretary of the Government of India as its executive head, who is assisted by joint secretaries, deputy secretary and a large administrative staff.
- **Department of Health and Family Welfare:** It was created in 1966 within the Ministry of Health and Family Welfare. The secretary to the Government of India is the overall in charge of health and family welfare. He is assisted by an additional secretary, commissioner and one joint secretary.

Functions

The functions are described in the Seventh Schedule of Article 246 of the Constitution of India under the following lists:

- Union list
- Concurrent list

Functions under union list: The functions described under the union list are the responsibility of central government:

- International health relations and administration of port quarantine.
- Administration of central institutes such as All India Institute of Hygiene and Public Health Kolkata, National Center of Disease Control, Delhi.
- Promotion of research through research centers and other bodies.
- Regulation and development of medical, pharmaceutical, dental and nursing profession.
- Establishment and maintenance of drug standard.
- Census and collection and publication of other statistical data.
- Immigration and emigration.

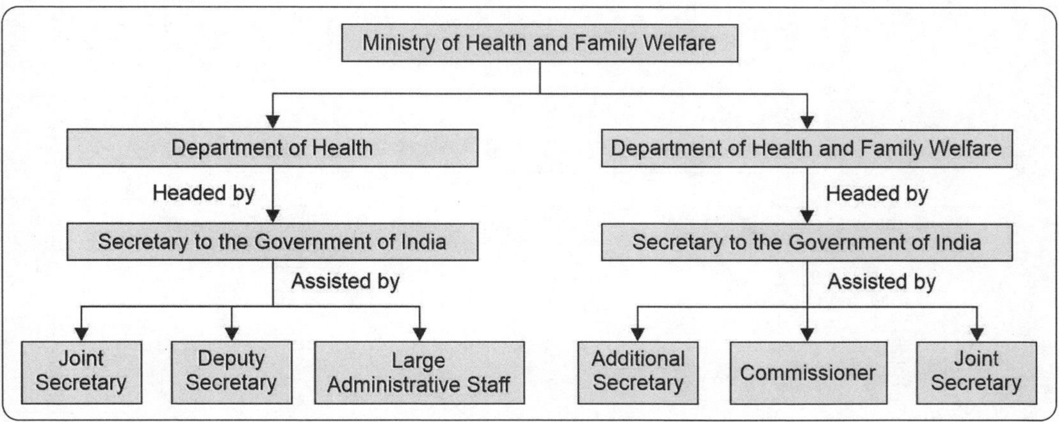

Figure 1.3: Organization of Union Ministry of Health and Family Welfare

- Regulation of labor in the working of mines and oil fields.
- Coordination with states and with other minister for promotion of health.

Functions under concurrent list: The functions described under the concurrent list are the responsibility of both the union list and the state list. These are as under:

- Prevention of extension of communicable diseases from one unit to another
- Prevention of adulteration of food stuffs
- Control of drugs and poisons
- Vital statistics
- Labor welfare
- Ports other than major
- Economic and social planning
- Population control and family planning.

Directorate General of Health Services

Organization

The Directorate General of Health Services (DGHS) is the principal adviser to the union government in both, medical and public health matters. He is assisted by an additional DGHS, a team of deputies and large administrative staff. The DGHS is having three main units, i.e., the medical unit, includes medical care and hospital, public health and general administration (Fig. 1.4).

Functions

The functions are divided into general functions and specific functions (Fig. 1.5). These are described here:

General Functions

- Survey
- Planning
- Coordination
- Programming
- Appraisal of all health matters in the country

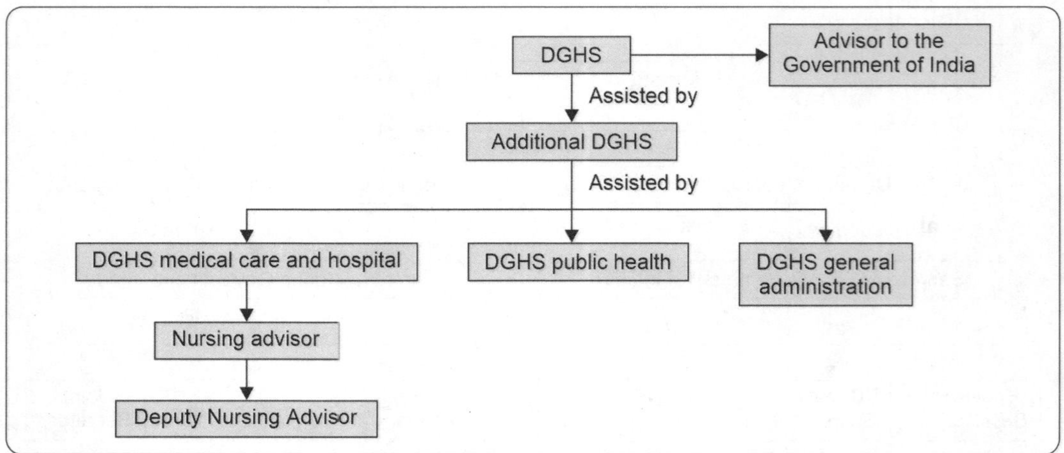

Figure 1.4: Organization of Directorate General of Health Services

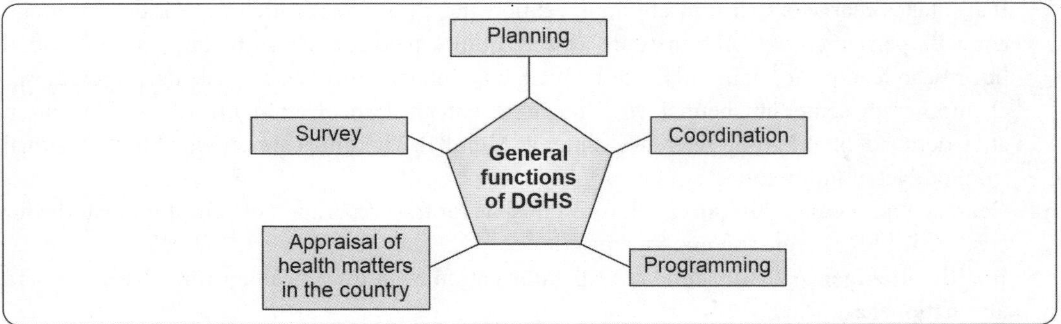

Figure 1.5: General functions of Directorate General of Health Services
Abbreviation: DGHS, Directorate General of Health Services

Specific Functions

- **International health relations and quarantine:** All the major ports, i.e., Kolkata, Visakhapatnam, Chennai, Kochi, Mumbai, Kandla and international airports are directly controlled by DGHS.
- **Control of drug standards:** Drugs control organization is the part of DGHS and it is headed by the drug controller. Its primary function is to lay down and enforce standards and control the manufacture and distribution of drugs through both central and state government officers. The Drug Act (1940) vests the central government with the powers to test the quality of important drugs.
- **Medical store depots:** The union government runs medical stores at Mumbai, Chennai, Kolkata, Karnal, Guwahati and Hyderabad. These depots supply drugs to the central government and various state governments. These depots also handle the supplies from foreign agencies.
- **Postgraduate training:** DGHS is also responsible for national institutes which provide postgraduate training to various categories of health personnel. Some of the institutes are mentioned as under:
  - All India Institute of Hygiene and Public Health, Kolkata
  - All India Institute of Mental Health and Neuroscience, Bengaluru
  - National Tuberculosis Institute, Bengaluru
  - Central Research Institute, Kasauli
  - National Institute of Communicable Diseases, Delhi
  - National Institute of Health and Family Welfare, New Delhi
  - RAK College of Nursing, New Delhi
- **Medical education:** The central directorate is directly in charge of the following medical colleges in India:
  - Lady Hardinge Medical College and Associated SSK and KSC Hospital
  - Maulana Azad Medical Collage
  - Medical colleges of Puducherry and Goa other than these colleges, there are many medical colleges in India which are guided and supported by the center.
- **Medical research:** The Indian Council of Medical Research founded in 1911 at New Delhi plays a significant role in aiding, promoting and coordinating scientific research on human diseases.

It also takes charge of their causation, prevention and cure. The research work is done through council's permanent research institute, research units, field surveys and a large number of ad hoc research enquiries financed by the council. It maintains cancer research center, tuberculosis, chemotherapy center at Chennai, virus research center at Pune, National Institute of Nutrition at Hyderabad, blood group reference center at Mumbai. The funds are provided to the council from budget of union ministry of health.

- **Central health education bureau:** It is responsible for the preparation of education material for creating health awareness among the people.
- **Health intelligence:** It disseminates all information regarding health to all the states and international agencies.
- **National medical library:** The main aim of this library is the advancement of medical health and allied sciences in addition to exchanging professional books, journals and medical reports, etc.
- Central government health schemes.
- National health programs.

Central Council of Health and Family Welfare

The Central Council of Health and Family Welfare is an advisory body. The main objective of this council is to maintain coordination between center and states for the implementation of programs and policies recommended by the central government pertaining to health.

Organization

Central Council of Health and Family Welfare was set up on 9th August 1952. The Union Minister is the chairman and the state health ministers are the members.

Functions

- Considering policies and recommendation pertaining to medical care, environment, nutrition, medical education and research.
- Preparing proposals for making laws in areas of medical and public health matters and to lay down the patterns of development for the country as a whole.
- Making plans for development of health in the entire nation.
- Preparing recommendation to the central government for providing grants and financial assistance to states for medical services and also review the work done through the utilization of grants in different areas.
- Cooperation between the center and state in health administration and also to establish necessary organization for better functioning.

Health Organization at the State Level

States are empowered to all matters related to health. There are 28 states in India. Each state has its own health administration on similar pattern as that of central level. The states are responsible for all the health-related services within the state. Some variations are found in the health organization at state level but the main characteristics of health organization at the state level are almost similar in all the states. The management system comprises the following (Fig. 1.6):

- State Ministry of Health
- State Health Directorate

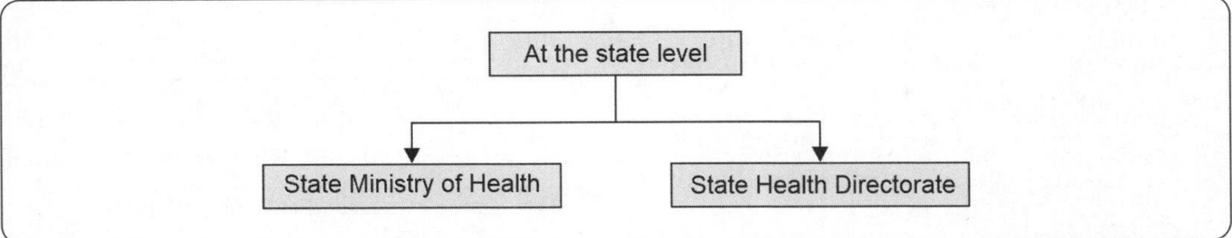

Figure 1.6: Health organization at state level

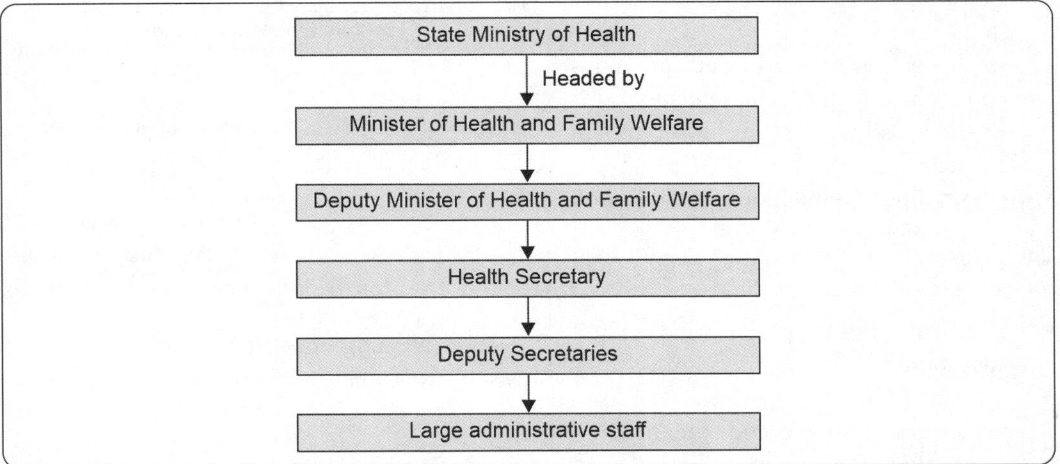

Figure 1.7: Organization of State Ministry of Health

State Ministry of Health

The Minister of Health and Family Welfare is the chief of the State Ministry of Health (Fig. 1.7). He is assisted by Deputy Minister of Health and Family Welfare. The health secretariat is the official organ of the State Ministry of Health and is headed, by Health Secretary, Deputy Secretary and large administrative staff. The Minister of Health and Family Welfare has the political vision and is overall responsible for all matters related to health. The Health Secretary is in charge of health department. He is an IAS Officer. He is assisted by Deputy Secretaries and other staff.

State Health Directorate

The State Health Directorate (Fig. 1.8) is the technical wing of State Ministry of Health and Family Welfare. It is headed by Director of Health and Family Welfare. He/she is the chief technical advisor to the state health ministry and the government on all matters related to health, family welfare services, public health and family planning. In some states, the director of health and family welfare is known as director of medical and health services. He is assisted by deputy director and assistant directors. The Deputy and Assistant Directors are of two types. The regional and functional. The regional directors inspect all branches of public health irrespective of their specialty whereas the functional directors are specialists in particular branch of public health such as maternal and child health (MCH), family planning, nutrition, tuberculosis and health education, etc.

Functions

The functions of State Health Directorate (Fig. 1.8) are as follows:

- State ministry of health is responsible for making plans and programs in health services at state level.
- Providing infrastructure
- Evaluation
- Assisting in planning for health services in the states.
- Implementing national health programs and evaluating their achievements.
- Providing all types of health services in the state.
- Controlling sanitation and food adulteration.
- Encouraging maternal and child health activities.
- Improving nutrition program and medical education.
- Training of health personnel, i.e., nurses, female health workers and other health workers.
- Controlling rural and urban health services through District Medical Officer.
- Collecting vital statistics.
- Providing feedback to the State Health Ministry regarding health.
- Following the directives of Union Ministry of Health/State Health Ministry.

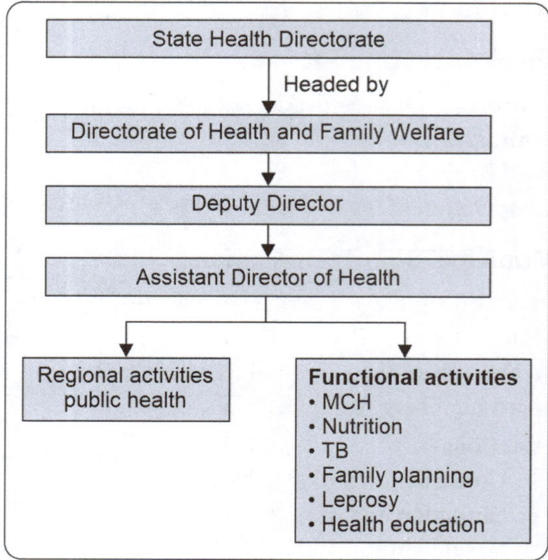

Figure 1.8: Functions of State Health Directorate

Abbreviations: MCH, maternal and child health; TB, tuberculosis

Health Organization at the District Level

The district is the basic unit of administration in India under a Collector. There are 806 districts (year 2024) in India. The districts vary widely in area and population. The following are the administration units within each district:

1. Subdivisions
2. Tehsils (Talukas)
3. Community development blocks
4. Municipalities and Municipal corporations
5. Village Panchayats

Most districts are divided into two or more subdivisions, each is under the supervision of an Assistant Collector or Subcollector. Further, each subdivision is divided into Tehsils (Talukas), which is under the charge of a Tehsildar. A Tehsil usually comprises 200–600 villages. The rural areas of districts have been organized into blocks known as community development blocks which was launched in 1952. The concerned area may or may not coincide with a Tehsil. The block comprises approximately 100 villages with population ranging from 80,000 to 1,20,000 is under the charge of a Block Development Officer. After blocks there are village Panchayats. The village Panchayats are unique, basic democratic units of Indian Administration and are institutions of local self-government.

Urban Administration

These are organized into the following:

Town Area Committee

Towns are the areas between the village and city. These are neither village nor a city. Town area committee is under the administration of district collector. These are found in States of MP, UP, West Bengal, Kerala, Assam, J&K, and HP. They are like Panchayats. A town area committee covers a population of 5000–10,000 and it is responsible for maintaining sanitation in the area.

Municipal Board (Municipality)

It is constituted where the population of city or town ranges between 10,000 and 2 lakhs. Municipality has three components, i.e., (1) Chairman, (2) Board and (3) Municipal Commissioner or Executive Officer. Municipal board is headed by a chairman/president elected usually by the board members. The term of municipal board ranges from 3 to 5 years.

Functions

- Construction and maintenance of roads
- Sanitation and drainage
- Street lighting
- Water supply
- Maintenance of hospitals and dispensaries
- Education
- Registration of birth and death

Municipal Corporation

It is constituted when the population of city is >2 lakhs. It is headed by mayors. It has got a council. Councilors are elected from different wards of the city. Corporation has different committees of councilors. Its term is of 5 years. At administrative level, the executive agency includes Chief Executive Officer (CEO) also called commissioner, the secretary, an engineer and the health officer.

Functions

The functions of municipal corporation are similar to the municipal board but on much large scale and includes the following:

- Health and sanitation of the city
- Construction and maintenance of roads
- Safe drainage system
- Street lighting
- Safe water supply
- Maintenance of hospitals and dispensaries
- Education
- Registration of birth and death

Health Organizations

During 1946, the Bhore Committee recommended integrated, preventive and curative health services at all levels. This unified health authority is in each district, since "Health" is a state subject there is no uniform "Model" of district health organization in India. Each state developed its own pattern to suit its policy and convenience. Under the multipurpose health worker scheme, the states have been suggested to have an integrated set-up at the district level by having a CMO with 3 deputy CMOs (Fig. 1.9), i.e., existing civil surgeon, district health officer and district family welfare officer.

With each of the deputy CMOs being in charge of one-third of the district for all:

- The health
- Family welfare
- MCH programs

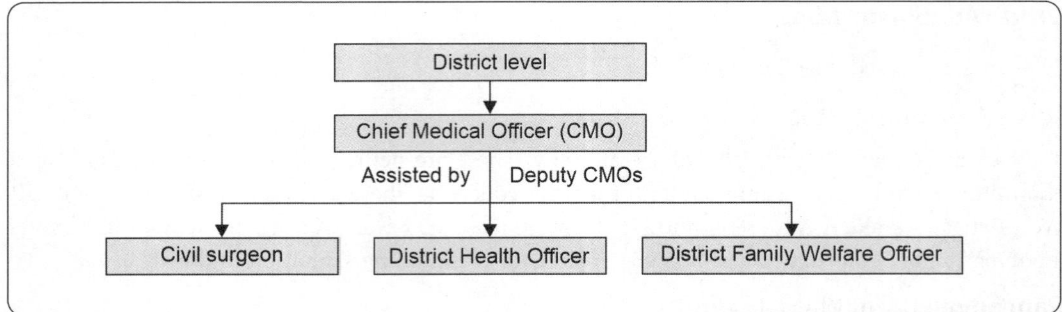

Figure 1.9: Integrated set-up at the district level

At the district level, the District Health Officer also known as Chief Medical Officer is the in charge of health administration and all national health programs implemented in the district. He is assisted by three deputy CMOs. These three CMOs are appointed at subdivisional headquarters of the district each is given the responsibility of one third of district for all the health, family welfare and MCH programs. The working group on health for all by 2000 AD recommended that district hospitals should be converted into district health centers to provide preventive, promotive and curative services.

Rural Administration

Panchayati Raj System

Panchayati Raj System was introduced in 1957. This system links the villages to the districts to have people's participation and strengthen the administration at grassroots level: The Panchayati Raj System is comprised of three-tier structure of rural self-government to involve people at various levels of administration. The three institutions of Panchayati Raj are shown in Figure 1.10.

1. Panchayat at village level
2. Panchayat Samiti at block level
3. Zila Parishad at district level

Panchayati Raj institutions are unique welfare agencies of our democratic pattern. Public welfare plans and developmental programs can be executed at the grassroots level. Panchayati Raj institutions strengthen the democracy at its root and ensure more effective and better community participation of the people in the government.

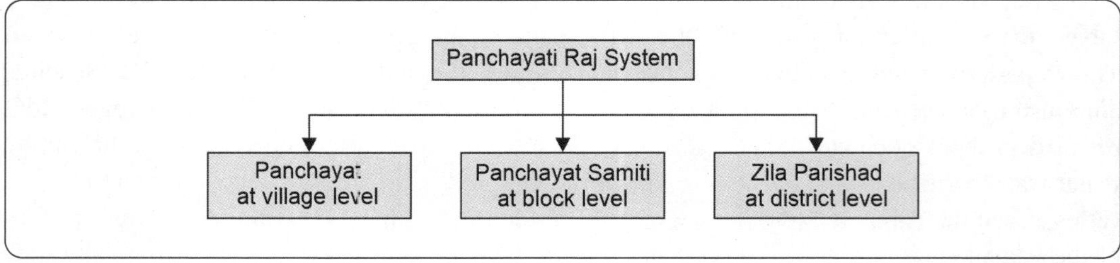

Figure 1.10: Three-tier system of Panchayati Raj

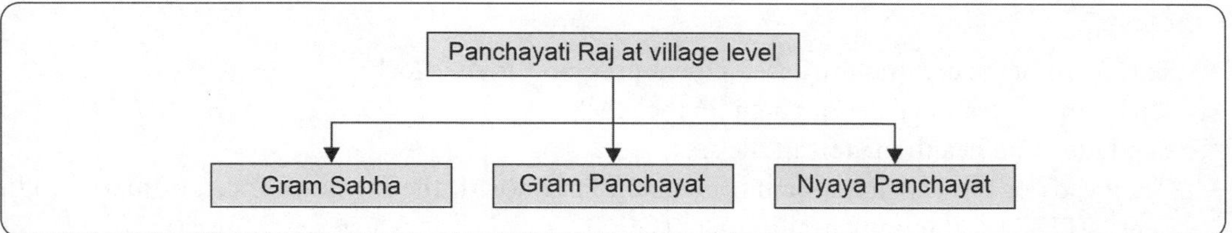

Figure 1.11: Structure of Panchayati Raj institution at village level

Panchayati Raj at Village Level

Panchayati Raj institution at village level (Fig. 1.11) comprises the following:

- Gram Sabha
- Gram Panchayat
- Nyaya Panchayat

Gram Sabha

It is the assembly of all the adults of the village who are registered voters of the village. They meet at least twice a year and discuss important issues and consider proposals pertaining to the various developmental aspects including health matters. Gram Sabha elects members of the Gram Panchayat.

Gram Panchayat

Gram Panchayat comprises 15–30 elected members, also known as Panch. It is the executive organ of Gram Sabha. Gram Panchayat covers a population of 5000–15000 or more. Gram Panchayat is headed by president or Sarpanch. It also has a vice president or Deputy Sarpanch and a Panchayat secretary. The members of the Gram Panchayat hold office for the tenure of 3–4 years.

Functions: The Gram Panchayat functions are very wide and covers the entire field of civic administration. Some of its functions are listed as under:

- Sanitation
- Public health
- Socioeconomic development of the village
- Planning and organizing various health activities in the villages

Nyaya Panchayat

It is comprised of five members from the Panchayat. It resolves the disputes between the two parties or groups or individuals of the village over certain matters on mutual consent. It solves the troubles of going to formal judicial system and thus creates harmony and peace among the members.

Panchayat Samiti at the Block Level

The Panchayat Agency at the block level is referred to as Panchayat Samiti. It is the local administration agency at the block level under Panchayati Raj. Block consists of 100 villages and a population about 80,000 to 1,20,000. The Panchayat Samiti consists of all Sarpanches of the village, Panchayats in the block, MLAs, MPs residing in the block area, representatives of women, schedule castes, schedule tribes and members of cooperative societies. The BDO is the ex-officio secretary of the Panchayat Samiti and takes care of its administration. He is the representative of the state government. Panchayat Samiti should meet at least once in a month.

Functions

- Execution of the community development programs in the block.
- Social and educational development in the block.
- Sanitation and health matters in the area.
- The heads of the Panchayat Samiti maintain liaison with the medical officer, primary health center (PHC), community health center (CHC), provide help whenever required.
- The BDO and his/her technical staff extend assistance and guidance to Gram Panchayats in carrying out developmental activities in these villages.
- The funds provided by the government at stage-I and stage-II development are channeled through Panchayat Samiti.

Zila Parishad at District Level

The Panchayati Raj Institution at the district level is known as Zila Parishad. Zila Parishad or Zila Panchayat is the agency of rural local self-government at the district level. The members of the Zila Parishad include all the heads of Panchayat Samiti in district, MLAs, MPs of district, representatives of schedule castes, schedule tribes, representatives of women and two persons related to rural development administration or public life. The number of members in Zila Parishad may be 40–70. The collector of the district is the nonvoting member. Zila Parishad is the supervising and coordinating agency for the development programs carried by the Gram Samities in the blocks of districts. The function of Zila Parishad may vary state-wise.

Summary

- Health system involves planning, organization and management so that the health services reach at the grassroots level and improve the health status of the people.
- Health system in India is organized at the central level, state level, district level and local level, i.e., rural and urban.
- Functions of Union Ministry of Health and Family Welfare include international health relations and administration of port quarantine, administration of central institution, promotion of research, regulation standards, maintenance of drugs, regulation of labor, immigration and emigration, publication of statistical data and coordination with states and with other ministers for health promotion.
- General functions of DGHS include survey, planning, coordination, programming and appraisal of all health-related matters. The specific functions are international health relations and quarantine, control of drug standards, medical education and research, central government health schemes, national health programs, central health education bureau, establishment of different units, etc.
- Functions of central council of health include broad outlines of health policy, proposal for legislation and cooperation between central and state administration.
- The district is divided into two or more subdivisions each under the charge of an assistant collector or sub collector. Each subdivision is divided into Tehsils (Talukas) which is under the charge of Tehsildar. Rural areas are divided into blocks headed by BDO.
- At district level, health organization consists of CMO with three deputy CMOs, i.e., Civil Surgeon, District Health Officer and District Family Welfare Officer.
- Block development officer and his/her staff assist and guide Gram Panchayat to carry out development activities.
- Heads of Panchayat Samiti maintain liaison with the medical officer, primary health centers and community health centers in order to provide help as and when required.

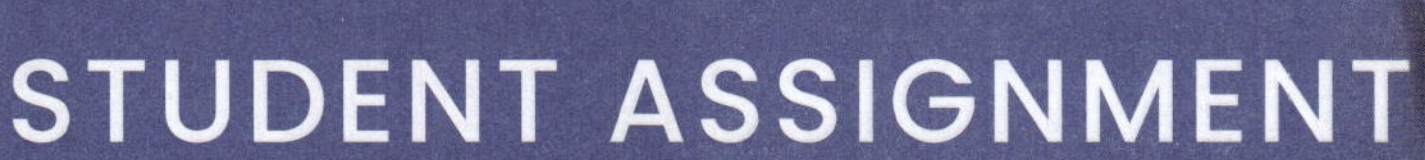

STUDENT ASSIGNMENT

LONG ANSWER TYPE QUESTIONS

1. Describe the organization of health system in India.
2. Explain the official organs of health system at the central level; discuss the functions of Directorate General of Health Services.
3. What is the organizational set up of health system at the state level and what are the functions of state health directorate?
4. Describe the organization of health system at the district level. How the health services are administered at district level?
5. When the community development program was implemented and how it is executed in rural and urban areas?

SHORT ANSWER TYPE QUESTIONS

1. Write about the Panchayati Raj System or local self-government in rural area.
2. What do you understand by the Panchayat Samiti at the block level? What are its functions?
3. Write about the central council of health and enlist its functions.
4. Write short notes on the following:
    a. Gram Panchayat
    b. Panchayat Samiti
    c. Nyaya Panchayat
    d. Zila Parishad
    e. Gram Sabha

MULTIPLE CHOICE QUESTIONS

1. **Which of the following is not the official organ of health system at the central level?**
    a. Ministry of Health and Family Welfare
    b. Directorate of National Health Programs
    c. Directorate General of Health Services
    d. Central Council of Health and Family Welfare

2. **Which of the following factor affects the community health?**
    a. Environment and lifestyle
    b. Socioeconomic and political factors
    c. Healthcare delivery system
    d. All of these

3. **The functions of central council of health include:**
    a. Broad outlines of health policy
    b. Proposal for legislation
    c. Grant distribution
    d. All of these

4. **The functions of district health officer at district level are:**
    a. Health administration
    b. National health programs
    c. Family welfare program
    d. All of these

5. **Community health is also called:**
   a. Public health
   b. Community medicine
   c. Public medicine
   d. All of these

6. **The functions of union list include the following except:**
   a. Economic and social planning
   b. Publication of statistical data
   c. Immigration and emigration
   d. Maintenance of drug standards

7. **Which of the following level is not the main link of the health system?**
   a. Central level
   b. Regional level
   c. State level
   d. Local or peripheral level

8. **Which of the following is not in concurrent list?**
   a. Control of drugs and poisons
   b. Population control and family planning
   c. Regulation and development of medical pharmaceutical, dental and nursing profession
   d. Prevention of adulteration of food stuff

9. **Panchayati Raj at the village level comprises:**
   a. Gram Sabha
   b. Gram Panchayat
   c. Nayaya Panchayat
   d. All of these

10. **Which of the following is not true regarding health system in India?**
   a. Autonomy to the states was given by the Government of India Act 1953.
   b. Bhore Committee in 1946, recommended that medical and public health organization should be integrated to have single administrative officer.
   c. The districts are divided into tehsils, municipalities and Panchayats for the purpose of administration.
   d. Ministry of Health and Family Welfare comprises health secretaries, deputy secretaries and administrative staff.

11. **Urban areas are organized according to their range of population into:**
   a. Town area committees
   b. Municipal boards
   c. Municipal corporation
   d. All of these

12. **At district level, CMO is assisted by:**
   a. Civil surgeon
   b. District health officer
   c. District family welfare officer
   d. All of these

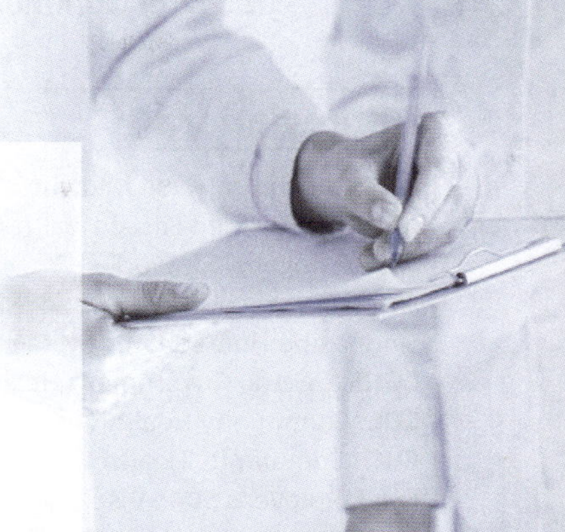

2

Healthcare Delivery System

LEARNING OBJECTIVES

After the completion of the unit, the readers will be able to:
- Describe the healthcare concept in India.
- Explain the healthcare services in India.
- Discuss the nurse's role in healthcare services.

UNIT OUTLINE

- Introduction
- Concepts of Healthcare
- Healthcare System
- Trends in Healthcare or Changing Concepts
- Healthcare Model
- Primary Healthcare in India
- Community Health Centers
- Community Development Program
- Healthcare Agencies
- Public-Private Partnership
- Indigenous System of Medicine
- Voluntary Health Services
- National Health Programs
- Nurses' Role in Healthcare Services

KEY TERMS

Basic health services (UNICEF/WHO): A network of coordinated, peripheral and intermediate health units capable of effectively performing, a selected group of functions, essential to the health of an area and ensuring the availability of competent professional and auxiliary personnel to perform these functions.

Comprehensive healthcare: Provision of integrated preventive, curative and promotive health services (from "womb to tomb") to every individual residing in a defined geographical area.

Healthcare: Multitude of services referred to as individuals, families and communities by the health professionals for the purpose of promoting, maintaining, monitoring or restoring health.

Primary healthcare (Alma-Ata Conference 1978): An essential healthcare made universally accessible to individuals and acceptable to them, through their full participation and at a cost the community and country can afford.

Abbreviations

ANM: Auxiliary Nurse Midwife
ASHA: Accredited Social Health Activist
AWW: Anganwadi Worker
AYUSH: Ayurveda, Yoga and Naturopathy, Unani, Siddha and Homeopathy System of Medicine
CGHS: Central Government Health Scheme
CHC: Community Health Center
CHO: Community Health Officer
ESI: Employees State Insurance Scheme
FHW: Female Health Worker
HFA: Health For All
HWCs: Health and Wellness Centers
ICDS: Integrated Child Development Services
IPHS: Indian Public Health Standard
ISM: Indian System of Medicine

IUD: Intrauterine Device
LHV: Lady Health Visitor
MCH: Mother and Child Healthcare
MTP: Medical Termination of Pregnancy
NIN: National Institute of Naturopathy
NRHM: National Rural Health Mission
ORS: Oral Rehydration Solution
PHC: Primary Health Center
PPP: Public-Private Partnership
RNTCP: Revised National Tuberculosis Control Program
SC: Subcenter
TB: Tuberculosis
TBA: Traditional Birth Attendant
VHG: Village Health Guide

INTRODUCTION

Healthcare services are a multitude of services provided to the individuals, families and communities by the healthcare agency for the purpose of promoting, preventing, curing, rehabilitating and restoring the health. Since health has been declared as a fundamental human right so, it is the responsibility of the government to provide healthcare services to its people in equal measures. The national governments are trying to expand and improve their health services. The present concern is not only to provide the adequate health services to the whole population but also to secure an acceptable level of health for all. This can be accomplished through the application of primary healthcare program both in developed and developing countries.

CONCEPTS OF HEALTHCARE

The present concept is that it is not limited to the medical care. It extends beyond this limit since health is influenced by a number of factors such as education, employment, food, housing, sanitation healthy lifestyle, protection against environmental hazards and communicable diseases. Therefore, it is a multitude of services provided to the individuals, families and community by the agents of health services for the purpose of promoting, maintaining, monitoring and restoring health of a country. The social policy throughout the world is to build up health system based on primary healthcare to meet the health needs of the people. There are two major themes in the delivery of health services:

1. The health services should be able to meet the health needs of the entire population and not merely the selected groups. It should cover the full range of preventive, curative and rehabilitative services.
2. It is realized that the best way to provide healthcare at the grassroots level to the underserved rural and urban poor, is to develop an affective "primary healthcare services" supported by an appropriate referral system.

To provide universal healthcare services, the participation of the community is an essential component. In this approach, whole system of healthcare, i.e., treatment, promotion of health and prevention from disease is taken under consideration. In present system of healthcare services, there is a shift from medical care to healthcare and from urban population to the rural population. Medical care is one component of the total healthcare system and it refers to the services directly provided by the physician or as a result of physician's instructions to the sick people mainly in the hospital or may be domiciliary care.

HEALTHCARE SYSTEM

It is not possible to define a fixed role of health services, since the socioeconomic pattern of one country differs from another. The health services are delivered by a healthcare system which is carefully planned and scheduled. This is done to meet the needs of an entire population and make health services accessible to them at a cost which the country can afford, with full participation of the people. To achieve the comprehensive healthcare, health services are organized at three levels.

Levels of Healthcare System

In the healthcare system, the health services are organized at three levels. These are primary, secondary and tertiary levels. These levels represent different types of care involving varying degree of complexity and supported by a referral system. These levels are described as under:

Primary Level

Primary level is the first level of contact between the individual, family and community with the national health system, where primary healthcare or an essential healthcare is provided.
- As it is the first level of care, hence, it is close to the people and accessible.
- Most of the health problems are dealt in a satisfactory manner and are resolved here.
- In an Indian context, the primary care is provided through subcenters and primary health centers by an agency of health workers which include ANM, ASHA, Anganwadi workers, village health guides. It also includes trained *dais*, medical officers and other staff at primary health center level as given in the model of primary level of care (Fig. 2.1).
- Besides providing primary healthcare, the village health team bridges the cultural and communication gap between the rural population and organized health centers.
- Since India has opted for 'Health For All' by 2000 AD, primary healthcare system has been reorganized and strengthened to make the primary healthcare delivery system more effective.

Secondary Level

The next higher level of care is secondary level or an intermediate level of care. At this level, more complex problems are dealt:
- The specialist services and investigation facilities are available here.
- This level of care comprises essentially curative services and is provided at district hospitals and community health center.
- This level serves as a first referral level in the health system. Model of secondary level of healthcare is shown in Figure 2.2.

Tertiary Level

The tertiary level of care is more specialized than the secondary level of care.

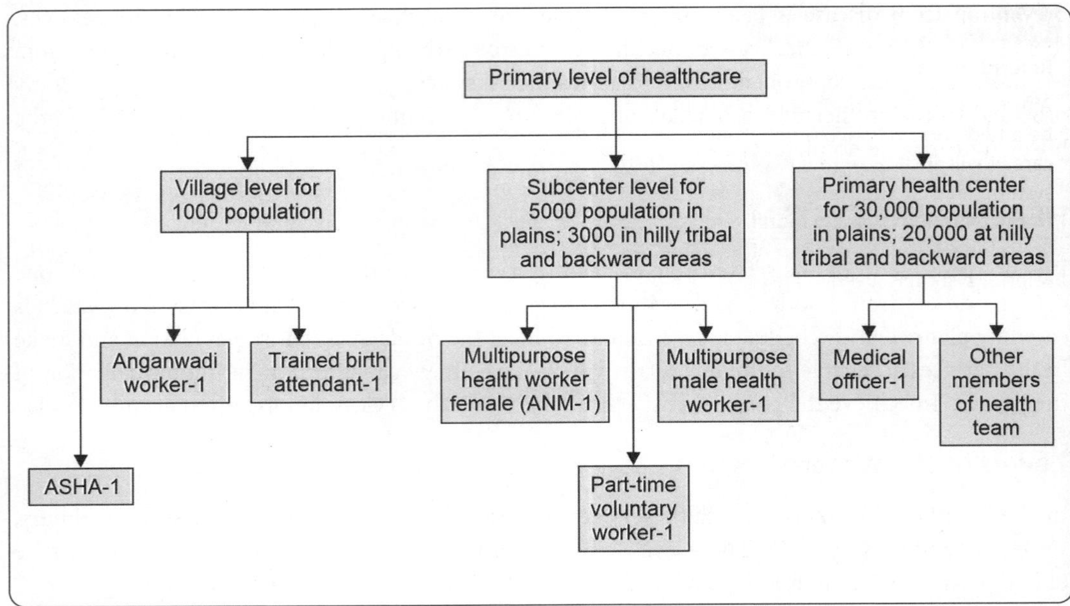

Figure 2.1: Model of primary level of healthcare

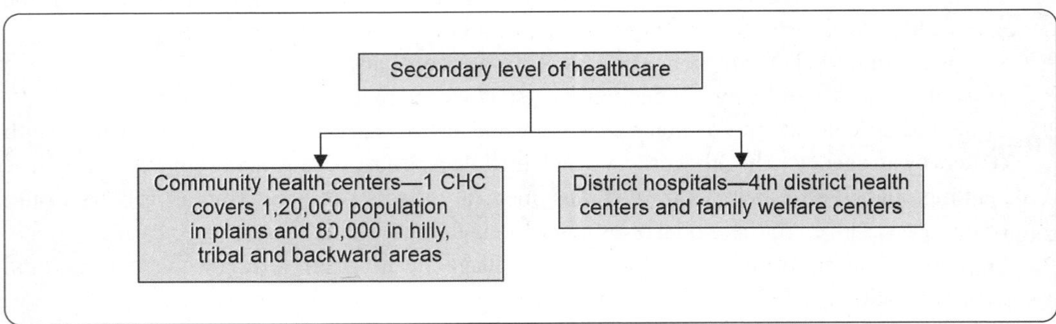

Figure 2.2: Model of secondary level of healthcare

- The specific facilities and highly specialized health workers are available to provide specialized healthcare.
- This level of care is provided by the regional or central level institution, such as medical colleges, hospitals, all India institutes, regional hospitals, specialized hospitals and other apex institutions.
- In addition, the tertiary level supports and complements the action carried out at primary and secondary level of care.
- The tertiary level institutions, in addition to providing tertiary level of care also serve as teaching institutions. The training and medical education is provided to the various categories of health workers.
- The planning, management and research work are also executed at this level.

Nursing Considerations

Referral System

A fundamental and necessary function of healthcare system is to provide a sound referral system. It must be a two-way exchange of information and returning patients to those, who referred them for follow-up care. It will ensure continuity of care and inspire confidence of the consumer in health system. This referral system needs to be strengthened to ensure smooth functioning of the health system. Patients are referred from community, health center to district hospitals and state level hospitals. After treatment again, they are referred back to the parent hospital/health center for follow-up care. The diagram representation of referral system is given in Figure 2.3.

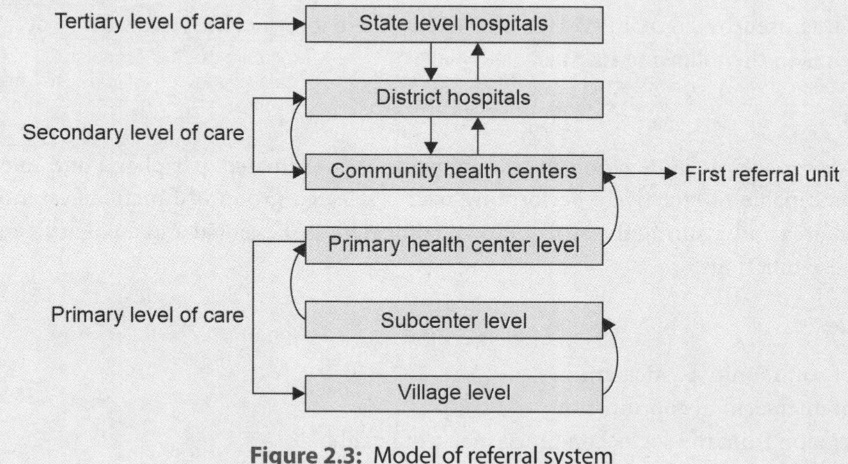

Figure 2.3: Model of referral system

TRENDS IN HEALTHCARE OR CHANGING CONCEPTS

With political independence, there was a national commitment to improve health in developing countries. Against this background different approaches came into existence as given here:

- Comprehensive healthcare
- Basic health services
- Primary healthcare

Comprehensive Healthcare

The Bhore Committee in 1946, used this term of comprehensive healthcare. The committee meant provision of integrated preventive, curative and promotional health services from 'womb to tomb' to every individual residing in a defined geographical area.

Criteria for Providing Comprehensive Healthcare

- It provides adequate preventive, curative and promotive health services.
- It should be as close to the beneficiaries as possible.
- It should be widest cooperation among the people, the services and profession.
- It should be available to all, irrespective of their capacity to pay.

- It should specially look after the vulnerable and weaker section of the community.
- It creates and maintains a healthy environment both in homes and in workplaces.

This concept of Bhore Committee formed the basis of national health planning in India and led to the establishments of a network of primary health centers, but was not able to provide comprehensive healthcare due to under staffing and lack of adequate supply of equipment and medicine. Moreover, it was not able to cover the whole population under its jurisdiction and the coverage of services, did not extend beyond 2–5 km of radius.

Basic Health Services

This term was used by UNICEF/WHO in 1965, in their joint health policy. They defined basic health services in the following manner.

Definition

'Basic health services' is understood to be a network of coordinated, peripheral and intermediate health units capable of effectively performing over a selected group of functions essential to the health of an area and assuring the availability of competent professional and auxiliary personnel to perform these functions.

Drawbacks

- Lack of community participation
- Lack of intersectoral coordination
- Dissociation from the socioeconomic aspects of health.

Primary Healthcare

This new concept came into existence in 1978, following an international conference at Alma-Ata (USSR), this is known as "primary healthcare". It has all the aspects of primary healthcare delivery proposed by Bhore Committee in 1946. It is now espoused worldwide by international agencies and national government. Before Alma-Ata Conference, the primary healthcare was regarded synonymous with basic health services, first contact care, easily accessible care, services provided by generalist, etc. Alma-Ata International Conference gave primary healthcare a wide meaning.

Definitions

"Primary healthcare is an essential healthcare made universally accessible to individuals and acceptable to them, through their full participation and at a cost the community and country can afford."

                                                          —WHO

According to Alma-Ata Conference (1978), "Primary healthcare is essential healthcare based on practical, scientifically sound and socially acceptable method and technology. This method should be universally accessible to individuals and families and also in the community, as their full participation would be required. Also, it should be available at the cost which the community and the country can afford in order to maintain the spirit of self-determination at every stage of their development".

Concepts

In the light of above definitions, it should be:
- Affordable to the country and community
- Universally accessible to all citizen of the country
- Available to all irrespective of rural, urban, rich or poor communities
- Socially acceptable based on practical and scientifically sound technology
- Accountable to healthcare agencies of the country.

Goals

The main goal of primary healthcare is to fulfill the global commitment of HFA by 2000 AD and achieve an improved state of health and quality of life for all people attained through self-reliance, thus placing people's health in people's hands.

Strategy

To strengthen the existing infrastructure of healthcare system by training people and increasing the strength of healthcare workers so that health services can reach to rural areas and at grassroots level.

Objectives

- To reduce the incidence of communicable and noncommunicable diseases.
- To sustain the population growth as per the available resources.
- To reduce the mortality and morbidity rate among infants and preschool children.
- To improve the level of healthcare in the community.
- To extend essential health services in rural areas and underserved sectors.
- To improve basic sanitation.

Elements of Primary Healthcare

There are eight essential elements of primary healthcare as mentioned here:
1. **Health education:** Educating people about health and existing health problems. In order to control and prevent these health problems, certain measures are formulated and people are made aware of the health facilities available to them so that it could be utilized when required.
2. **Nutrition:** Good nutrition is essential for the health and for the growth and development of children. People should be encouraged to pay attention to a balanced diet and knowledge must be provided regarding preparation of food and preserving the nutrients present in diet.
3. **Water and sanitation:** Adequate supply of safe drinking water and sanitation is necessary for good health and is an important factor for the environment.
4. **Mother and child health including family planning:** The mother and children are the most vulnerable group to suffer with health problems and accounts for large percentage of population. Protection of mother and child from illness and other risks would ensure good health of family and community. The family planning services include spacing of children and adopting small family norms will check the population growth.

5. **Immunization against major infectious diseases:** Protection from major infectious diseases of children by providing immunization to them, this involves providing vaccine to them against poliomyelitis, diphtheria, tetanus, measles, tuberculosis, hepatitis B along with other vaccines, which can prevent harmful infectious diseases.
6. **Prevention and control of locally endemic diseases**: To reduce the morbidity rate. An example of this, is malaria control.
7. **Treatment:** Appropriate treatment of general diseases and injuries by using appropriate technology.
8. **Provision of essential drugs:** Ensuring easy availability of drugs.

Principles

There are five principles of primary healthcare given by WHO, which are listed as follows:
1. Equitable distribution
2. Community participation
3. Appropriate technology
4. Focus on prevention
5. Intersectoral coordination

Equitable Distribution

The health services and resources should be equally distributed to all irrespective of their ability to pay. It should be available to all, without any discrimination of caste, creed, and gender, religion, rich, poor, urban or rural. According to this principle, the primary healthcare should be available to all individuals, families and community. It is based on the social justice. The people living in the rural areas are main target of the primary healthcare.

Community Participation

Without the involvement of community, it is difficult to achieve the goal of primary healthcare. There must be continuing efforts to seek involvement of the community in planning, implementation and maintenance of health services. The local health workers from the village, such as village health guide, Anganwadi workers, ASHA and trained *dais* are providing health services by overcoming cultural and communication barriers, this is done in such a way that it becomes acceptable to the community.

Appropriate Technology

The technology used in primary healthcare should be scientifically sound, safe, socially acceptable, suitable to local requirement and within the financial limits and should be locally available. Use of ORS is an example for the treatment of diarrhea.

Focus on Prevention

The main focus of primary healthcare is on prevention of disease and promotion of health rather than the treatment and it is one of the constituents of health services. Health education is also stressed by the primary healthcare.

Intersectoral Coordination

For the successful implementation of primary healthcare, coordination of other sectors is necessary, such as agriculture, sanitation, housing, nutrition, public works, communication and education.

In order to meet current needs and emerging challenges, a number of working groups were constituted in 1996 to comprehensively review the existing health situation in totality.

The areas included are:

- Communicable diseases
- Health system and biomedical research development
- Indigenous system of medicine
- Environmental health
- Health education and information education and communication (IEC)
- Women's empowerment
- Requirement for supportive and diagnostic services in primary, secondary and tertiary care.

Responsibilities of Nurses in Primary Healthcare

The successful implementation of primary healthcare lies with community health nursing. Therefore, the community health nursing system should be developed and strengthened so that nurses can effectively discharge their responsibilities related to primary healthcare. In 1984, the expert committee of WHO recommended the following responsibilities for nurses so that they could take care of primary health:

- Assessing the health level of individuals and community.
- Ensuring active participation of community and encouraging the individuals to participate.
- Providing treatment in emergencies and taking care of the general health.
- Referring the patients to the specialist following the referral system.
- Keeping an eye on the epidemics.
- Providing training and supervision of health workers.
- Coordination with other health programs.
- Providing health education on preventive, promotive and curative aspects of health.
- Maintaining the progress of primary healthcare.

HEALTHCARE MODEL

A various number of models of healthcare delivery systems are developed with a view to provide healthcare services. These services should be reasonably inexpensive and basic or essential requirements of rural population must be chosen. One of the simplest models is shown as in Figure 2.4.

The components of the model are:

- **Inputs:** Include health status or health problems and resources.
- **Healthcare services:** Comprises protective preventive, promotional and curative and rehabilitative services.
- **Healthcare system:** Comprises public and private system, along with voluntary and indigenous system.
- **Outputs:** Involves improved health status of the community, expressed in terms of lives saved, cases treated, diseases prevented, and deaths averted for prolonged life expectancy.

Inputs

Inputs involve considering the health status or health problems of the community. They represent the health needs and health demands of the community. The resources, such as manpower required

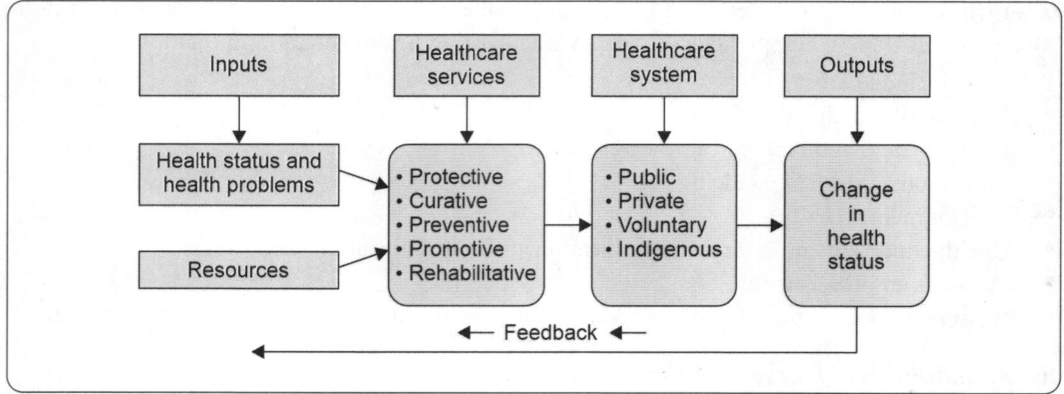

Figure 2.4: Model of healthcare delivery system

for maintaining good health, finance, equipment and supplies are limited, so, the health needs of vast population may not be fulfilled. In order to fulfill the requirements of health needs, it is essential to set a careful planning and good managerial skills are required for this purpose.

Health Status and Health Problems

The first requisite for any planned effort to develop healthcare services is the assessment of health status and health problems or community diagnosis. The data required to judge the health status and health problems comprises the following:

- Morbidity and mortality statistics.
- Demographic conditions of the population.
- Environment conditions which influence the health status.
- Socioeconomic factors which have a direct effect on health.
- Cultural background, attitudes, beliefs and practices which effect health.
- Medical and health services available.
- Other services available.

The health status and health problem can be analyzed in the light of above data. Then the problems are ranked according to the priority. On priority basis the resources are allocated. The current demographic and mortality profile and health problems in India are discussed as follows:

Demographic Profile

Population explosion is one of the biggest problems, which the country is facing. The demographic profile is characterized by the following:

- Large population based.
- High fertility, both in terms of birth rate and family size.
- Low or declining mortality.
- Young population which is below the age of 25 years is approximately 50% of the total population.
- According to the latest data, the literacy rate in India has improved from 77% to 85.91% in 2024 all over India, and it explains the decline in birth rate, which has been so slow.
- Dependency ratio 48.1 per 100 as per the census 2022, that is every economically productive member has to support almost one dependent.

Mortality Profile

The death rate has steadily declined from 21 (1965) to 7.473 (2024). The life expectancy at birth has risen considerably, since 1951. It is estimated as 70.62 years (2024), which shows a decline in mortality rate from a number of infectious diseases. This involves decline in the cases of cholera, tuberculosis and malaria.

Health Problems

Major health problems in India are listed here:

- Communicable disease problems
- Noncommunicable disease problems
- Nutritional problems
- Environmental sanitation problems
- Medical care problems
- Population problems
- Resources

Communicable disease problems: The diseases which are considered of great importance, have been listed here:

- **Malaria:** It continues to be a major health problem in India. Though the total cases have declined compared to previous years, but malaria cases have increased in states like, Madhya Pradesh, Chhattisgarh, Jharkhand, Odisha, Andhra Pradesh and Maharashtra.
- **Tuberculosis:** India accounts for one-fifth of incidence of tuberculosis in the world. The emergence of HIV/TB coinfection and multidrug-resistant TB has increased the severity and magnitude of the disease. In March 2006, RNTCP has achieved nationwide coverage.
- **Diarrheal disease:** It constitutes one of the major causes of morbidity and mortality, especially in children below five years of age.
- **Acute respiratory infection:** It is also one of the major causes of mortality and morbidity in children under-five years of age.
- **Leprosy:** It is another public health problem in India.
- **Filariasis:** It is an endemic disease, in almost 250 districts of 22 States and 5 UTs. The population at risk is over 600 million.
- **AIDS:** It is relatively stable in India.
- **Others:** Kala-azar, meningitis, viral hepatitis, Japanese encephalitis, and enteric fever and helminthic infections are among the other important communicable diseases in India. These can be easily treated and prevented with minimum input of resources.

Noncommunicable disease problems: Noncommunicable diseases are estimated to account for 60% of all deaths in 2024. Especially, diabetes mellitus, cardiovascular diseases, cancer, strokes, lung disease, and cataract are major health problems due to aging population and environmentally driven change in behaviors.

Nutritional problems: The specific nutritional problems are:

- Protein-energy malnutrition (PEM)
- Nutritional anemia
- Low birth weight
- Xerophthalmia due to deficiency of vitamin A
- Iodine deficiency disorders.
- **Others:** Other important nutritional problems include lathyrism and endemic goiter in certain parts of the country.

Environmental sanitation problems: The environmental sanitation problems are of great concern, but are very difficult to tackle. These problems are multifaceted and multifactor. The sanitation problems suffered in the country are:

- Lack of soft water
- Excreta disposal
- Besides this, the 'new' problems are emerging out from population explosion, urbanization and industrialization leading to pollution in air, water and food.
- As for the year 2015, safe water is available to 97% of urban and 93% to rural population
- Adequate waste disposal facilities are available to 63% urban and 28% to rural population.

Medical care problems: The medical care problems in India are concerned with the health services, which are curative in nature and hospital-based. About 80% of health facilities are concentrated in urban area and that too is not equally distributed. The rural population of India, which constitutes about 72%, where the health facilities are meager and unevenly distributed. The major health problem in India is the inequitable distribution of availability of health resources among the urban and rural areas.

The "Health for all by 2000 AD" movement and primary healthcare approach laid stress on equity, intersectoral coordination and community participation which are required in order to redress these imbalances.

Population problems: The main problem India is facing of population explosion. Population explosion has inevitable consequences on all aspects of development, especially employment, education, housing, healthcare, sanitation and environment. The government has set a goal to achieve 1% population growth rate by the year 2000 AD, which was not attained. The population size and structure represent the single most important factor in health and manpower planning.

Resources: Resources are needed to meet the health needs of vast community. The basic resources for providing healthcare are:

- Health manpower
- Money and material
- Time

Healthcare Services

Purpose

The purpose of healthcare services is to improve the health status of the population and national development.

Millennium Goals

The goals to be achieved in the light of HFA, by 2000 AD were the following:

- Reduce the mortality and morbidity
- Increase the life expectancy
- Decrease the population growth rate
- Improve the nutritional status
- Provide basic sanitation
- Improve the literacy rate
- Reduce the level of poverty

- Increase food production
- Health manpower requirement and resources development
- The resources must be distributed according to the needs of the community
- Health services should be comprehensive, accessible, and acceptable. It should provide scope for community participation and must be available at a cost the community and country can afford.

Healthcare System

The healthcare system (Fig. 2.5) is intended to deliver healthcare services. It constitutes management sector and involves organizational matters. It operates in the context of socioeconomic and political framework of the country. In India, there are five major sectors or agencies which provide healthcare and they differ from each other by the health technology applied and source of funds in operation. The health sectors in India are:

- **Public Health Sector (Fig. 2.6):** The public health sector is a government sponsored system. It is financed by public funds generated through taxes. Services are provided to the rural and urban areas by 3-tier system, i.e., at block level, district level and state level.

  Public health sector includes the following:

  - **Primary healthcare:**
    - Subcenters
    - Primary health centers
  - **Hospitals/health centers:**
    - Community health center
    - Specialist hospitals
    - Rural hospitals
    - Teaching hospitals
    - District hospital/health center
  - **Health insurance schemes:**
    - Employees state insurance
    - Central government health schemes
  - **Other agencies:**
    - Defense services hospital
    - Railway hospitals
- **Private health sector:**
  - Private hospitals, polyclinics, nursing homes and dispensaries
  - General practitioner and clinics.

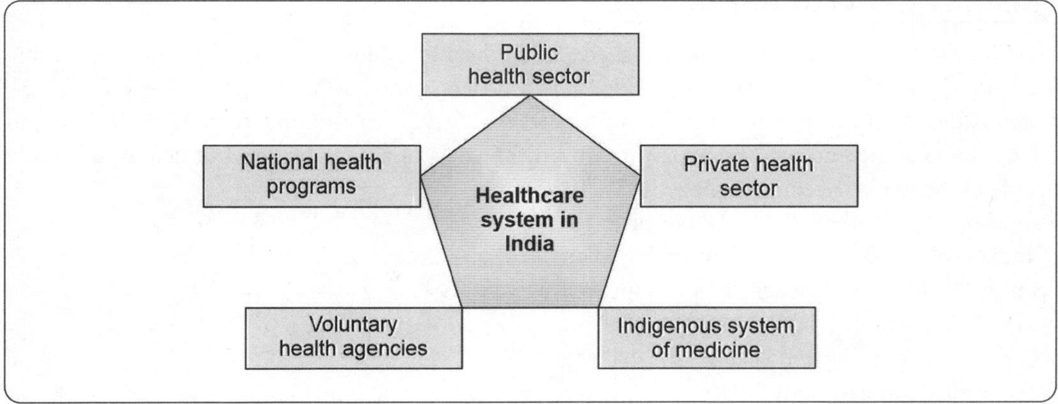

Figure 2.5: Model of healthcare system in India

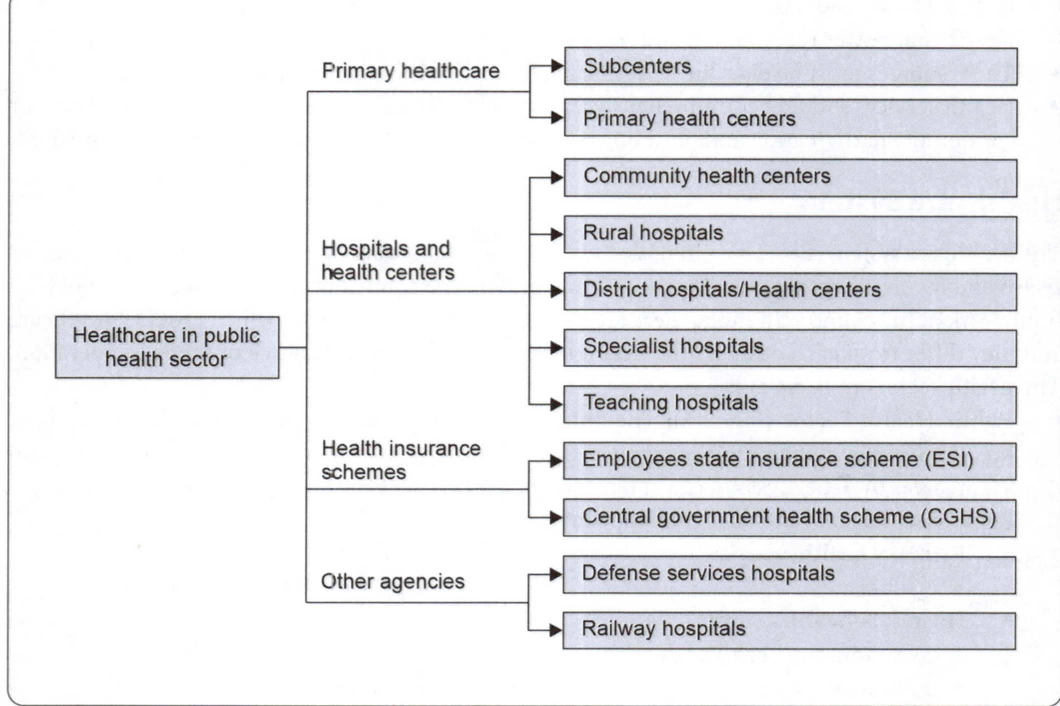

Figure 2.6: Healthcare system in public sector

- **Indigenous system of medicine (AYUSH):**
  - Ayurveda and Siddha
  - Unani and Tibbi
  - Homeopathy
  - Unregistered practitioners
- **Voluntary health agencies**
- **National health programs**

PRIMARY HEALTHCARE IN INDIA

In 1977, the Government of India launched a rural health scheme with the principles of placing the people's health in people's own hands. It is a 3-tier system of healthcare delivery (Fig. 2.7), which is based on the recommendation of the heels of Srivastava Committee in 1975. In 1978, an international conference at Alma-Ata introduced the goals of acceptable level of health for all the people of the world. Keeping in view the WHO goal of health for all by 2000 AD, Government of India evolved national health policy based on primary healthcare approach. It was approved in 1983. This policy laid down the plan of actions for reorienting and shaping the existing rural health infrastructure. Steps were taken to implement national health policy objectives

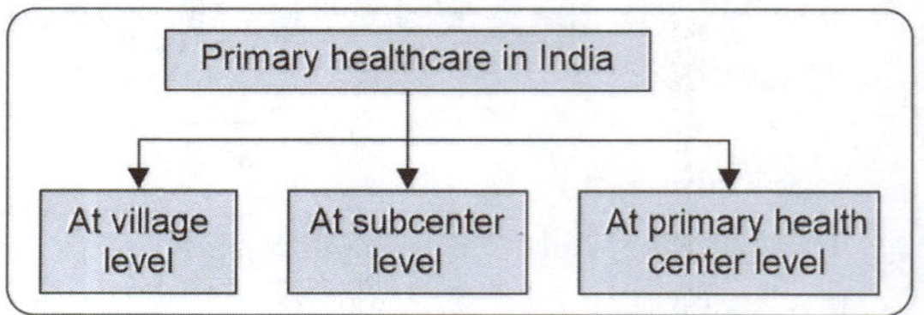

Figure 2.7: Three-tier system of primary healthcare in India

and implementing the primary healthcare approach. During last decade, further development of rural health infrastructure took place in view to implement national health policy 2000 and more recently national rural health mission with formulation of Indian public health standard.

National Health Policy 2017

National Health Policy 2017, recommended strengthening the delivery system of primary healthcare and announced Ayushman Bharat Program, a flagship scheme of Government of India to achieve the vision of Universal Health Coverage (UHC). The initiative has been designed to meet Sustainable Development Goals (SDGs) and its underlying commitment which is to "Leave no one Behind".

Ayushman Bharat

This program was announced in 2018 by Government of India and an attempt to move from sectoral and segment approach of the health services delivery to a comprehensive need based healthcare service. The scheme aims to undertake path breaking intervention to holistically address the healthcare service system covering prevention, promotion and ambulatory care of primary, secondary and tertiary level of care. Ayushman Bharat has two components:
1. Health and wellness centers
2. The second component is the Ayushman Bharat Pradhan Mantri Jan Arogya Yojana (AB-PMJAY)
1. Health and wellness center: In February 2018, Government of India announced the creation of 1,50,000 health and wellness centers by transforming existing subcenters and primary health centers as the base pillar of Ayushman Bharat. These centers are to deliver Comprehensive Primary Healthcare (CPHC) bringing healthcare closer to the homes of people. They cover both maternal and child health services and noncommunicable disease including free essential drugs and diagnostic services.

   Health and wellness centers are envisaged to deliver an expanded range of services to address the primary healthcare needs of the entire population in that area expanding access, universality and equity close to the community. The emphasis of health promotion and prevention is designed to bring focus on keeping people healthy by engaging and empowering individuals and communities to choose healthy behaviors and make changes that reduce the risk of developing chronic diseases and mortalities. There are about 1,60,000 HWCs functioning in India and gradually all existing SC and PHC will be transformed into HWCs. The first health and wellness center was inaugurated on 14th April 2018 in Bijapur district of Chhattisgarh.
2. The second component of Ayushman Bharat Program is Ayushman Bharat Pradhan Mantri Jan Arogya Yojana (AB-PMJAY) which provides health coverage up to ₹5 lakh per family per year to about 12 crore poor and vulnerable families identified on the basis of socioeconomic cast census data for secondary and tertiary care hospitalization. PMJAY covers 3 days of prehospitalization and 15 days post hospitalization expenses such as diagnostics and medicines. There is no restriction of family size, age, or gender. All pre-existing conditions are covered from day one. To promote wellness and healthy lifestyle activities and lifestyle modification like increased physical activities such as cyclothon and marathon are encouraged. Eating right and safe.
   - For cessation of smoking and drugs, deaddiction centers are opened
   - Yoga sessions are being conducted at these centers on regular basis.

- The meditation centers, laughter clubs and gyms are being opened.
- Through annual health calendar, planned activities at these centers on health conditions of the day has increased the awareness and preventive measures for keeping good health.

Primary healthcare is a 3-tier system of healthcare:
1. At village level
2. At subcenter HWC (SC-HWC) level
3. At primary health center HWC (PHC-HWC) level

At Village Level

One of the basic principles of primary healthcare services is the universal coverage and equitable distribution of health services. That is healthcare must reach to the farthest of the rural areas and everyone should have access to it. At village level (Fig. 2.8), this policy is implemented through the following schemes:
- Training of local *dais*
- ICDS Scheme (Anganwadi workers)
- Accredited Social Health Activist (ASHA)

Training of Local Dais

The deliveries were handled by untrained *dais* in rural areas. A scheme for training of local *dais* was initiated during 1977. It was implemented in 156 districts in 18 states/UTs of India. The districts were selected on the basis of the safe delivery (being <30%). The aim was to train at least one *dai* in every village for 1000 population. The objective was to make the delivery safe.

Training Period

- *Dais* are given training for 30 working days at primary health center or subcenter.
- The training is conducted for 2 days in a week at subcenter or primary health center and in the remaining 4 days they accompany the ANM to the village.
- They are required to conduct 2 deliveries under the guidance and supervision of female health worker.
- Each *dai* is paid ₹300/- during the training.
- After completion of training, each *dai* is provided with a delivery kit and a certificate.
- They are entitled to ₹150/- delivery provided; the case is registered with subcenter or primary health center. Trained *dais* is also known as traditional birth attendants (TBA) in the country.

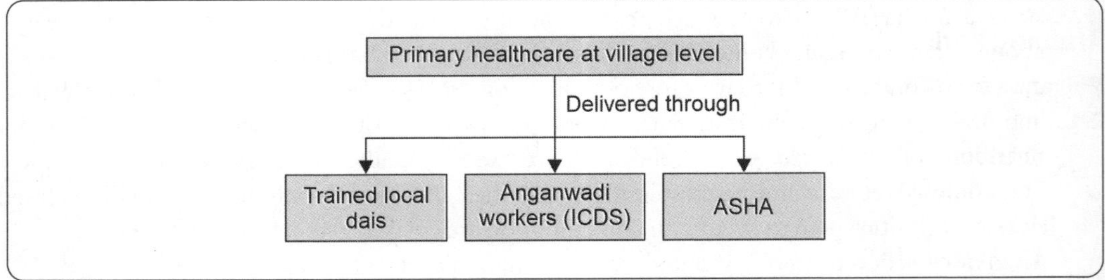

Figure 2.8: Delivery of primary healthcare at village level

To reduce neonatal mortality, the trained birth attendants like ANM, and staff nurses are preferred as compared to traditional birth attendant who is not having professional education and is illiterate. The training of local *dais* is given less importance except very remote and hard to reach area. Since the aim is to have 100% institutional delivery under the National Health Mission, primary healthcare is reaching to rural and remote areas. People are becoming aware of hospital facilities. Moreover, Government of India has provided incentives for institutional deliveries under the various schemes. Due to advancement in education and services of ASHA, ladies prefer institutional deliveries. Though the services of local *dais* are also utilized for motivation to attend prenatal clinics, for immunization and family planning services, etc.

Functions

Dais have vital role in providing domiciliary services in rural areas:
- Conduct every pregnant woman for registration
- Attend every prenatal clinic
- Ensure immunization of pregnant woman and newborn babies
- Motivate eligible couple
- Report about birth and death in the area to the subcenter or primary health center
- Provide essential newborn care
- Provide postnatal care to the delivery cases.

According to National Health Mission 2013, the Government of India adopts the goal of universal institutional delivery, as the Skilled Birth Attendants (SBAs) are more effective in lowering maternal and neonatal mortality rate than Traditional Birth Attendants (TBA) who is not having professional knowledge and is illiterate with the foundation of NRHM in 2005, gradually the primary healthcare became accessible to 70% of the rural population of India. With the awareness about the safety of hospital delivery. Due to increased access to hospitals, the institutional delivery has become a trend. In addition, the government has provided incentives like JSY and JSSK to achieve 100% institutional deliveries. Therefore, RCH-II program excluded *dais* as skilled birth attendant (MOHFW). This marginalization of *dais*, included a gradual half of *dai* training and provision of *dai* kit. Thus, the *Dai* training program is discontinued, but it is still existing in very remote and rural areas of some parts of the country. Secondly, ASHA and women are benefitted by institutional delivery.

ICDS Scheme (Anganwadi Workers)

"Angan" literally means a courtyard. Under the Integrated Child Development Scheme (ICDS), there is one anganwadi worker for 1000 population. There are about 100 anganwadi workers in each ICDS project. They are part-time workers.

Training Period

Anganwadi workers are selected from the community, they are expected to serve. They undergo training for 4 months on the following aspects of health:
- Nutrition
- Child development, i.e., health check-up of children at various stages of development
- Health education
- After training they are paid salary as per the government policies, at present ₹5000 to 8000 per month and it varies in each state.

Duties

- Health checkup of children including maintenance of growth chart
- Supplementary nutrition
- Immunization
- Informal education of preschool children
- Health education
- Care of lactating mothers, adolescent girls and women of reproductive age (15–40) and children under 6 years of age.
- Referral services
- Anganwadi along with ASHA are the community's primary link with health services and all other services for young children.

Accredited Social Health Activist (ASHA)

The post of ASHA was created under national rural health services, also known as NRHM. There is one ASHA for 1000 population.

Selection of ASHA

- ASHA is selected from the same community.
- She should be married/divorcee/widow.
- She should be between the ages of 25 and 45 years.
- She should have minimum education up to 10th standard.
- She should have good knowledge of communication and leadership.
- She is volunteer worker. Central Government pays her ₹3000/month and salary from State Government is incentive based paid salary ₹3000/month by central government, and salary from state government is incentive based. The list of incentive-based payment from state is presented as follows:

ASHA incentive for routine and recurrent activities		
Sl. no.	**Activities**	**Incentive in Rs./Case**
1.	Mobilizing and attending Village Health and Nutrition Days or Urban Health and Nutrition Days	₹200/session
2.	Conveying and guiding monthly meetings of VHSNC/MAS	₹150
3.	Attending monthly meetings at Block PHC/UPHC	₹150
4.	a. Line listing of households done at beginning of the year and updated every 6 months	₹300
	b. Maintaining village health register and supporting universal registration of births and deaths to be updated on the monthly basis	₹300
	c. Preparation of due list of children to be immunized on monthly basis	₹300
	d. Preparation of list of ANC beneficiaries to be updated on monthly basis	₹300
	e. Preparation of list of eligible couple on monthly basis	₹300

Contd...

ASHA Incentives under National Health Program		
I	**Maternal Health**	
	JSY financial package	
1.	a. For ensuring antenatal care for the woman	₹300 for Rural areas and ₹200 for Urban areas
	b. For facilitating institutional delivery	₹300 for Rural areas and ₹200 for Urban areas
2.	Reporting Death of women (15–49 years age group) by ASHA to PHC Medical Officer	₹200 for reporting within 24 hours of occurrence of death by phone
3.	Mobilization of HRPs under E-PMSMA	₹300 per ASHA to mobilize high-risk pregnant woman to facility for follow-up @ ₹100/-per visit for maximum up to 3 visits
4.	Healthy outcome for HRPs under E-PMSMA	₹500 after ensuring survival of baby and mother duo after 45 days of delivery.
5.	Identification of HRPs and their healthy outcome during Postnatal Period under optimization of PNC	₹250 after ensuring survival of baby and mother duo after 45 days of delivery
II	**Child Health**	
1.	Home visit for the newborn and postpartum mother (2), six visits in case of institutional delivery (days 3, 7, 14, 21, 28 and 42), seven visits in case of home deliveries (days 1, 3, 7, 14, 21, 28 and 42)	₹250
2.	Home visits of young child for strengthening of health and nutrition of young child through home visits (recommended schedule- 3, 6, 9, 12 and 15 months) -(₹50 × 5 visits)	₹50/visit with total ₹250/ child for making 5 visits
3.	Ensuring quarterly follow-up of low-birth-weight babies and newborns discharged after treatment from Specialized newborn care units.	₹50/Quarter-from the 3rd month until 1 year of age
4.	Child death review for reporting child death of children under 5 years of age	₹50
5.	Week-1 and 2-ASHA incentive for prophylactic distribution of ORS to families with under-five children	₹1 per ORS packet for 100 under-five children or ₹100 per ASHA
III	**Immunization**	
1.	Full immunization for a child under 1 year	₹100
2.	Complete immunization per child up to two years age (all vaccination received between 1st and 2nd year of age after completing full immunization after one year)	₹75
3.	Mobilizing children for OPV immunization under Pulse Polio Program	₹100/day
4.	DPT Booster at 5–6 years of age	₹50
5.	Mobilization of children for routine immunization	₹150/session

Contd...

IV	Family planning	
1.	Ensuring spacing of 2 years after marriage	₹500
2.	Ensuring spacing of 3 years after birth of 1st child	₹500
3.	Ensuring a couple to opt for permanent limiting method after 2 children	₹1000
4.	Counseling, motivating and follow-up of the cases for Tubectomy	₹200 in 11 states with high fertility rates (UP, Bihar, MP, Rajasthan, Chhattisgarh, Jharkhand, Odisha, Uttarakhand, Assam, Haryana, and Gujarat) ₹300 in 146 MPV districts ₹150 in remaining States
5.	Counseling, motivating and follow-up of the cases for Vasectomy/NSV	₹300 in 11 states with high fertility rates (UP, Bihar, MP, Rajasthan, Chhattisgarh, Jharkhand, Odisha, Uttarakhand, Assam, Haryana, and Gujarat) 400 in 146 MPV districts ₹200 in remaining States
6.	Female postpartum sterilization	₹300 in 11 states with high fertility rates (UP, Bihar, MP, Rajasthan, Chhattisgarh, Jharkhand, Odisha, Uttarakhand, Assam, Haryana, and Gujarat) and 400 in 146 MPV districts
7.	Escorting or facilitating beneficiary to the health facility for the PPIUCD insertion	₹150/case
8.	Escorting or facilitating beneficiary to the health facility for the PAIUCD insertion	₹150/case
Mission Parivar Vikas (MPV) extended in all districts of the seven high focus States (UP, Bihar, Jharkhand, MP, Chhattisgarh, Rajasthan and Assam) as well as six North-Eastern States of the country.		
9.	Injectable Contraceptive—MPA (Antara Program) and a nonhormonal weekly centchroman pill (Chhaya)—Incentive to ASHA	₹100 per dose
10.	Mission Parivar Vikas Campaigns Block level activities—ASHA to be oriented on eligible couple survey for estimation of beneficiaries and will be expected to conduct eligible couple survey—maximum four rounds	₹150/ASHA/round
11.	Nayi Pahel—an FP kit for newlyweds- an FP kit would be given to the newlywed couple by ASHA (in initial phase ASHA may be given 2 kits/ASHA)	₹100/ASHA/Nayi Pahel kit distribution
12.	Saas Bahu Sammelan—mobilizes Saas Bahu for the Sammelan—maximum four rounds	₹100/meeting

Contd...

V	Adolescent Health	
1.	Distributing sanitary napkins to adolescent girls	₹1/ pack of 6 sanitary napkins
2.	Organizing monthly meetings with adolescent girls pertaining to menstrual hygiene	₹50/meeting
3.	Incentive for support to peer educator (for facilitating selection process of peer educators)	₹100/PE
4.	Incentive for mobilizing adolescents for Adolescent Health Day	₹200/AHD
VI	Participatory Learning and Action- (In selected 10 states that have low RMNCH+A indicators – Assam, Bihar, Chhattisgarh, Jharkhand, MP, Meghalaya, Odisha, Rajasthan, Uttarakhand and UP)	
1.	Conducting PLA meetings—2 meetings per month *Note*: Incentive is also applicable for AFs @₹100/- per meeting for 10 meetings in a month	₹100/ASHA/per meeting for 2 meetings in a month
VII	Nutrition	
1.	Referral of SAM children to NRC and follow-up of SAM children after discharge from NRC	₹300 per SAM child/ASHA. Break-up as below: ₹100 for referral and ₹200 for follow-up
2.	For mobilizing and ensuring every eligible child (1–19 years out-of-school and nonenrolled) is administered Albendazole.	₹100/ ASHA/Biannual
3.	Mother's Absolute Affection (MAA) Program Promotion of Breastfeeding—Quarterly mother meeting	₹100/ASHA/ Quarterly meeting
4.	Anemia Mukt Bharat	
4a.	ASHA incentive for mobilizing children and ensuring compliance of IFA for 6–59 months children	₹100/month/ASHA
4b.	ASHA incentive for mobilizing and ensuring compliance of IFA for WRA	₹50/month/ASHA
VIII	National Tuberculosis Elimination Program	
1.	Honorarium to treatment supporter to be disbursed upon completion or cure of TB patient for Drug Susceptibility TB patients	₹1000
2.	For treatment and support to drug resistant TB patients	₹5000 (₹2000 for IP and ₹3000 for CP) for Drug Resistant TB patients (including shorter regimen, MDR and XDR TB patients
3.	Incentives to informant for notification	₹500 for referral of presumptive TB patient to public health facility and diagnosis as TB
4.	Incentive to ASHA/Community Health Volunteers for ensuring seeding of bank account details of TB patients in Nikshay portal within 15 days of treatment initiation for enabling DBT Payments under NTEP	₹50/notified TB patient for seeding of bank account details on the Nikshay portal

Contd...

5.	Incentive to ASHA/Community Health Volunteers for supporting treatment adherence and completion of TB preventive treatment among eligible individuals	₹250/- per individual for successful completion of TB preventive treatment
6.	Mobilization of beneficiary through ASHA or other mobilizers for additional adult BCG beneficiaries	₹150 per session, two mobilizers will be present at each session site (ASHA/AWW/link worker). Each mobilizer may be paid ₹75 with a maximum limit of ₹150 per session site
7.	ASHA incentive for due list preparation (for monthly updating of due list of beneficiaries for adult BCG vaccination)	₹300/month × 3 months (if mop-up is required). This amount may be paid to the ASHA. If no ASHA is identified or available, the same may be paid to the link worker/AWW, subject to a total ceiling of ₹300
8.	ASHA incentive for house-to-house survey, before the campaign.	₹300 once for the campaign. This amount may be paid to the ASHA. If no ASHA is identified or available, the same may be paid to the link worker/ AWW, subject to a total ceiling of ₹300
IX	**National Leprosy Eradication Program**	
1.	Referral and ensuring compliance for complete treatment in paucibacillary cases of leprosy	₹250/ case (for early detection) ₹200/ case (for late detection, any visible disability) ₹400/ case, for Paucibacillary (PB) case treatment completion
2.	Referral and ensuring compliance for complete treatment in multibacillary cases of Leprosy—for 33 States	₹250 per case (for early detection) ₹200 per case (for late detection, any visible disability) ₹600 per case for multibacillary (MB) case treatment completion
3.	ASHA Incentives for Leprosy Case Detection Campaign (LCDC)	Search activity incentives for ASHA- ₹75 per day for 14 days, a total amount of ₹1050 for 14 days. ASHA incentives are given two times in a year if LCDC is done twice in a year in few States/UTs.
X	**National Vector-Borne Disease Control Program**	
A.	**National Malaria Control Program**	
1.	Preparing blood slides or testing through RDT	₹15/slide or test
2.	Providing complete treatment for RDT positive Pf cases	₹200/confirmed case for ensuring complete treatment.
3.	Providing complete radical treatment to positive Pf and Pv case detected by blood slide, as per drug regime	
4.	For referring a case and ensuring complete treatment	₹300

Contd...

B.	**Lymphatic filariasis**	
1.	For one timeline listing of lymphedema and hydrocele cases in all areas of nonendemic and endemic districts	₹200
2.	For annual mass drug administration for cases of Lymphatic filariasis	₹200/day for maximum 3 days to cover 50 houses 250 person.
C.	**Acute Encephalitis Syndrome/Japanese Encephalitis**	
1.	Referral of AES/JE cases to the nearest CHC/DH/Medical College	₹300/ case
D.	**Kala-Azar elimination**	
1.	Involvement of ASHAs during the spray rounds (IRS) for sensitizing the community to accept indoor spraying	₹100/- round during indoor residual Spray, i.e., ₹200 in total for two rounds
2.	ASHA Incentive for referring a suspected case and ensuring complete treatment.	₹500/notified case
3.	Incentive to ASHAs for referring Post Kala-Azar Dermal Leishmaniasis (PKDL) case	₹500/- case (₹200/- at the time of diagnosis and ₹300/- after treatment completion)
E.	**Dengue and Chikungunya**	
1.	Incentive for source reduction and IEC activities for prevention and control of Dengue and Chikungunya in all States	Incentive @ ₹200/- (1 Rupee per house for maximum 200 houses per month). The time period for involvement of ASHAs may be throughout the year. However, total amount should not be exceeding from ₹2400/- per ASHA/year.
F.	**National Iodine Deficiency Disorders Control Program**	
1.	ASHA incentive for salt testing	₹25 a month for testing 50 salt samples
XI	**Incentives under Comprehensive Primary Healthcare (CPHC) and Universal NCDs Screening**	
1.	Maintaining data validation and collection of additional information- per completed form/family for NHPM – under Ayushman Bharat	₹5/form/family
2.	Filling-up of CBAC forms of every individual—onetime activity for enumeration of all individuals, filling CBAC for all individuals 30 or >30 years of age	₹10/- form/per individual as one time incentive
3.	Follow-up of patients diagnosed with Hypertension/ Diabetes and three common cancers for initiation of treatment and ensuring compliance	₹50/- case/Biannual
4.	Delivery of new service packages under CPHC component	₹1000/ASHA/PM (linked with activities)

Contd...

XII	Drinking Water and Sanitation	
1.	Motivating Households to construct toilet and promote the use of toilets.	₹75 per household
2.	Motivating households to take individual tap connections	₹75 per household
XIII	ASHA Certification	
1.	Incentive award in cash for ASHAs and ASHA facilitators who have certified in two independent certificates: RMNCHA+N Expanded Service Package from NCDs to palliative care	₹5000 for all ASHAs and ASHA facilitators who successfully receive certification by NIOS in two independent certificates: RMNCAH+N Expanded package of new services from noncommunicable diseases to palliative care Total incentive: ₹5000 × 2 (two independent certificates) = ₹10,000/- (Introduced in 2022)
XIV	Facilitating Creation and Seeding of ABHA ID in Various IT Portals	
1.	Incentive for ASHAs for each ABHA account created and seeded in various IT portals of MoHFW	₹10 for ASHAs for each ABHA account created/seeded (2022)

Roles and Responsibilities of ASHA

ASHA is a health activist in the community who creates awareness on health. Her responsibilities are listed here:

- Create awareness and provide instructions to the community about health, nutrition, personal hygiene and sanitation.
- Counsel the woman on safe pregnancy, delivery, breastfeeding and complementary feeds and immunization, contraception and prevention of common infections, including infections of reproductive tract and care of the young child.
- Counsel the woman to adopt small family norms.
- Depot holder for essential medicines like ORS, iron and folic acid tablets, chloroquine tablets, oral pills, condom and disposable delivery kit.
- Mobilize the community to access health services at the subcenter and primary health center.
- Escort pregnant women requiring treatment.
- Provide primary medical care for minor ailments, such as fever, diarrhea and first-aid for minor injuries.
- Provide directly observed treatment short course (DOTS) under national tuberculosis control program.
- Inform about birth and death in the village and outbreak of unusual health problems to subcenter and primary health center.
- Promote construction of household toilets under total sanitation campaign.
- Work with village health and sanitation committee of the Gram Panchayat to develop a comprehensive village health plan.

Roles and Integration of ASHA with Anganwadi Worker

Anganwadi worker guides ASHA in preparation of the following activities:
- Organization of health days—once or twice a month. On health days women, adolescent- girls and children from the village will be mobilized for orientation on health related issues, such as importance of nutritious food, personal hygiene, care during pregnancy, importance of antenatal check-up, institutional delivery, care of newborn baby, postnatal care, home remedies for minor ailment and importance of immunization.
- Anganwadi workers will inform ANM to participate and guide organization of health day at Anganwadi center.
- Anganwadi and ANM will act as a resource person for the training of ASHA.
- IEC activities by displaying posters and folk dances, such activities can sensitize the beneficiaries on health-related issues.
- Anganwadi workers will be depot holder for drug kits and issuing it to ASHA.
- AWW will update the list of eligible couple and children under the age of 1 year in the village with the help ASHA.
- ASHA will take initiative to bring the beneficiaries from the village on specific days of immunization and for health check-ups on health days to anganwadi center.
- ASHA will also support the Anganwadi Worker (AWW) in mobilizing pregnant and lactating women and infants for nutrition supplement.

Roles and Integration of ASHA with Auxiliary Nurse Midwife (ANM)

ANM will guide ASHA in the following activities:
- ANM will hold weekly/fortnightly meeting with ASHA and discuss the activities undertaken during the week/fortnight.
- ANM will also guide ASHA in case, she had faced any difficulties during the execution of the activities.
- Anganwadi workers and ANM will act as resource person for the training of ASHA.
- ANM will inform ASHA regarding date and time of outreach session and will guide for bringing the beneficiaries to the outreach session.
- ANM will participate and guide ASHA in organization of health days at Anganwadi Center.
- ANM will take help of ASHA in updating the registration of eligible couples of the concerned village.
- ANM will utilize ASHA in motivating pregnant women for coming to subcenter for initial checkups.
- ASHA will also help ANM in bringing the eligible couple to subcenter for adopting small family norms.
- ANM will guide ASHA in motivating pregnant women for taking full course of iron and folic acid tablets and tetanus toxoid injections.
- ANM will orient ASHA on the dose, schedule and side effects of oral pills.
- ANM will educate ASHA on dangerous signs of pregnancy and labor so that she can timely identify and help beneficiaries in getting further treatment.
- ANM will inform ASHA on date, time and place for training schedule and ensure that during the training, she gets compensation for performance and TA/DA for attending the training.

At Subcenter HWC (SC-HWC) Level

According to National Health Policy 2017, these subcenters are being converted into health and wellness centers HWC (SC-HWC), to provide comprehensive primary healthcare. It is the first peripheral health unit between the community and health services in rural area. It covers a population of 5,000 in plains and 3,000 in hilly, tribal and backward areas.

Staffing Pattern of Subcenter

The subcenter HWC is manned by the following members:

Community Health Nursing Officer - CHO	1	
Health worker female	1	(If the deliveries at subcenter are 20 or more, another ANM to be out sourced)
Health worker male	1	
ASHA	1	Part time or full time to be out sourced
Safai Karamchari	1	To be out sourced
Total	**5**	In addition to the above staff, the subcenter will have support of ASHA/TBA/AWW

Functions of SC-HWC

The team of SC-HWC will deliver expanded range of services:
- Field visits
- Mother and child care including family welfare services
- Immunization and supervision of *dais*
- IUD (intrauterine device) insertion
- Simple laboratory investigations, such as urine testing for sugar and albumin
- Adolescent healthcare—education, counseling and referral
- Training and supervision of *dais*
- Birth and death registration
- Joint health activities with anganwadi and ASHA
- Assistance to school health services
- Water quality monitoring
- Promotion of sanitation a including use of toilet and appropriate garbage deposal
- Community assessment
- Curative services for minor ailments such as fever, diarrhea, animal and snake bite. Prompt referral if needed
- Coordinate services of anganwadi, ASHA, village health sanitation and nutrition committee
- Coordinate with other agencies and sectors
- Disease surveillance
- Involvement in national health programs
- Record of vital events

Supervision of SC-HWC

The work at SC-HWC is supervised by male and female health assistant.

At Primary Health Center HWC Level

Primary health centers are being converted into PHC-HWCs by strengthening existing facilities to provide comprehensive primary healthcare. Primary health center (PHC-HWC) is the first central-point between the village community and medical officer. It is the first structural unit of public health services for rendering primary healthcare services and healthcare in peripheral area. The Bhore Committee in 1946 gave this concept of primary health center as the basic health unit, which is provided to the people. This is regarded as possible, with an integrated curative and preventive healthcare to the rural population with emphasis on preventive and promotive aspects of health. Primary health centers were started in 1952 as a part of community development program. The Alma-Ata declaration of "health for all by 2000 AD" through primary healthcare approach and National Health Policy (1983), proposed the reorganization of primary health centers. Based on this proposal, one primary health center for 30,000 rural populations in plains and 20,000 rural populations in hilly, tribal and backward areas were created for more affective health coverage.

Staffing Pattern at Primary Health Center

The staffing pattern at primary health center (PHC) is as follows:

Staffing pattern at PHC	Existing	IPHS recommendation
Medical officer	1	3 Mo 1 from AYUSH
Pharmacist	1	2
Nurse midwife	1	5 for 24 hours
Health worker female (ANM)	1	1
Block extension educator	1	1
Health assistant male	1	1
Health assistant female (LHV)	1	1
Upper division clerk (UDC)/storekeeper	1	1
Lower division clerk (LDC)/junior assistant	1	1
Laboratory technician	1	2
Driver (if vehicle available)	1	Optional
Class IV workers	4	4
Accountant cum data entry operator	–	1
Total	**15**	**24/25**

The number and qualification of staff at PHC-HWC would continue as defined in the Indian Public Health Standard. This health team delivers healthcare services in each PHC for 30,000 populations in plains and 20,000 in hilly, tribal and backward areas. There are Six subcenters under each PHC.

Functions of Primary Health Center - HWC

The functions of primary health center PHC-HWC (Fig. 2.9) in India is to provide expanded service and to cover all the essential elements of primary healthcare. These are as under:
- Medical care

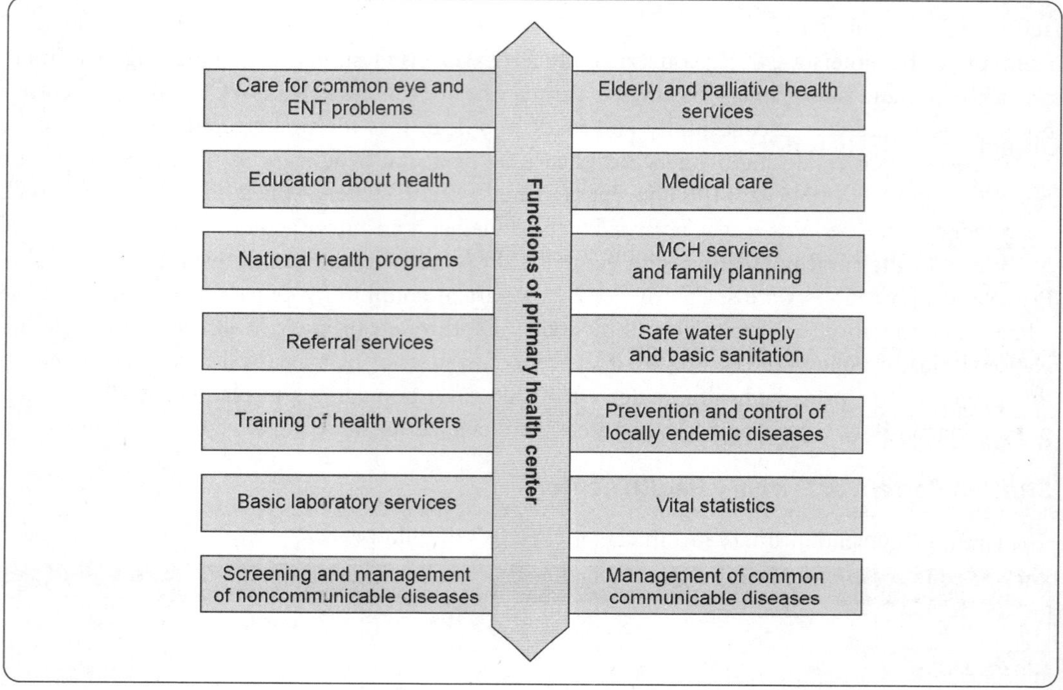

Figure 2.9: Functions of primary health center

- MCH services including family planning
- Neonatal and child healthcare services
- Safe water supply and basic sanitation
- Prevention and control of locally endemic disease
- Management of common communicable diseases
- Screening, prevention, control and management of noncommunicable disease
- Care for common ophthalmic and ENT problems
- Basic oral healthcare
- Elderly and palliative healthcare services
- Emergency medical services
- Screening and basic management of mental health ailments
- Collection and reporting of vital statistics
- Education about health
- National health programs establishment and awareness
- Referral services
- Training of health guide, health worker, local *dais* and health assistants
- Basic laboratory services.

Indian Public Health Standards of Primary Health Center

The Indian Public Health Standards (IPHS) have been revised in 2012. This has been done by keeping in view the resources available with respect to functional requirement for PHC along with minimum standards, such as building, manpower, equipment, instruments, drugs and other facilities. The standards prescribed are for a PHC covering population of 20,000 to 30,000 with 6 beds as all the block level PHCs are ultimately to be converted into CHC with 30 beds providing specialist services.

Objectives of IPHS for PHC

- To provide comprehensive primary healthcare to the community through the primary health centers.
- To achieve and maintain an acceptable standard of quality care.
- To make the services more responsive and sensitive to the needs of the community.

COMMUNITY HEALTH CENTERS

Community health centers (CHCs) were established by the Government of India under the Minimum Needs Program (MNP). The community health centers provide secondary level of healthcare in rural health services. As on 31st March 2014, 5363 community health centers were established by upgrading the primary health centers. Each community health center covers a population of 1,20,000 in plains and 80,000 in hilly and tribal areas. Each community development block has one community health center with 30 beds and specialists in surgery, medicine, obstetrics and gynecology and pediatrics with X-rays and laboratory facilities. A new nonmedical post has been created called CHO to strengthen the preventive and promotive aspect of healthcare. The community health officer is selected from the supervisory category of staff at PHC and district level, he must possess minimum 7 years of experience in rural health programs. Some states have not accepted this and opted for second medical officer. One community health center is referral unit for 4 primary health centers. The specialists at community health center may refer patients directly to state level hospitals as may be necessary without the patient having to go first to the subdivisional or district hospital. Community health centers are maintained by state government under the Minimum Needs Program (MNP). The specialized services provided at CHC are:

- Surgery
- Medicine
- Obstetrics and gynecology
- Pediatrics
- Dental and eye

Staffing Pattern at Community Health Center

In order to provide round the clock services, the revised IPHS staff pattern is as follows:

Staffing pattern at CHC		Existing	
Specialist medical officers	4	Physician	1
		Surgeon	1
		Obstetrician and Gynecologist	1
		Pediatrician	1
Nurse midwives	7		
Dresser	1		
Pharmacist	1		

Contd...

Staffing pattern at CHC		Existing
Lab technician	1	
Radiographer	1	
Ward boys	2	
Safai karamchari	3	
Aya	1	
Peon	1	
Dhobi	1	
Mali	1	
Chowkidar	1	
Total	**25**	

Staffing as per IPHS Pattern

Sl. no.	Personnel	Strength	Desirable qualification
1.	Block health officer	1	Senior most specialist among the below mentioned speciality (Physician, Pediatrician, Obstetrician and Gynecologist, Anesthetist, Public Health, Ophthalmologist)
2.	General surgeon	1	MS/DNB (General surgery)
3.	Physician	1	MD/DNB (General medicine)
4.	Obstetrician and gynecologist		MD/DNB/DGO (OBG)
5.	Pediatrician	1	MD (Pediatrics/DNB/DCH)
6.	Anesthetist	1	MD (Anesthesia) DNB/DA or certificate course in anesthesia for 1 year
7.	Public health manager	1	MD (PSM)/MD (CHA)/MD community medicine or postgraduation degree with MBA
8.	Eye surgeon	1 (for every 5 CHC)	MD/MS/DOMS/DNB/(Ophthalmology)
9.	Dental surgeon	1	BDS
10.	General duty medical officer	6 (at least 2 female doctors)	MBBS
11.	Specialist of AYUSH	1	Postgraduate in AYUSH
12.	General duty medical officer of AYUSH	1	Graduate in AYUSH
	Total	**15/16**	

Supporting Manpower

Personnel	Strength
Staff nurse	19
Public health nurse	1
ANM	1
Pharmacist/compounder	3
Pharmacist AYUSH	1
Lab technician	3
Radiographer	2
Ophthalmic assistant	1
Dresser (certified by Red Cross/St Johnson Ambulance)	2
Ward boys/nursing orderly	5
Safai Karamchari	5
Chowkidar	5
Dhobi	1
Mali	1
Aya	5
Peon	2
OPD attendant	1
Registration clerk	2
Statistical assistant/data entry operator	2
Accountant/admin assistant	1
OT technician	1
Total	**64**

Functions of CHCs

- Routine and emergency surgery
- Routine and emergency medical care
- 24 hours, delivery services including surgical intervention like cesarean section
- Essential and emergency obstetric care
- Newborn care
- Routine and emergency care of sick children
- Blood storage facilities
- Essential laboratory services
- Safe abortion center
- Full range of family planning services including laparoscopic surgery
- All national health programs
- Other emergency measures like tracheostomy, foreign body removal and nasal packing, etc.
- Referral services.

COMMUNITY DEVELOPMENT PROGRAM

Community Development Program started in 1952 as a part of Nation's five-year plans so that the social, cultural and economic progress of the rural areas can be achieved through multidisciplinary approach.

Objectives

The major objectives are to eradicate poverty, diseases and ignorance through community efforts and awakening the interest of rural populations in improving their living conditions.

Activities

- Identification of health needs of the community
- Agricultural development
- Improvement of communication
- Health education
- Rural sanitation
- Improvement of housing, arts, crafts, cottage industries
- Improvement of health
- Animal husbandry
- Cooperative marketing
- Special programs for women and children, such as anganwadi, participation of the villagers in implementing the planned health schemes.

HEALTHCARE AGENCIES

Rural Hospitals

The rural dispensaries are now proposed to upgrade to primary health centers. There are good number of PHCs located in Tensile/subdivisional headquarters which also have hospitals.

District Hospitals/Health Centers

The district hospitals provide services to the urban communities. These hospitals are also referral units for the rural communities. There is a proposal to convert district hospitals into district health centers. The difference between district hospital and district health center (Table 2.1) is given as follows.

TABLE 2.1: Differences between district hospital and district health center

District hospital	District health center
The services provided in the hospitals are mostly curative	The health center provides integrated preventive, promotive and curative health services
Hospitals have no catchment area. Patients may come from any part of the country	It has definite area and population
The health team consists of only curative staff, i.e., doctors, nurses and compounders, etc.	The health team is an optimum "mix" of medical and paramedical workers

Specialist Hospitals

The specialist hospitals provide specialized services to the urban and rural population, such as neurological hospital, orthopedic hospital, cardiac center, TB hospital and maternity hospital, etc.

Teaching Hospitals

These hospitals provide training to the doctors, nurses and various categories of paramedical staff in addition to provide specialist services to the people. Few examples include the medical college hospitals like PGI, AIIMS, etc.

Health Insurance Schemes

There is no Universal Health Insurance in India. It is limited to the industrial worker and their families. The central government employees are also covered by the health insurance under the banner "Central Government Health Scheme" (CGHS).

Employees State Insurance Scheme (ESI)

The ESI Scheme was introduced in India on the principles of contribution by the employer and the employees. It was started under the Parliament Act in 1948 to provide medical benefits in cash and kind during sickness, employment injury, maternity benefits and pension for dependents on the death of worker because of injury. The Act covers employees drawing wages not exceeding ₹21,000/- per month.

Central Government Health Scheme

The Central Government Health Scheme (CGHS) was introduced in 1954 first at New Delhi to provide comprehensive healthcare to the central government employees. Later on, it was extended to other cities not only to the employees, but to their family members also. It was implemented to the autonomous organization employees, members of parliament, retired central government servants, widows receiving family pension, governors and retired judges. The scheme is based on the principles of cooperative effort by the employees and employer for mutual advantage.

Facilities at CGHS

The facilities at CGHS are:
- Outpatient care
- Supply of necessary drugs
- Lab and X-ray investigations
- Domiciliary visits
- Hospitalization at government as well as private hospital
- Referral services
- Pediatric services
- Obstetric services
- Family welfare services
- Emergency treatment
- Supply of optical and dental aids.

Autonomous Institute

Under this category some institutes receive aid from central government, but except few important matters, all other decisions are made by the institution itself. Some of the autonomic institutes are All India Institute of Medical Science (AIIMS), New Delhi, National Institute of Mental Health and Neuroscience (NIMHANS) Bengaluru and Postgraduate Institute (PGI), Chandigarh. These institutes provide direct referral services to the rural and urban communities.

Other Agencies

There are defense services hospitals and railway hospitals.
- **Defense services hospitals:** These hospitals are financed by central government and provide services to the defense employees and their families.
- **Railway hospitals:** These hospitals are managed by central government and provide services to the railway employees and their families.

Private Sector

In private sectors, there are specialty hospitals, super specialty hospitals, medical college hospitals, dispensaries and health clinics. The people who can afford heavy expenses are taking the facilities of healthcare from these hospitals. But, these hospitals provide only curative services. However, poor and weaker section cannot avail their facilities.

Mission/Religious Hospitals

These types of institutions are charitable and run by the trust or mission. They provide medical services either free or at minimum rate. They are present mainly in urban areas but also provide care to the rural area through camps.

General Practitioner and Clinics

These are private agencies run by the general practitioners. They also provide healthcare to the people who can afford or cannot reach the government hospitals or health centers.

PUBLIC-PRIVATE PARTNERSHIP

Public-private partnership (PPP) is an important aspect to achieve the objectives of health as per population policy 2000 and RCH-II and National Rural Health Mission. Public-private partnership is an essential tool toward implementing the programs. A large number of population of the country avail the health services of private sector, but there was no formal channel for better use of resources available in the private sector. To utilize better services of private sector a technical advisory group (TAG) has been constituted, which suggested concepts, guidelines and fund flow mechanism for public-private partnership.

Objectives of PPP

- Improving the healthcare delivery.
- Monitoring the growth of private sector and directing it.

- Exchanging skills and specialties between the public and private sector.
- Enhancing the quality of RCH services.
- Providing access to essential RCH.
- Improving and mobilizing the additional resources and its proper allocation.
- Widening the range of services.
- Increasing community ownership.
- Improving the health management.

Benefits of PPP

- Economize the services by fixing the standardization.
- Utilizing the existing capacity of health system.
- Creating competition and improving quality choice and availability of RCH and other services to the poor.
- Creating synergy between the public and private system.
- Focusing more on primary healthcare and providing good quality services to the vulnerable groups on affordable prices.
- Flexibility in action by developing models involving PPP.
- Mobilization of resources through donations, etc.

INDIGENOUS SYSTEM OF MEDICINE

The indigenous system of medicine (ISM) or Indian system of medicine is an ancient system of medicine which was practiced in India. The western system of medicine got support and was flourished in India during the British rule. The Indian government after independence continued with the same system of medicine which is inherited from the British Government. The Indian medical traditions include folk medicine and classical medical system. The folk medicine implies local health traditions which are practiced in rural and tribal communities. Folk medicine is practiced by indigenous *dais*, bone setters who deal with the joint problems or fractured bones. Housewives treat the minor ailment at home and some traditional doctors provide herbal treatment for all types of common ailments. The classical stream of Indian medicine is theory-based healing in which knowledge about complete body is provided along with instructions on all branches of medicine and surgery, which is documented in several regional manuscripts. But, its practice is noninstitutional, only few governments and private institutions provide institutional services.

The practice of indigenous system of medicine provides medical care to the rural population. Most of the practitioners are local resident and remain very close to the people socially and culturally. The services of indigenous system are provided through outdoor patients' departments, dispensaries and hospitals. The interest of indigenous system has regenerated after the declaration of health for all by 2000 AD and National Health Policy 1983. It is envisaged to involve ISM and homeopathy in National Healthcare delivery system, including reproductive and child health. The NHP 1983 also envisaged the private practitioners of ISM and included their involvement in preventive and promotive aspects of health. Lots of efforts have been made to strengthen the indigenous system of medicine in the public sector of healthcare in both rural and urban areas.

The ISM includes Ayurveda, siddha, and homeopathy.

Ayurveda

The documentation of Ayurveda dates back to Veda period, i.e., 5000 BC. The word "Ayurveda" means science of life.

Ayur   – life
Veda   – science

The origin of Ayurveda is linked with the origin of universe. The Ayurveda takes holistic view of health comprising of four integrated components, i.e., physical, mental, social and spiritual, affecting one another. The health is considered prerequisite for achieving the goal of life for dharma, artha, kama and moksha. Universe as well as human body is made up of five basic elements collectively called Pancha Mahabhutas. These are:

1. Akash (ether)
2. Vayu (air)
3. Agni (fire)
4. Aapa (water)
5. Prithvi (earth)

The 6th mandatory component is Atman (life spirit) without which life ceases.

As per Ayurveda, health is a state of equilibrium of normal functions of Doshas, Dhatus, Malas and Agni with delighted body, mind and soul. The distortion of the equilibrium results into disease. Father of Ayurvedic medicine is Charaka (Charaka Samhita—the treatise of medicine) and Sushruta (Sushruta Samhita—the treatise of surgery).

Diagnosis and Treatment

To diagnose a disease, various factors such as age, sex, temperament, sleep, rest, work pattern and diet are considered. The treatment includes preventive measure, such as personal hygiene, regular daily routine, rest, sleep, balanced, diet and curative treatment.

So, the diagnosis is based on health history, examination of pulse, urine, faces, tongue and eyes, etc.

The Government of India has established a National Institute of Ayurveda in Jaipur (on February 1976), to establish a high standard of training and research in all aspects of Ayurveda system of medicine.

Siddha Medicine System

Siddha is one of the oldest systems of medicine in India. Father of siddha medicine is Agastya. Siddha means achievement. Siddha medicine was practiced by "Sidharas" who aimed at to maintain perfect health in order to achieve 'siddhi'—a heavenly bliss. Siddha is practiced in Tamil speaking parts of India.

Basic Philosophy

The basic philosophy of siddha is that there is an intimate link between man and environment. It believes that all objects of universe including man are composed of five elements, i.e., earth, water, fire, air and space or ether. Food is the basic building material of the body which gets processed into humors of body tissues and waste products. The equilibrium of humors is considered health and its disturbance or imbalance leads to disease or sickness.

Diagnosis and Treatment

The causative factors of disease are identified by examination of pulse, eyes, color of the body, tongue, status of digestive system, urine and study of voice. The treatment taken into account, tests the patients as a whole, i.e., age, sex, race, habits, mental status, diet, appetite, physical condition, habits and environment.

Siddha medicine makes use of elements, like mercury, silver, arsenic, lead, and sulfur, etc. It also includes minerals, plants and animals parts. This system of medicine is effective in treating chronic rheumatic problems, anemia, peptic ulcer, bleeding piles, liver and skin diseases. Siddha system of medicine is therapeutic in nature.

UNANI System of Medicine

The Unani system of medicine has its origin in Greece before Christ under the patronage of Hippocrates (377–460 BC) and Galen. It was introduced in India by the Arabs and Persians around eleventh century. This system though originated in Greece, but was taken to various countries such as Arabia, China, Syria and India. It was in great demand among the people. Through this system ailment was treated using naturally occurring herbs and ingredients of animals and marine origin.

This system is not only therapeutic, but also deals with prevention of disease and promotion of health.

Diagnosis and Treatment

Diagnosis is done by feeling pulse, observation of urine, stool, color of skin and gait. Treatment seeks restoration of the body as a whole to its original state. It is carried out at 4 forms, i.e., pharmacy therapy, diet therapy, regimental therapy and surgery.

Pharmacy therapy makes use of drugs. Regimental therapy has 12 methods for specific and complicated disease and includes cupping, leeching, venesection, and sweating and hammam (bath). These are drugless therapies and found to be effective in diabetes, blood pressure, obesity, arthritis, migraine, etc. This system has emphasized on developing defense mechanism of the body and advocates six essentials, i.e., rest, sleep, psychic movements, wakefulness, evacuation and retention. Unani practitioners recommend immunization against diseases, balanced diet and general health habits.

Homeopathy System of Medicine

Homeopathy is based on the law of "Similia Similibus Curentur", or "let likes be treated by likes" which means that any substance capable of producing artificial symptoms on healthy individual can cure the same symptoms in a natural disease. Similar, observations were made as early as 400 BC by physician from the time of Hippocrates. But, these observations were thoroughly examined and concluded by German physician, Dr Samuel Hahnemann, during the 17th century. Dr Samuel Hahnemann is known as father of homeopathy. He was struck with the view that the effect of certain drugs when taken during healthy conditions, produced symptoms that the drug was known to cure in sickness. Example of this law—*cinchona* bark which contains quinine made the person ill with symptoms that exactly mimicked intermittent fever, which is now called malaria. He wondered about the reason behind working of *cinchona* against intermittent fever and discovered that it caused symptoms, which were indistinguishable from intermittent fever in a healthy human.

Based on this experiment, Hahnemann noted that no two substances produced exactly the same set of symptoms; rather each provoked its own unique pattern of symptoms. Further, the symptoms were not just confined to the physical plane. Every substance tested also affected the mind and emotions apart from the body. Therefore, Hahnemann began to treat the sick people based on the principle, "let likes be treated by likes".

Diagnosis and Treatment

Homeopathy has effective treatment for individuals with chronic diseases, such as diabetes, arthritis, bronchial asthma, skin, allergy and immunological disorders, behavioral disorders, mental diseases and for several other diseases. The services are rendered by private practitioners working in government and nongovernment dispensaries, outpatient's department of hospitals; clinics, etc. There are more than one hundred homeopathy medical colleges all over the country, which teach graduate and undergraduate programs in homeopathy. A national institute of homeopathy has been established in Kolkata, in order to set high standards of training and research in homeopathy.

Naturopathy and Yoga

Naturopathy

Naturopathy system is based on the application of simple laws of nature and it is closely associated to Ayurveda because both share the same fundamental principles. The naturopathy system pays adequate attention to eating and living habits, adoption of purificatory measures, use of hydrotherapy, cold packs, mud packs, baths, massage and variety of measures based on various innovations depending upon the disease and its root causation. Naturopathy helps promote physical, mental, emotional, social and spiritual health by self-regulation of life activities on a normal and natural basis. It requires strong will power, efforts and proper discipline to follow naturopathic way of life. In fact, some elements of naturopathy are practiced in all system of medicine all over the world, such as diet regulation, life activities, steam baths, cold packs, etc.

National Institute of Naturopathy was established in Pune. During 1984 with the purpose of promotion and propagation of naturopathy throughout the country and to encourage research in the field of naturopathy treatment to cure chronic ailment, prevention of disease and promoting health.

Yoga

Yoga is an ancient science. It has been described in Vedas. It was propounded by Patanjali about 2500 years ago. It is a science which helps to coordinate body and mind effectively. Yoga promotes mental, physical, social and spiritual health. It also helps in prevention and treatment of various psychosomatic disorders, i.e., psychic and physical disorders. There are eight components of Yoga listed as under:

1. Restraint in every sphere of life
2. Austerity in every sphere of life
3. Maintaining physical posture
4. Breathing exercises
5. Restraining of sense of organs
6. Contemplation
7. Meditation
8. Samadhi

The yogic practices help to improve personal and social behaviors and improve individual's resistance and ability to endure stressful situation, improves physical health and prevention of psychosomatic disorder by improving circulation of oxygenated blood in the body restraining the sense organs, thereby including tranquility and serenity of mind and body.

There are a number of postures and yogic exercises described, which help to improve health, prevent disease and cure illness. Meditation is one of the eight elements of yoga. It is a mental exercise in which one directs one's mind inwardly by shutting one's sense organs to external stimulation and can direct the mind to perform more useful functions. Yoga is becoming very popular. It is now being introduced in the schools through the ministry of human resource development in phased manner. It has also been introduced in many private schools.

VOLUNTARY HEALTH SERVICES

The voluntary health services are provided by many voluntary health agencies in India. Those agencies which provide voluntary health services are described as under:

Indian Red Cross Society

Indian Red Cross Society (IRCS) was established in 1920 and has 400 branches all over India. It has been executing programs for promotion of health, prevention of disease and mitigation of suffering among the people.

The main activities of Indian Red Cross Society are:

- **Relief work:** The Red Cross Society mobilizes its resource immediately to rescue people during natural calamities such as, earthquakes, floods, epidemics and droughts.
- **Milk and medicine supplies:** Many orphanage homes, schools, maternal and child welfare centers, dispensaries and hospitals receive milk powder, medicines, vitamins and other supplies.
- **Armed forces:** Care of the sick and wounded is the primary obligation of Red Cross. It has got Red Cross home in Bengaluru for permanently disabled ex-servicemen.
- **Maternal and child welfare services:** There is a bureau of maternity and child welfare which provides technical advice and financial aids to its branches and to others, who are interested in improving maternity and child welfare services and working for child welfare.
- **Family planning:** Several states in India are running family planning clinics under the auspices of Indian Red Cross.
- **Blood bank and first aid:** Some of the branches started blood banks; St John Ambulance Association of India which is a part of Red Cross has trained lakhs of men and women in first aid, home nursing and allied subjects.

Hind Kusht Nivaran Sangh

- The Hind Kusht Nivaran Sangh (HKNS) was established in 1950. Its headquarters is in New Delhi. It provides financial assistance to various leprosy homes and clinics. It also provides health education through publication of posters.
- Training of medical workers and physiotherapist is also imparted by this agency
- It conducts research and field investigations on leprosy.
- It has got branches all over India and works in close association with government and other agencies.
- It organizes all India Leprosy Worker's Conference and is responsible for the publication of "Leprosy in India" (which is a quarterly journal).

Indian Council for Child Welfare

- The Indian Council for Child Welfare was founded in 1952 and is affiliated with International Union for Child Welfare
- Its services are devoted to secure indian children
- It has branches in all states and districts all over India
- It provides opportunities and facilities by law and other means. It also helps children to develop physically, mentally, socially and spiritually a good health in a normal manner and in conditions of freedom and dignity.

Tuberculosis Association of India

The Tuberculosis Association of India (TAI) was established in 1939. It has got branches in all the states of India.

Activities

- Organizing TB seal campaign every year to raise funds.
- Training of doctors, health visitors and social workers in antituberculosis work.
- Promotion of health education and consultation and conferences.
- The institutions under the management of association are: The New Delhi Tuberculosis Center; The Lady Linlithgow Sanatorium at Kasauli, the King Edward VII Sanatorium at Dharampur and the Tuberculosis Hospital at Mehrauli.

Bharat Sevak Samaj

- Bharat Sevak Samaj (BSS) was formed in 1952
- It is nonpolitical and nonofficial organization
- It helps people to achieve health by their own actions and efforts
- Its branches are in all states and districts in India
- Its important activity is to improve sanitation in villages.

Central Social Welfare Board

The Central Social Welfare Board (CSWB) was set up by the Government of India in 1953. It is an autonomous organization under the general administrative control of ministry of educations.

Functions

- Surveying the needs and requirements of voluntary welfare organization in the country.
- Promoting and setting up social welfare organization on a voluntary basis.
- Rendering of financial assistance to deserving existing organization and institutions.
- Providing a scheme in urban areas to the lower middle-class women with the help of industrial cooperative (tailoring, sewing, match box and candle making, etc.) to supplement their family.

Kasturba Memorial Fund

- Kasturba Memorial Fund was created in 1944; after the death of Kasturba Gandhi.

- The main objective of this fund is to raise the standard of women, especially in the villages through Gram Sevikas.
- It has branches in all the states of India except J&K.
- The trust is actively engaged in various projects of the country.
- It promotes charitable activities for the welfare of mothers and children.

Family Planning Association of India

The Family Planning Association of India was formed in 1949 with its headquarters in Mumbai.

Activities

- Propagating family planning in India
- Association has branches all over the country and clinics which are running with grants in aid from the government.
- Several hundreds of doctors, health visitors and social workers have been trained on the aspect of family planning.
- Association has done commendable work in propagating family planning in India.
- Headquarters is answerable to enquiries on family planning.

All India Women's Conference

- The All India Women's Conference was originated in 1926 and has branches all over the country
- It is the only women's voluntary welfare organization in India
- Most of the branches are running MCH clinics, medical centers, adult education centers, milk centers and family planning clinics
- It teaches craft to the mothers
- It organizes Balwadis

All India Blind Relief Society

- It was established in 1946 with a view to coordinate different institutions working for the blind.
- It organizes eye relief camps and other facilities for the betterment of the blind.

Professional Bodies

There are:
- Indian Medical Association
- All India Licentiates' Association
- All India Dental Association
- Trained Nurses' Association of India

These are the voluntary agencies of men and women who are qualified in their respective fields of specialties and possess registered qualification. These professional bodies:
- Conduct annual conference
- Publish journals
- Arrange scientific sessions and exhibitions
- Foster research

- Set up standard of professional education.
- Organize relief camps during periods of natural calamities.

The health services in India have their origin with voluntary group, such as missionaries from abroad who came and established services for women, children and leprosy patients. Even today, voluntary health agencies play a vital role in the health programs in India.

NATIONAL HEALTH PROGRAMS

After independence, the Indian government has taken several steps to improve the health of the people. The national health programs are prominent among these measures. The national health programs have been launched by the central government for the control and eradication of communicable disease, improvement of environmental sanitation, raising the standard of nutrition, control of population and improving the health of rural India.

The topic is discussed separately in Unit 6

NURSES' ROLE IN HEALTHCARE SERVICES

Nurses play key roles in the delivery of healthcare services to the communities (Fig. 2.10). Healthcare is a multitude of services rendered to the individuals, families and communities by the healthcare professionals for the purpose of promoting, maintaining, monitoring and restoring health, so the health services are comprehensive in nature and it includes the following:

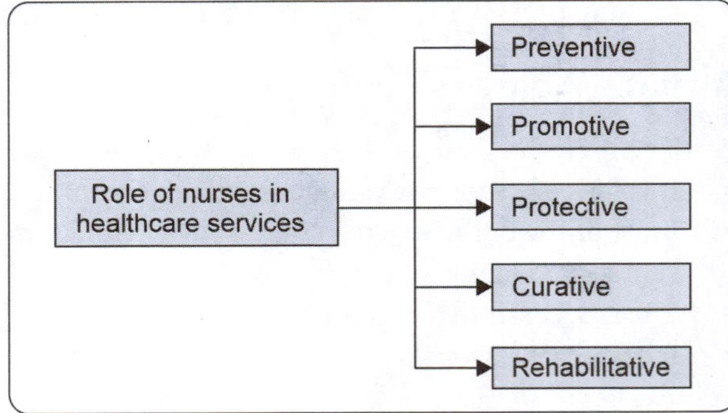

Figure 2.10: Role of nurses in healthcare services

- Preventive
- Promotive
- Protective
- Curative and
- Rehabilitative services.

It is the responsibility of nurses to provide all types of health services to the communities.

Preventive Services

Preventive services are the prime responsibility of nurses to educate the people on preventive aspects of disease by giving health education on personal hygiene, sanitation, nutrition, immunization, adopting healthy lifestyle and family planning.

There are four levels of prevention:

1. **Primordial prevention:** This is the new concept recommended by WHO. In this prevention, the efforts are directed toward discouraging people from adopting harmful lifestyle through individual and mass education. Primordial prevention is concerned with helping people to develop healthy lifestyle such as eating healthy food, having adequate rest, sleep, regular exercise, avoiding the use of tobacco, alcohol and drugs. Teaching children to be honest in their dealings

so that they do not develop adult health problems like obesity, heart disease, hypertension and cancer, etc.

2. **Primary prevention:** Actions taken prior to the onset of disease which remove the possibility of disease occurrence. It is aimed at intervention before pathological changes have begun. The specific interventions are as follows:

    - **Health promotion:** By promoting the health of the individuals and community, the number of diseases such as typhoid fever, tuberculosis, cholera and nutritional deficiencies can be prevented. The measures adopted to promote health are as follows:
        - Health education
        - Personal hygiene
        - Environmental sanitation
        - Adequate rest, sleep and regular exercise
        - Good nutritional intake, balanced diet, healthy food habits and drinking plenty of water.
    - Provision of adequate housing, healthy and safe working condition
    - Attention to personality development
    - Periodic health screening and selective examination
    - Marriage counseling and sex education
    - Genetic counseling
    - **Specific protection:** Specific protection refers to those measures which are directed to intercept causative agents of a particular disease or a group of diseases can be prevented before these agents can cause disease in population. The specific protection includes the following:
        - Specific immunization
        - Use of specific nutrients to prevent deficiency diseases
        - Protection against industrial and other accidents
        - Protection from environmental and occupational hazards
        - Controlling air and sound pollution
        - Protection from allergens
        - Protection from carcinogens
        - Use of prophylactic and supportive drugs
        - Control of quality and safety of foods
        - Chemoprophylaxis.

The community health nurse works in community and close to the individuals and families and can educate the people about health promotion and specific protection, while implementing primary healthcare.

3. **Secondary prevention:** It may be defined as "action which halts the progress of disease at its incipient stage and prevents complications." The secondary prevention focuses on individuals who are experiencing health problems and are at risk for developing complications. The aim of secondary prevention is early diagnosis and prompt treatment.

    - **Early diagnosis:** Early diagnosis of secondary prevention are as follows:
        - Case finding measures.
        - Screening survey.
        - Periodic examination and selective examination.

- **Prompt treatment:** The aim of prompt treatment is to:
  - Arrest the disease process and shorten the duration
  - Prevent the complications
  - Help to reduce morbidity and mortality in certain diseases. Here, the nurse can identify the signs and symptoms of the disease or health problems and refer the people for early diagnosis and prompt treatment to hospitals or health centers.
4. **Tertiary prevention:** It is the fourth level of prevention and may be defined as the measures available to reduce or limit impairment and disabilities, minimize suffering caused by existing departure from good health and to promote patient's adjustment to irremediable conditions Here, the nurse provides the services in psychosocial, vocational and medical components of rehabilitation measures which are taught to the community through health education.

Promotive Services

Promotive services include the process of enabling people to increase control over their health and thereby improve their health. To provide promotive services, the community health nurse focuses on:
- Health education
- Environmental modification
- Nutritional intervention
- Modification of healthy lifestyle, etc.

Health Education

Through health education, the community health nurse arouses interest in general public, patients, community leaders and decision makers. Adequate education is given to the public so that necessary precautions are taken in time. Health education is cost-effective and creates awareness about health in general public.

Environmental Modification

It includes:
- Provision of safe water supply
- Sanitary latrines and safe disposal of water
- Control of insects and rodents
- Improvement of housing.

Nutritional Intervention

- Educate the community about importance of balanced diet
- Menu planning
- Prepare food and how to conserve nutrients
- Prepare food for vulnerable group, i.e., children, pregnant women, adolescent and geriatrics
- Bring awareness about child feeding programs and food fortification.

Lifestyle and Behavioral Changes

- Focus on good lifestyle pattern.

- Make the people to participate in the community activities and programs.
- Encourage people regarding healthcare activities and services. Prepare them to take care of themselves and their family members.

Protective Services

The aim of protective services is to avoid disease all together and bring awareness among the people regarding health protection.

Specific Protection

- Immunization
- Use of specific nutrients
- Protection against occupational hazards
- Control of environment pollution
- Safety of food, drugs and cosmetics.

Health Protection

Health protection includes the provision which ensures normal mental and physical functioning of individual along with other individuals in the community. It is wider than the specific protection and covers literacy, good rest, exercise and sleep, etc.

Curative Services

Early Detection and Treatment

These help in prognosis as well as in preventing the further occurrence of complications or disabilities. Early curative services also shorten the period of communicability (TB, leprosy STD, etc.), and also reduce the morbidity and mortality.

Mass Treatment

In this, we can control certain diseases, which help in interrupting disease transmission. Giving the total mass treatment, e.g., juvenile mass treatment or selective mass treatment.

Rehabilitative Services

Rehabilitative services are defined as the combined and coordinated, use of medical, social, educational and vocational measures for training and retraining the individuals to the highest possible level by functional ability. These include all the measures aimed at reducing the disabling and handicapping conditions. Rehabilitation medicine has emerged in recent years as a medical specialty. The variety of disciplines links and provides the services to gain optimum health to the individual, such as:

- Physical medicine or physiotherapy
- Occupational therapy
- Speech therapy
- Audiology
- Psychology
- Education and social work
- Vocational guidance and placement services.

Must Know

Branches of Rehabilitation

- Medical rehabilitation—Restoration of function.
- Vocational rehabilitation—Restoration of the capacity to earn a livelihood.
- Social rehabilitation—Restoration of family and social relationship.
- Psychological rehabilitation—Restoration of personal dignity and confidence.
  Nurses play vital role in providing all these services to the individuals, families and community.

Summary

- Healthcare services are a multitude of services provided to individual, families and community by the healthcare agency for the purpose of promoting, preventing, caring and restoring the health of individuals.
- The concept of the healthcare is to provide universal healthcare at the grassroots level to the underserved rural and urban poor through a primary healthcare approach with full participation of the community to achieve the goal of "health for all" by 2000 AD.
- There are three levels of healthcare: (1) Primary (2) Secondary and (3) Tertiary.
- The Bhore Committee (1946) used the term 'comprehensive healthcare' which means provision of integrated preventive, curative and promotive services from 'womb to tomb' to every individual residing in a defined geographical area.
- The term 'Basic healthcare' was used by UNICEF/WHO in 1965 in their joint health policy. It is a network of coordinated, peripheral and intermediate health units, capable of effectively performing a selected group of functions essential for the health.
- Primary healthcare concept came into existence in 1978 following an international conference at Alma-Ata. It has all the aspects of primary healthcare delivery proposed by Bhore Committee in 1946 and is now espoused worldwide by international agencies and national government.
- National health programs are launched by the central government for the control and eradication of communicable disease, improvement of environmental sanitation, raising the standard of nutrition, control of population and improving rural health.
- Nurses play a vital role in providing healthcare services to the community by virtue of their profession, and provide integrated health services.

LONG ANSWER TYPE QUESTIONS

1. Explain the concept and trends of healthcare in India.
2. Explain the groups of healthcare system. Describe the healthcare system in public sector.
3. Give an account of primary healthcare at the village level.
4. Describe primary healthcare at the subcenter level and the primary health center level.
5. What are the activities of community health center? Write the staffing pattern at community health center.
6. Enumerate the various voluntary health agencies in India. Describe the activities of Indian Red Cross Society.
7. Describe the services of community health nurse in public healthcare sector.
8. Enumerate the goals to be achievement in the light of Health for All (HFA) by 2000 AD.

SHORT ANSWER TYPE QUESTIONS

1. What are the elements of primary healthcare?
2. Name the principles of primary healthcare.
3. Give a diagrammatic representation of model of healthcare delivery system.
4. Write an account of national health problems.
5. Write about the Public-private partnership.
6. Write short notes of the following:
   a. ESI
   b. CGHS
   c. Anganwadi worker
   d. ASHA
   e. VHG
   f. Ayurveda
   g. Siddha
   h. Homeopathy

MULTIPLE CHOICE QUESTIONS

1. **Which committee has used first the term "comprehensive healthcare"?**
   a. Kartar Singh Committee
   b. Bhore Committee
   c. Kothari Committee
   d. None of these

2. **In which year the Alma-Ata conference gave the definition of primary healthcare?**
   a. 1970
   b. 1978
   c. 1987
   d. 1990

3. **The delivery of healthcare services in rural areas is:**
   a. 3-tier system
   b. 2-tier system
   c. Indigenous system
   d. All of these

4. **Placing people's health in people's hands is the principle of:**
   a. Rural health scheme
   b. Urban health scheme
   c. Both a and b
   d. None of these

5. **The Village Health Guide Scheme was started in the year:**
   a. 1919
   b. 1986
   c. 1977
   d. 2001

6. **The concept of Primary Health Centers was given by:**
   a. Bhore
   b. Srivastava
   c. Kothari
   d. None of these

7. **Primary health centers were started in which year as a community development program:**
   a. 1946
   b. 1952
   c. 1977
   d. 1978

8. **Indian Red Cross Society was established in the year:**
   a. 1920
   b. 1926
   c. 1947
   d. 1950

9. **Hind Kusht Nivaran was formed in the year:**
   a. 1920
   b. 1948
   c. 1950
   d. None of these

10. **Indian Council for Child Welfare was formed in:**
    a. 1950
    b. 1952
    c. 1962
    d. 1977

11. **Tuberculosis association of India was established in the year:**
    a. 1933
    b. 1939
    c. 1950
    d. 1952

12. **All India women's conference was established in:**
    a. 1926
    b. 1939
    c. 1950
    d. 1957

13. **One CHC is a referral unit for:**
    a. 3 PHC
    b. 4 PHC
    c. 2 PHC
    d. 6PHC

14. **One PHC provides health cover to:**
    a. 4 subcenter
    b. 3 subcenter
    c. 6 subcenter
    d. 2 subcenter

15. **The father of homeopathy system of medicine was:**
    a. Charaka
    b. Sushruta
    c. Siddha Agastya
    d. Dr Samuel Hahnemann

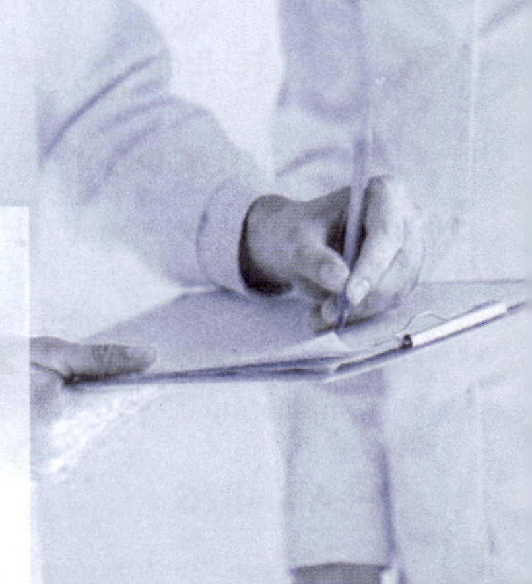

3

Health Planning in India

LEARNING OBJECTIVES

After the completion of the unit, the readers will be able to:
- Discuss health planning in India.
- Describe the progress made during the Five-Year Plans.
- Explain the health committees reports and recommendation.

UNIT OUTLINE

- Introduction
- Planning
- Health Planning
- National Health Planning
- Twenty Point Program
- Planning Commission
- Health Sector Planning
- National Development Council
- Five-Year Plans
- Health Committees and Reports
- National Health Policy

KEY TERMS

NITI Aayog: National institute for transforming India to replace Planning Commission.

Planning: An organized, conscious and continual attempt to select the best available alternative to achieve specific goals.

Abbreviations

DOTS: Directly Observed Therapy (Short Course)
ESI: Employee's State Insurance Scheme
IMCD: Integrated Mother and Child Development – Service Scheme
IMR: Infant Mortality Rate
MMR: Maternal Mortality Rate
MNP: Minimum Needs Program

NDC: National Development Council
NHP: National Health Policy
NRHM: National Rural Health Mission
NURM: National Urban Health Mission
RCH: Reproductive and Child Health
ROME: Reorienting Medical Education
TFR: Total Fertility Rate

INTRODUCTION

The central government through the Council of Health and Family Welfare and various Committee recommendations has shaped health policy and planning in India. It has directed this through the Five-Year Plans through which it executes its decisions. Health planning and policy seek to create a group of mutually interacting bodies to produce goods and services to meet the health needs of a population.

PLANNING

Planning is the foremost and pervasive function of administration and management. Planning is a decision-making process, which helps in developing a framework for allocation of resources. Planning means making a decision in advance about what is to be done, when, where, how and by whom. Therefore, a plan is a determined course of action. Planning and management are essential components of any organization. Planning is for tomorrow and management is for today. Planning and management have acquired greater attention during past few decades. Planning is defined as an organized, conscious and continual attempt to select the best available alternatives to achieve specific goals.

Purpose of Planning

The following are the purposes of planning:
- To match the limited resources with many problems.
- To eliminate wasteful expenditure or duplication of expenditure.
- To develop the course of action to accomplish a defined objective.

The increasing demand for healthcare services with limited resources for a large population in India, requires for careful planning and management of health services. In order to achieve high standards of healthcare services in India, it becomes essential that higher planning and management is implemented.

Steps of Planning

The planning includes the following steps:
- Plan formulation
- Execution
- Evaluation

Planning Team

Planning is a matter of teamwork and consultation. Planning team consists not only of specialists who are good at planning the fieldwork but also requires specialists who have specialization in other fields such as economics, statistics, sociology and management, etc.

Conditions Required for Planning

The conditions required for planning include the following:
- Laws and regulations to facilitate planning.
- Planning and organization of all socioeconomic planning at policy level.
- Administrative capacity.

Sources of Basic Information for Planning

The basic information can be generated from:
- Policy data
- Demographic data
- Economics data
- Health status data
- Environmental health data
- Data on health service resources and facilities
- Health manpower data
- Unit cost data
- The expansion of health service depends upon the status and their resource.

HEALTH PLANNING

Health planning is a part of national development planning. Health planning is necessary for the economic utilization of material, manpower and financial resources. The purpose of health planning is to improve the health services of the country. Health services are primarily the responsibility of the states. Only certain activities are performed by the central government. For this it is essential that there should be national policies which are widely accepted and agreed. This would ensure coordination at all levels of government and proper planning. A good health planning will enable the country to establish a healthcare system which will be socially acceptable, medically sound and cost-effective for every citizen of the country. The cycle of planning is shown in Figure 3.1.

Factors Affecting Health Planning

Health planning has been an important part of the Five-Year Plans. Health services depend upon health needs and demands of the community and the resources available to meet these needs.

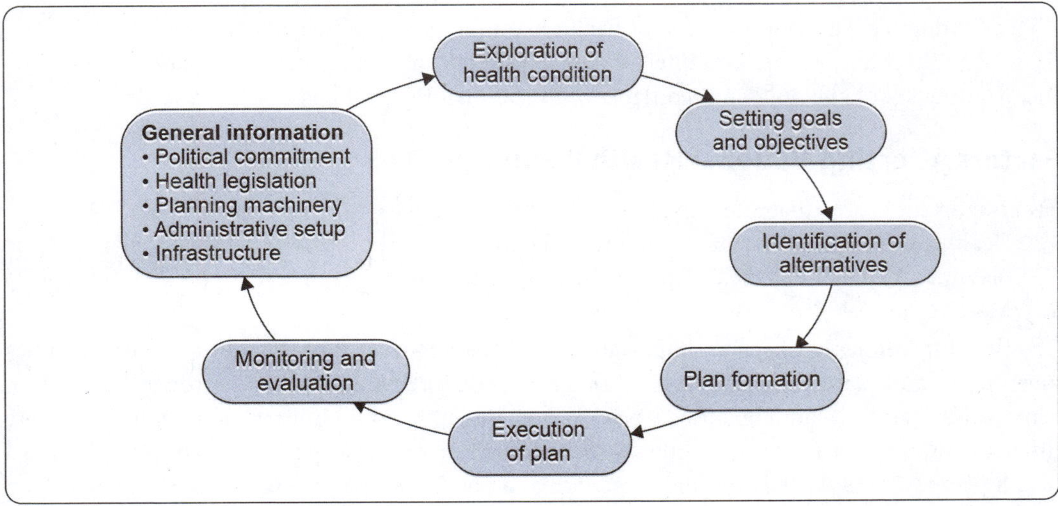

Figure 3.1: Cycle of planning

Health Needs and Demands

Planning is important to meet the health needs and demands of the people. The health needs are defined as "deficiencies in health that call for preventive, curative, control or eradication measures." Community needs such as medical care, safe water supply, adequate nutrition, immunization, environmental sanitation are all essential requirements. The health needs seen by people are not exactly the same as seen by experts. Some needs may not be perceived at all; others may be vaguely perceived and still other may awaken only on contact with new ways of life. In democratic society, people's needs may be presented at demands.

Resources

Resources include manpower, money, material, skill, knowledge, technologies and time need available for the performance or support of action directed toward specified objective. The resources can be readily wasted if there is no proper planning and management.

NATIONAL HEALTH PLANNING

National Health Planning has been defined by WHO as "the orderly process of defining community health problems, identifying unmet needs and surveying the resources to meet them, establishing goals which have high priority are realistic, feasible and projecting administrative action to accomplish the process of the proposed program."

After independence, planning has been done at the central, state, district, block and village level. Most of the planning process has been initiated through successive Five-Year Plans which have been providing a thorough infrastructure framework to state government in order to develop their services, infrastructure and policies for socioeconomic development. Health planning is a part of the overall socioeconomic development. This planning is done based on the reports submitted by various committees which have been set up by the Government of India to review the existing health condition and resources, etc. After looking at the report certain measures are recommended to improve healthcare. The health survey and development—committee popularly known as— Bhore Committee has been the basis for health planning in India after Independence.

As national health planning is an integral part of general, social and economic planning therefore, the planning should be done in accordance with National Health Policies.

Factors Affecting National Health Planning

Two important factors that affect the health planning in India:
1. Health planning is performed as an integral part of general process of national socioeconomic planning. The first Five-Year Plan began on April 1, 1951.
2. Most of the health work is carried out at the state level.

Health planning has been an important part of the Five-Year Plan. Planning Commission has given important place to health services in all Five-Year Plans. For better coordination between center and state, a planning bureau was started under Union Ministry of Health. There are different divisions of health planning for the performance of specific heath care plan. National health planning was started after independence as a part of development. The first Five-Year Plan was started on April 1, 1951. Since then, 12 Five-Year Plans and several annual plans have been completed. In the past 70 years, different aspects of economic development have been focused and the nation has made quite a large progress due to health awareness and education.

Objectives of National Health Planning

In each plan, different objectives were set, but the main objectives are as follows:
- Control of communicable diseases
- Environment and occupational health
- Healthcare services
- Healthcare for women and children
- Implementation of population policy and rapid stabilization of population
- Improving nutritional status of the population with special focus on vulnerable groups
- Development of human resources for health
- Health economics
- Health education and IEC
- Noncommunicable diseases
- Indian System of Medicine and Homeopathy (ISMH)
- Health system research and development.

TWENTY POINT PROGRAM

The Government of India initiated a Twenty Point Program as an agenda to promote social justice and economic growth. The Twenty Point Program has been described as the cutting edge of the plan for the poor.

Objectives of Twenty Point Program

- Eradication of poverty
- Raising productivity
- Reducing inequalities
- Removing social and economic disparities
- Improving the quality of life

High Yield Points

At least eight out of twenty point are related to health directly or indirectly. These are:
- **Point 1:** Attack on rural poverty
- **Point 7:** Safe drinking water
- **Point 8:** Health for all
- **Point 9:** Two child norm
- **Point 10:** Expansion of education
- **Point 14:** Housing for people
- **Point 15:** Improvement of slums
- **Point 17:** Protection of the environment

PLANNING COMMISSION

The Planning Commission has given an important place to health services in all Five-Year Plans. Planning Commission is the apex body in the field of national planning. It was set up by the Government of India in 1950 to make an assessment of the material, capital and human resources of the country and to draft developmental plans for the most effective utilization of these resources. In 1957, the Planning Commission was provided with a perspective planning division, which makes projections into the future over a span of 20–25 years, involving planning for future years to come. The Planning Commission is an advisory body. The membership of the commission is highly distinguished. The commission consists of a chairman, a deputy chairman and 5 members. The prime minister of India is the chairman from the very beginning.

The Planning Commission works through three major divisions; these are:
1. Program advisors
2. General secretariat
3. Technical division

These three divisions are responsible for scrutinizing and analyzing various schemes and projects to be incorporated in the Five-Year Plans. Over the years, the Planning Commission has been formulating successive Five-Year Plans. By its terms of reference, the Planning Commission also reviews from time to time, the progress made in various directions and to make recommendation to government on problems and policies relevant to the pursuit of rapid growth and balanced economic development. The planning process was decentralized toward decentralized districts planning by the year 2000.

NITI Aayog

Government of India on January 1, 2015 replaced the Planning Commission with NITI Aayog. The role of the NITI Aayog is to provide critical, directional and strategic input into the development process. The Aayog acts as a think tank which provides government at the central and state levels with relevant strategies and technical advice across the spectrum of key elements of strategic policy. In addition, NITI aayog monitors and elevates the implementation of program and also focuses on technology upgradation and capacity building.

The seven pillars of the NITI Aayog include Pro-activity, Pro-people, Participation, Empowering, Inclusion of all, Equality, and Transparency.

> **Recent Updates**
>
> NITI Aayog has taken initiative on blockchain usages in e-governance and has conceptualized the tech stack as 'IndiaChain'. IndiaChain is the name given to NITI Aayog's ambitious project to develop a nationwide blockchain network.

HEALTH SECTOR PLANNING

Since "health" is an important contributory factor in the utilization of manpower. The Planning Commission gave considerable importance to health programs in the Five-Year Plans. In order to achieve its required purpose, the planning in health sector has been divided in to the following subsectors:

- Water supply and sanitation
- Control of communicable diseases
- Medical education, training and research
- Medical care including hospitals, dispensaries and primary health centers
- Publish health services
- Family planning
- Indigenous system of medicine

All the sectors receive due consideration in the Five-Year Plans. However, emphasis has changed from plan to plan depending upon priority needs of the people and technical considerations. The health plan is implemented at various levels, i.e., center, state, district, block and village.

Steps of Health Planning

The steps of planning in health sector (Fig. 3.2) include:

1. **Assessments of health situation:** The first and foremost step in health planning is to know the existing health-related problems in the population. To estimate the health needs and determine the demands of the people.
2. **Set goals and objectives:** After knowing the health-related problems, needs and demands of the population; specific goals and objective have to be outlined. The objectives should be specific, achievable, timely, measurable and realistic.
3. **Capacity building, reviewing the health resources:** After setting the goals and objectives, we have to assess our resources within the capacity of organization. We need money to train health manpower, building and purchasing equipment material, supplies and drugs.
4. **Fixing priorities:** According to available resources, the first priority is given to tackle those problems which are more hazardous to health. Second priority is assigned to less hazardous problems.
5. **Implementation:** After setting the priority, the plan is put into action. Definite time is given to complete the action. Roles and responsibilities are delegated to staff involved in monitoring and supervision. A definite schedule and timetable are drafted, so that the plan can be brought into action.
6. **Evaluation:** After implementation, evaluation is done to know the desired results. A systematic workout is planned on how to achieve better outcome and improvement in services.

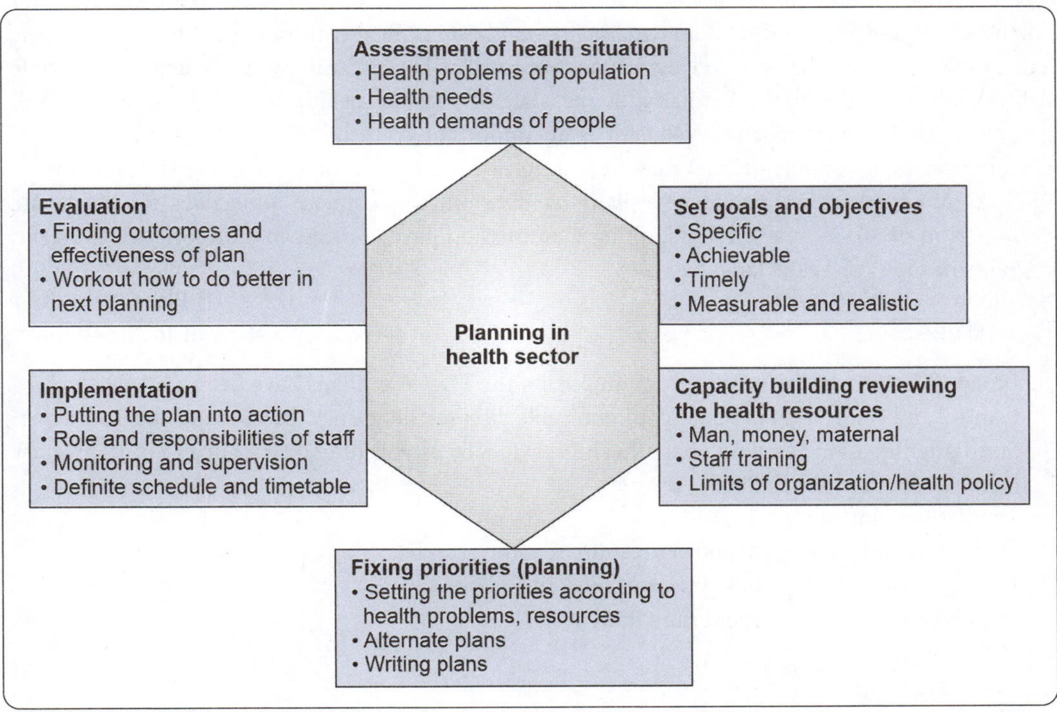

Figure 3.2: Steps of planning in health sector

NATIONAL DEVELOPMENT COUNCIL

National Development Council (NDC) was established to review the working of the national plan from time to time and to consider important social and economic aspects in the planning. The NDC's membership includes the Prime Minister, the Chief Minister of the states, and the members of the Planning Commission. The ministers of the central government who are concerned with economic and social development, are also invited to participate in the meeting of the council. This runs parallel to the planning at national level. The states prepare their own draft plans for submissions to their legislatures and to the Planning Commission.

Functions

- It is an advisory body
- It reviews the working of the national plan from time to time
- It considers important questions of social and economic policy effecting national development
- It recommends measures for the achievement of the aims and targets set out in the plan.

FIVE-YEAR PLANS

The Five-Year Plans were conceived to rebuild rural India, to lay foundation of industrial program and to secure the balanced development of all parts of the country. In 1950, Planning Commission was constituted to help government to plan an integrated development plan for the entire country within the available resources for defined period of 5 years for its socioeconomics program. In 1952, a Central Council of Health was established to have close collaboration between the center and the states and to coordinate and maintain standards of health throughout the country. The Central Health Council is headed by Union Minister of Health and Family Welfare, with state health minister as members. Similarly, at the state level, state health council with state health minister as chairman. Recognizing health is an important contributory factor in the utilization of manpower and to uplift the economic condition of the country, the Planning Commission in 1957 was provided with a perspective planning division, which makes objectives for the future over a period of 20–25 years. The Planning Commission gave considerable importance to health programs in the Five-Year Plans.

Objectives

The broad objectives of the health program during the Five-Year Plans have been:
- Control and eradication of major communicable diseases, deficiency diseases and choric diseases.
- Strengthening of medical and basic health services by establishing district health unit, primary health center and subcenters
- Population control
- Development of health manpower resources and research
- Development of indigenous system of medicine
- Improvement of environment sanitation
- Drug control
- Safe water supply

These objectives differed in each Five-Year Plan depending upon the priority needs of people, technical consideration and available resources.

First Five-Year Plan (1951–1956)

Aims

The following were the aims in the first Five-Year Plan:
- To fight against diseases, malnutrition and unhealthy environment.
- To build up health services for rural population, mothers and children in order to improve general health status of people.

Priorities

- Safe water supply
- Sanitation
- Control of malaria
- Healthcare of rural population
- Health services for mothers and children
- Education, training and health education
- Self-sufficiency in drugs and equipment
- Family planning and population control

Health Outlay

A sum of ₹140 crores was allocated for health program, which was 5.9% of the total outlay for the entire development for the first Five-Year Plans.

Major Developments

The major development took place to meet the identified priority area and objectives as mentioned in Table 3.1.

TABLE 3.1: Major developments during first Five-Year Plan

Years	Major developments
1951	BCG vaccination program to prevent and control tuberculosis.
1952	• Primary health centers were set up to provide health services in rural areas • Auxiliary Nurse Midwife training was started to function in a network of subcenters and primary health centers in the rural areas, to provide comprehensive maternal and child health services and family welfare services under the supervision of lady health visitors/ public health nurses at the block level • The central council of health was constituted • A pilot project of Community Development Program was launched in 55 project areas on 2nd October to get rid of poverty, ignorance and ill health (the 3 ills) in society
1953	• National Malaria Control Program was launched • National Family Planning Program was launched • A committee was set up to draft a Model Public Health Act for the country • National Smallpox Eradication Program was launched • Community Development Program was extended to national level on 2nd October

Contd...

Years	Major developments
1954	• National Water Supply and Sanitation Program was initiated • Central Government Health Scheme started in Delhi • National Leprosy Control Program was started • Prevention of food Adulteration Act was enacted • VDRL Antigen production center was set up in Kolkata • Shetty committee was constituted by the Government of India on May 19, 1954 • Central Social Welfare Board was set up
1955	• National Filaria Control Program was launched • Filaria training center was set up in Ernakulum (Kerala) • National TB sample survey was started • Central Leprosy Teaching and Research Institute was started in Chengalpattu, Chennai. • Minimum marriage age for boys 18 years and girls 15 years was prescribed by Hindu Marriage Act.

Second Five-Year Plan (1956–1961)

Aims

- To expand existing health services to bring them within the reach of all people.
- To promote the progressive improvement of nation's health.

Priorities

- Establishment of institutional facilities for rural and for urban population
- Development for technical manpower
- Control of communicable diseases
- Water supply and sanitation
- Family planning and other supporting programs

Major Developments

The major developments achieved during second Five-Year Plan are presented in Table 3.2.

TABLE 3.2: Major developments during the second Five-Year Plan

Years	Major developments
1956	• Family planning director was appointed at the center • Draft Model Public Health Act was prepared by a committee and published • Central Health Education Bureau was established under the Ministry of Health • Trachoma control pilot project was initiated • Demography training and research center was started in Mumbai • Tuberculosis chemotherapy center was set up in Chennai
1957	• The demography research centers were established in Delhi, Calcutta (now Kolkata) and Madras (now Chennai)

Contd...

Years	Major developments
1958	• National Malaria Control Program was converted into National Malaria Eradication Program • National TB survey completed • Leprosy Advisory Committee was constituted • Three tier structure was recommended as self-governing bodies at villages, district and tehsils
1959	• Mudaliar Committee was appointed to survey the progress made after recommendations of Bhore Committee and suggestions for future development and extension of health program • National TB institute was started in Bangalore (now Bengaluru) • The first Panchayati Raj was introduced in Rajasthan • A central expert committee was constituted under the ICMR to study the problem of smallpox and cholera in India. Committee recommended programs and their eradication
1960	• Pilot project of smallpox eradication was started • National Nutrition Advisory Committee (NNAC) was constituted • School Health Committee was formed to assess the existing health and nutrition status of school children and to improve it • Vital statistics were transferred from Directorate General of Health Services (DGSH) to the Registrar General of India, Ministry of Home Affairs

Third Five-Year Plan (1961–1966)

Aims

To remove the shortage and deficiencies which were observed at the end of second Five-Year Plan in the field of health. These shortcomings were pertaining to institutional facilities especially in rural areas, shortage of trained personnel and supplies, lack of safe drinking water in rural areas and an inadequate drainage system.

Priorities

- Safe water supply in village and sanitation, especially the drainage program in the urban areas.
- Expansion of institutional facilities to promote accessibility especially in rural areas.
- Eradication of malaria and smallpox and control of various other communicable diseases.
- Family planning and supporting services for improving health status of people.
- Development of manpower.

Major Developments

The major developments during third Five-Year Plan are given in Table 3.3.

TABLE 3.3: Major developments during third Five-Year Plan

Years	Major developments
1961	• The central bureau of health intelligence was established • Mudaliar Committee report was submitted and published
1962	• National Smallpox Eradication Program and National Goiter Control Program were launched. • School Health Program was started. • District TB Program was conceptualized. • Central Family Planning Institute was established in Delhi.

Contd...

Years	Major developments
1963	• Applied nutrition program started by Government of India with aid from WHO, UNICEF and FAO. • Chadha Committee recommended a norm of one basis health worker for every 10,000 of population for multipurpose work. • National institute of communicable diseases was established in Delhi • Safe Drinking Water Board (SDWB) was set up • Extended Family Program was launched • National Trachoma Program was initiated
1964	• National Institute of Health Administration and Education, Delhi was started in this year • Shantilal Shah Committee was set up to study the legislation of abortion
1965	• Reinforced extended family program was launched • Direct house to house BCG vaccination was initiated • Director of ICMR introduced Lippes loop as safe and effective method for family planning

Annual plan (1966–1969)

Year 1966

A separate department of family planning was set up in the Union Ministry of Health to coordinate family planning program at the center and states.

Year 1967

- Mukherjee Committee was appointed to review the working of malaria eradication program.
- The Central Council of Health recommended compulsory payment by patients attending hospital, i.e., minimum charge of 10 paisa per patient and 25 paisa per day of hospital stay.
- A committee was set up on small family norms to recommend suitable incentives for those accepting small family norms and practicing family planning.

Year 1968–69

- A bill on registration of birth and death was reinforced by parliament for compulsory registration of birth and death.
- A Medical Education Committee was appointed to study the various aspects of medical education within the framework of national needs and resources.

Fourth Five-Year Plan (1969–1974)

This plan could not be started soon after the third Five-Year Plan due to some political reasons. It was started in 1969. So, annual plans were made which carried the same objectives from 1966 to 1969.

Aims

- To strengthen primary health center network in the rural areas for undertaking preventive, curative and family planning services.
- To take over the maintenance phase of communicable diseases.

Priorities

- Strengthening of primary health centers, subdivisional hospitals and district hospitals.
- Intensification of control programs.
- Expansion of medical and nursing education, training of paramedical personnel to meet the minimum technical manpower requirement.

Major Developments

The major developments during fourth Five-Year Plan are tabulated in Table 3.4.

Fifth Five-Year Plan (1974–1979)

Aims

- To provide a minimum level of integrated health MCH, family planning, nutrition and immunization services to all the people, with special reference to vulnerable groups, especially children, pregnant women and nursing mothers.
- To remove imbalances in respect of medical facilities and strengthening the health infrastructure in rural and tribal areas.

TABLE 3.4: Major developments during fourth Five-Year Plan

Years	Major developments
1969	• The Nutritional Research Laboratory was expanded to National Institute of Nutrition • Comprehensive legislation for control of river water pollution from domestic and industrial wastes was drafted • Central Birth and Death Registration Act (1969) was promulgated • The report of medical education committee was submitted
1970	• The population council of India was set up • All India Hospital (postpartum) Family Planning Program was launched • The Demography Training and Research Center in Mumbai was changed to International Institute for Population Studies
	• Registration Act of Birth and Death came into force • The drugs (price control) order was promulgated.
1971	• The medical termination of pregnancy bill was passed by parliament • Expert committee was appointed for control of air pollution • Family pension scheme for industrial worker was initiated
1972	• The Medical Termination Act was implemented • National Nutritional Monitoring Bureau was set up by the ICMR at the National Institute of Nutrition in Hyderabad. Regional units were also established in the states • The national services bill to compel medical personnel below 30 years of age to work in villages was passed • The committee on "multipurpose worker" under health and family planning was set up, headed by Kartar Singh
1973	• The National Program of Minimum Needs Program (MNP) was formulated • A scheme for setting up 30-bedded rural hospitals serving four primary health centers was conceptualized • Kartar Singh Committee submitted its report

Priorities

The priorities of fifth Five-Year Plan were based on the Minimum Needs Program as mentioned here:

- Increasing accessibility of health services in rural areas.
- Correcting regional imbalances.
- Further development of referral services by removing deficiencies in district and subdivisional hospitals.
- Integration of health, family planning and nutrition services.
- Intensification of the control and eradication of communicable diseases, especially malaria and smallpox.
- Qualitative improvement with education and training of health personnel.

Major Developments

The major developments during fifth Five-Year Plan are mentioned in Table 3.5.

TABLE 3.5: Major developments during fifth Five-Year Plan

Years	Major developments
1974	• Reports of evaluation committee suggested revised strategy for National Malaria Eradication Program • Prevention and Control of Water Pollution Act was passed by parliament • The year 1974 was declared as World Pollution Year by United Nations • A group on medical education and support manpower popularly known as Srivastava Committee, was set up in November 1974
1975	• India became smallpox-free on July 5, 1975 • The revised strategy of National Malaria Eradication Program was accepted by the government • Integrated Child Development Scheme was launched on October 3, 1975. • Children Welfare Fund was set up • The ESI Act was amended • In 1975, Cigarette Regulation Act was enacted by the parliament to provide for certain restrictions in relation to trade and commerce and production and distribution of cigarettes. • Srivastava Committee submitted its report with regard to medical education and manpower support.
1976	• National Program for Prevention of Blindness and Visual Impairment was initiated • Prevention of Food Adulteration Act, 1975 was amended and passed • Indian Factories Act of 1948 was amended • A new policy for population was announced by the government • The Central Council of Health proposed a three-tier plan for medical care in villages
1977	• WHO adopted the goal of "Health for All" by 2000 AD. India was one of the member countries in that assembly • Rural Health Scheme was launched on the basis of Kartar Singh and Srivastava Committee report • Training of community health workers was initiated • The (ROME) scheme was started • Revised Modified Plan of Malaria Eradication was implemented • The 42nd Amendment of the constitution, i.e., "Population Control and Family Planning" as the subject of concurrent list was made.

Contd...

Years	Major developments
1978	• Alma-Ata declared "Primary Healthcare Strategy" to achieve the goal of "Health For All" by the year 2000 AD. India was one of the signatories to this declaration • Air pollution bill was initiated in Lok Sabha • Expanded Program on Immunization, launched by WHO against six killer diseases was started • Child Marriage Restraint Act was approved by parliament, with minimum age for boys at 21 years and for girls at 18 years
1979	• The declaration of Alma Ata on primary healthcare strategy was endorsed by WHO • The offices of Health and Family Planning were merged to formulate regional offices of Health and Family Welfare

Sixth Five-Year Plan (1980–1985)

Aims

To workout alternative strategy and plan of action for primary healthcare as a part of national health system, which is accessible to all sections of society and especially to those living in tribal, hilly, remote, rural areas and urban slum.

Priorities

- Rural health services
- Control of communicable and other diseases
- Development of rural and urban hospital and dispensaries
- Improvement in medical education and training
- Medical research
- Drug control and prevention of food adulteration
- Population control and family welfare including MCH
- Water supply and sanitation
- Nutrition

Major Developments

The major developments during sixth Five-Year Plan are mentioned in Table 3.6.

TABLE 3.6: Major developments during sixth Five-Year Plan

Years	Major developments
1980	• WHO declared eradication of smallpox from the world • The working group on health was constituted by the Planning Commission under the chairmanship of health secretary Shri Kripa Narain on July 18
1981	• The 1981 census was undertaken • Primary healthcare strategy—health for All was evolved by WHO and adopted by member countries of WHO • India committed itself to the goal of providing safe drinking water and adequate sanitation for all by 1990, under the international drinking water supply and sanitation decade 1981–1990 • The Prevention and Control of Air Pollution Act of 1981 was enacted.

Contd...

Years	Major developments
1982	• The National Health Policy was announced and placed in the Parliament • The 20-Point Program was announced
1983	• The National Leprosy Control Program was changed into National Leprosy Eradication Program • National Guinea Worm Eradication Program was started • National Health Policy was approved by the Parliament • National Plan of Action against Avoidable Disablement as "Impact India" was initiated • Medical Education Review Committee submitted its report
1984	• The ESI (Amendment) Bill was passed by the Parliament • The Workmen's Compensation (Amendment) Act, 1984 came into force

Seventh Five-Year Plan (1985–1990)

Aims

To plan and provide primary healthcare and medical services to all with special consideration of vulnerable group and those who are living in tribal, hilly and remote rural areas so as to achieve goal of Health For All (HFA) by 2000 AD.

The plan emphasized on community participation, intersectoral coordination and cooperation.

Priorities

• Health services in rural, hilly and tribal areas under Minimum Needs Program (MNP)
• Medical education and training
• Control of emerging health problems especially in the area of noncommunicable diseases
• MCH and family welfare
• Medical research
• Safe water supply and sanitation
• Standardization integration and application of Indian system of medicine

Major Developments

The major developments during seventh Five-Year Plan are mentioned in Table 3.7.

TABLE 3.7: Major developments during seventh Five-Year Plan

Years	Major developments
1985	• The Universal Immunization Program was launched on 19th November; the birthday of late Prime Minister Smt. Indira Gandhi • The Lepers Act of 1898 was revoked by the Parliament • A separate department of women and child development was established by the Minister of Human Resource Development
1986	• The 20-Point Program was modified • National AIDS Control Program was started • Juvenile Justice Act started functioning • The Parliament passed Mental Health Bill • Environment Protection (amendment), 1986 was promulgated

Contd...

Years	Major developments
1987	• Worldwide safe motherhood campaign was started by world bank • National Diabetes Control Program was launched • High Power Committee was appointed by the Government of India for nursing standards and to assess the working conditions of nurses, nursing education and related matters • New 20-Point Program was launched • The Factories (Amendment) Act 1987 came into force
1988–1989	• The ESI Amendment Act 1989 came into force
1989–1991	• 1989–1991 was a period of political instability in India and hence no Five-Year Plan was implemented. Between 1990 and 1992 there were only annual plans
1989	• High power committee on nursing and nursing profession published its report
1990	• Acute Respiratory Infection Control Program was started as a pilot project in 14 districts
1991	• Census was conducted

Eighth Five-Year Plan (1992–1997)

Aims

To continue reorganization and strengthening of health infrastructure and medical services accessible to all, especially to vulnerable group and those living in tribal hilly and remote areas.

Priorities

- Development of rural health
- Medical education and training
- Control of communicable diseases
- Strengthening of health services
- Medical research
- Universal immunization
- MCH and family welfare
- Safe water supply and sanitation

Major Developments

The major developments during eighth Five-Year Plan are mentioned in Table 3.8.

TABLE 3.8: Major developments during eighth Five-Year Plan

Years	Major developments
1992	• Child Survival and Safe Motherhood (CSSM) Program was started on August 20 • The infant milk substitute, feeding bottles and infant foods (regulation of production, supply and distribution) Act 1952 came into operation
1993	• A revised strategy for National Tuberculosis Program with Directly Observed Therapy (DOT) a community-based TB treatment and care strategy was introduced as a pilot project in phased manner

Contd...

Years	Major developments
1994	• The Panchayati Raj Act came into operation • The first Pulse Polio Immunization Program for children under 3 years was organized on 2nd October and 4th December by Delhi Government • Post Basic BSC Nursing Program (3 years), was launched by Indira Gandhi National Open University (IGNOU)
1995	• Integrated Child Development Scheme was changed to Integrated Mother and Child Development Services • Transplantation of Human Organs Act was enacted • Expert Committee on Malaria submitted its report on the guidelines for modified plan of action
1996	• Nationwide Pulse Polio Immunization was conducted on 9th December 1995 and 20th January which was repeated on December 7, 1996 and January 18, 1997 • Family Planning Program was made target free from April 1 • Prenatal Diagnostic Technique (Regulation and Prevention of Misuse) Act – 1994 came into force from January

Ninth Five-Year Plan (1997–2002)

The ninth Five-Year Plan could not commence on April 1, 1997 due to some political reasons.

Aims

The ninth plan continued with the same aim as that of eighth plan, which was mainly concerned with reorganization and strengthening of infrastructure as to provide primary healthcare services accessible to all, especially those living in the remote, rural, hilly and tribal areas.

Objectives

- To tackle communicable and noncommunicable diseases effectively so that there is sustained improvement in the health status of the population.
- Further intensify the efforts to improve the health status of population by optimizing coverage and quality care by identifying the critical gaps in infrastructure, manpower, equipment and essential diagnostic reagents and drugs, etc.

Priorities

- Control of communicable and noncommunicable diseases
- Efficient primary healthcare system as part of basic healthcare services to optimize accessibility and quality care
- Strengthening of existing infrastructure
- Improvement of referral system
- Strengthening of national vertical program
- Involvement of practitioners from indigenous system of medicine voluntary and private organization
- Intersectoral coordination

Approaches

- Providing efficient primary healthcare system as a part of basic services to improve accessibility and quality services.
- Strengthening of existing infrastructure at primary secondary and tertiary care setting and improvement of referral linkages.
- Development of human resources for health meeting the increased demand for specialized areas.
- Strengthening of MCH and family welfare program.
- Strengthening of existing program for control of communicable diseases and horizontal integration of ongoing vertical program at the district and below district level.
- Development and implementation of integrated noncommunicable diseases prevention and control program.
- Screening for common nutrition deficiencies especially in vulnerable group and rendering remedial services.
- Strengthening of occupational and industrial health programs.
- Disaster and emergency management at all levels of healthcare.
- Strengthening of food and drug safety programs.
- Strengthening of basic, clinical and health system research.
- Increasing the involvement of voluntary, private organization, and self-help group in the provision of healthcare.
- Intersectoral coordination in implementation of health programs.

Significant Events

- Reproductive and Child Health Program was launched in 1997.
- Government of India announced National Population Policy in 2000.
- National Malaria Eradication Program was renamed as National Antimalaria Program in 1999.
- Phase -2 of National AIDS Control Program was started.
- Census 2001 was completed.
- Government of India announced National Health Policy in 2002.
- Government of India announced National AIDS Prevention and Control Policy in 2002.
- The second National Family Health Survey (NFHS-2), was undertaken in 1998–1999.

Major Developments

The major developments during ninth Five-Year Plan are mentioned in Table 3.9.

TABLE 3.9: Major developments of ninth Five-Year Plan

Years	Major developments
1998	Annual Surveillances for HIV Infection started in the country.
2000	Government adopted the National Population Policy for Stabilizing the Population.
2001	Glaucoma and corneal research laboratories was inaugurated JP Narayan Trauma Center was inaugurated National Technical Committee on Child Health was constituted National Program for Control and Treatment of Occupational Diseases

Tenth Five-Year Plan (2002–2007)

During the tenth Five-Year Plan, the strategies were to improve the health status of the people by improving infrastructure and manpower, equipment, essential diagnostic reagents and drugs.

Objectives

- Reduction of poverty ratio by 5% point by 2007.
- Reduction in gender gaps in literacy and wage rates by at least 50% by 2007.
- Reduction in the decadal rate of population growth between 2001 and 2011 to 16.2%.
- Increase in literacy rates to 75% within the tenth plan period (2002–2007).
- Schooling to be compulsory for all children by the year 2003 and all children to complete five-year schooling by the year 2007.
- Reduction of infant mortality rate to 45 per 1000 live births by 2007 and to 28 per 1000 live births by 2012.
- Reduction of maternal mortality rate to 2 per 1000 live births by 2007 and 1 per 1000 live births by 2012.
- Increase in forest and tree cover to 25% by 2007 and 33% by 2012.
- All villages to have sustained access to potable drinking water within the plan period.

Major Developments

- Government of India announced National Health Policy, 2002.
- Government of India announced National AIDS Prevention and Control Policy, 2002.

Eleventh Five-Year Plan (2007–2012)

The eleventh Five-Year Plan provided an opportunity to restructure policies to achieve a new vision based on faster and inclusive growth.

Objectives

Income and Poverty

- Create 70 million new work opportunity.
- Raise real wage rate of unskilled workers by 20%.
- Reduce educated unemployment to below 5%.
- Increase agricultural GDP growth rate to 4% per year to ensure a broader spread of benefit.
- Accelerate GDP growth from 8% to 10% and then maintain at 10% in the 12th plan in order to double per capita income by 2016–17.
- Reduce the headcount ratio of consumption poverty by 10%..

Education

- Reduce dropout rates of children from elementary school from 52.2% in 2003–2004 to 20% by 2011–2012.
- Increase literacy rate for persons of age 7 years or above to 85%.
- Reduce gender gap in literary by 10%.
- Increase the percentage of each cohort going to higher education from present 10–15% by the end of the plan.

Health

- Decreasing maternal mortality ratio to one per thousand live births.
- Reducing infant mortality rate to 28 per thousand live births.
- Providing potable drinking water for all by 2009 and ensuring no slip back.
- Reducing malnutrition among children of age group 0–3 year to half its present level.
- Reducing anemia among women and adolescent girls by 50% at the end of the plan.
- Reducing total fertility rate to 2.1.
- Improving the health equity of NRHM and NUHM.
- Adopting system centric approach rather than centric approach.
- Integrating AYUSH in health system.
- Increasing the role of RMPs.
- Propagating indigenous and low-cost technology.
- Establishing e-health.
- Improving medical, paramedical nursing and dental education.
- Focusing on neglected areas such as older population, disabled and integrating disabled reduction, old healthcare.
- Enhancing efforts at diseases reduction.
- Providing focus on health system and biomedical research.

Women and Children

- Raise the sex ratio for age group 0–6 to 935 by 2011–2012 and to 950 by 2016–2017.
- Ensure that 33% of the direct and indirect beneficiaries of all government schemes are women and girl children.
- Ensure that all children enjoy the safe childhood without compulsion to work.

Infrastructure

- Ensure electricity connections to all villages and remote areas.
- Connect every village by telephone by 2007 and broadband connectivity by 2012.
- Ensure all weather road connection to all habitation with population 1000 and above and in hilly areas 500 and above by 2009 and ensure coverage of all significant habitation by 2015.
- Provide homestead site to all by 2012 and set up the pace of house construction for rural poor to cover all the poor by 2016–2017.

Environment

- Attain WHO standards of air quality in all major cities by 2011–2012.
- Increase forest and tree cover by 5 percentage.
- Treat all urban waste water by 2011–2012 to clean river water.
- Increase energy efficiency by 20 percentage by 2016–2017.

Twelfth Five-Year Plan (2012–2017)

The Twelfth Five-Year Plan targeted to strengthen initiatives taken in the eleventh Five-Year Plan and to expand the reach of healthcare and work toward the long-term objectives of establishing a system of universal health coverage in the country.

Objectives

- Reduction of infant mortality rate (IMR) to 25. India was projected to have an IMR of 36 by 2015 and 32 by 2017. An achievement of MDG to reducing IMR to 27 by 2015 required further acceleration of the historical rate of decline.
- Reduction of material mortality ratio (MMR) to 100 per lakh live births. At the recent rate of decline of 5.8% per annum India was projected to have MMR of 139 by 2015 and 123 by 2017. An achievement of MDG of reducing MMR to 109 by 2015 required an accelerated rate of decline.
- Reduction of total fertility rate (TFR) to 2.1. India was on the target to achieve TFR to 2.1 by 2017, to achieve replacement level of unity.
- Prevention and reduction of under nutrition in children under 3 years to half of NFHS-3 (2005–06) levels.
- Prevention and reduction of anemia among women aged 15–19 years to 28%. Anemia is one of the causes of maternal mortality and low-birth-weight babies. It is preventable and treatable by a very simple intervention. The prevalence of anemia was expected to be steeply reduced to 28% by the end of the twelfth plan.
- Raising child sex ratio in the 0–6 years of age group from 914 to 950. Child sex ratio is another indicator which has been showing a deteriorating trend and needed to be targeted on priority basis.

Thirteenth Five-Year Plan

There is no 13th Five-Year Plan for India. The Five-Year Plans were implemented by Nehru Government after the independence to bring social and economic development in the country. After the 12th Five-Year Plan which ended in 2017, there is no further Five-Year Plan.

NITI Aayog

Five-Year Plan has been replaced by National Institute for Transforming India (NITI Aayog). Its objectives are:
- Prevention and reduction of burden of communicable and noncommunicable diseases (including mental illness) and injuries. State-wise and national targets for each of these conditions are set by the Ministry of Health and Family Welfare as robust systems which are put in place to measure their burden.
- Reduction of poor household's Out-of-Pocket Expenditure (OOPE). OOPE on health is a burden for poor families. It leads to poverty and is a regressive system of financing. An increase in public health spending to 1.87% of GDP by the end of 12th plan, cost-free access to essential medicines in public facilities, regulatory measure proposed in the health plan are an likely to lead to increase in share of public spending. The twelfth Five-Year Plan also aimed to reduce Out-of-Pocket spending as a proportion of private spending on health.

HEALTH COMMITTEES AND REPORTS

A number of committees were appointed to provide guidelines for National Health Planning in India, dating back to the Bhore Committee in 1946. The purpose of appointing these committees was to review the existing health situations and recommend the further course of action in planning and formulating health policies to provide the best possible health services in the country. An important feature of health policies, plans and programs in India originated during the National Movement against colonial rule. The National Planning Committee (NPC) was set up in 1938.

The Alma-Ata declaration on Primary Healthcare and National Health Policy of the Government gave a new direction to health planning in India, making primary healthcare the central function and main focus of the national health system.

Timeline of Committees Involved in Healthcare

A brief description of the health committees which is important landmarks in the history of public health in India is given here:

- Bhore Committee – 1946
- Mudaliar Committee – 1962
- Chadha Committee – 1963
- Mukherjee Committee – 1966
- Jungalwalla Committee – 1967
- Kartar Singh Committee – 1973
- Srivastava Committee – 1975
- Mehta Committee – 1983
- Bajaj Committee – 1986
- Ramalingaswami Committee – 1992

Bhore Committee (1946)

Bhore Committee was appointed by British Government of India in 1943 under the chairmanship of Sir Joseph Bhore, to survey the existing health conditions and health organization in India and to make recommendations for the future development. The Bhore Committee is also known as "Health Survey and Development Committee". The committee had members who were pioneers of public health. They met regularly for two years and submitted its report in 1946.

Recommendations

The committee put forward for the first time comprehensive proposal for the development of a national program of health services in India. The important recommendations of the Bhore Committee were:

- Integration of preventive and curative services at all administrative levels
- Development of primary health centers in two stages:
    i. **Short-term measure:** One primary health center for population of 40,000. Each PHC to be manned by 2 doctors, 4 public health nurse, 1 nurse, 4 midwives, 4 trained *dai*, 2 sanitary inspectors, 2 health assistants, 1 pharmacist and 15 other class IV employees and secondary health center was also envisaged to provide support to PHC and to coordinate and supervise their functioning.
    ii. **Long-time measure:** It is also called 3 million plan of setting up primary health units with 75 bedded hospitals for each 10,000 and 20,000 population. Secondary units with 650 bedded hospitals, again regionalized around district hospitals with 2500 beds.

- Major changes in medical education, which include 3 months training in preventive and social medicine to prepare social physicians.
- Village health committee should be established for better coordination and support in the development program.
- District health board should be established, having representation from public and districts health officials.

Mudaliar Committee (1962)

During the second Five-Year Plan government of India appointed another committee with Dr Lakshmanswami Mudaliar as Chairman, known as "Health Survey and Planning Committee". This was popularly known as Mudaliar Committee. It was formed in 1959 to survey the progress made in the field of health (after the submission of Bhore Committee's report) and to make recommendations for future development and expansion of health services. The committee found that the basic health facilities have not reached even half the country and there was a gross misdistribution of hospital and beds in favor of urban areas. The committee also noticed that the quality of services provided were grossly inadequate with poor functioning, lack of referral services and gross understaffing due to insufficient resources.

Recommendations

The main recommendations of the Mudaliar Committee were:
- Strengthening of existing PHC and development of referral centers before new centers were established
- Strengthening of subdivisional and district hospitals
- Establishing mobile services units in rural areas
- People availing hospital facilities may be levied with a small fee. Poor people may be exempted
- All citizens may be provided with long-term health insurance policies
- Each primary health center should not serve >40,000 populations
- The preventive, promotive and curative health services should be provided at PHC
- Integration of medical and health services as recommended by Bhore Committee
- The functions of undergraduate course education may be continued and extended in the faculties of medicine, engineering agriculture and veterinary sciences.
- Constitution of All India Health Services on the pattern of Indian administrative services.
- The basic infrastructure of health services consisting of subcenters PHCs and district health organization.
- Upgrading the nursing sector into 3 grades of nurses: Basic Nursing (4-year degree program), General Nursing and Midwifery (3-year diploma program) and ANM (18-month training period).

Chadha Committee (1963)

This committee was appointed on April 1963 by Government of India under the chairmanship of Dr MS Chadha (Director General of Health Services), to study the arrangements necessary for the maintenance phases of National Malaria Eradication Program.

Recommendations

- The committee suggested that strict monitoring and vigilance of implementation of National Malaria Eradication Program should be the responsibility of general health services at all levels, i.e., basic health worker of PHC, CHC and Zila Parishad.
- The committee also recommended that the vigilance operations through monthly home visits should be implemented through basic health worker.
- One basic health worker (now multipurpose health workers) for every 10,000 populations was recommended.
- Basic health worker should visit house to house once in a month to implement malaria activities.
- The basic health worker should take additional duties of collection of vital statistics and family planning, etc.
- The family planning health assistants were to supervise 3–4 of the basic health workers.
- At the district level, the general health services were to take the responsibility for the maintenance phase.

Mukherjee Committee (1965)

After recommendation of Chadha Committee within a couple of year, it was found by some states that the basic health workers were not able to function effectively. As a result, the Malaria vigilance operations, had suffered and Family Planning Program could not be carried out satisfactorily. The subject came up for discussion at a meeting of the Central Council of Health in 1965. A committee under the chairmanship of Shri Mukherjee (secretary to the Government of India) was appointed to review the health system of different levels from the point of view of manpower and financial planning.

Recommendations

The important recommendations of the Mukherjee Committee are:
- Strengthening of administrative set up at different levels from PHC to state health service.
- The committee recommended separate staff for the Family Planning Program.
- The family planning assistants had to undertake family planning duties only.
- The basic health workers were to be utilized for purposes other than family planning.
- The committee recommended to delink the malaria activities from family planning so that the latter would receive undivided attention of its staff.

Mukherjee Committee (1966)

It was realized by the states that multiple activities of the mass programs like family planning, smallpox, leprosy, trachoma and National Malaria Eradication Program (maintenance phase) etc, were making it difficult for them to undertake these programs effectively because of shortage of funds. This matter came up for discussion at the meeting of central council of health held at Bangalore in 1966.

Recommendations

The council recommended that related questions may be examined by a committee of health secretaries, under the chairmanship of the Union Health Secretary—Shri Mukherjee. The committee worked out the details of Basic Health Service which should be provided at the block level and some consequential strengthening required at higher levels of administration.

Jungalwalla Committee (1967)

The Central Council of Health at its meeting held at Srinagar in 1964, taking a note on the importance and urgency of integration of health services and elimination of private practice by the government doctors. A committee was appointed on integration of "Health Services" under the chairmanship of Dr N Jungalwalla (Director of National Institute of Health Administrative and Education, New Delhi) to examine the various problems related to integration of health services, abolishment of private practice by doctors in government services and improvement in the service conditions of doctors.

Recommendations

The steps recommended for the integration of service at all levels of health organization in the country. The committee defined "integrated health services" as:
- A service with a unified approach for all problems, instead of a segmented approach for different problems:
    - Unified cadre
    - Common seniority
    - Recognition of extra qualification
    - Equal pay for equal work
    - Special pay for special work
    - Abolishing of private practice by government doctors
    - Improvement in their service conditions
- Medical care and public health programs should be under the charge of a single administrator at all levels of hierarchy.

Kartar Singh Committee (1973)

Government of India Constituted a Committee in 1972 under the chairmanship of Mr Kartar Singh (Additional Secretary Minister of Health and Family Welfare Planning, Government of India). The committee was known as "the Committee on Multipurpose Worker under Health and Family Planning."

Objectives

The committee was appointed to study:
- The structure for integrated services at the peripheral and supervisory levels
- The feasibility of having multipurpose, bi-purpose workers in the field
- The training requirements for such workers
- The utilization of mobile services units set up under family planning program for integrated medical, public health and family planning services operating in the field.

Recommendations

- The various categories of peripheral workers should be into a single cadre of multipurpose workers (male and female).

- The auxiliary nurse midwives (ANMs), were to be converted into multipurpose workers (MPW)—(f) female and basic health workers. Malaria surveillance workers, etc., were to be converted to multipurpose workers (MPW)—(m) male.
- The work of male and female MPWs was to be supervised by one health supervisor female and male respectively.
- The existing lady health visitors to be converted into female health supervisors.
- One primary health center (PHC) should cover a population of 50,000. It should be divided into 16 subcenter one subcenter for 3000–3500 populations. Each subcenter to be staffed by a male and a female health worker.

Srivastava Committee (1974–1975)

The Government of India formed a committee under the chairmanship of Dr JB Shrivastav in 1974. This was set up as a "Group on Medical Education and Manpower Support" popularly known as Srivastava Committee.

> **Mnemonics**
>
> The purpose of setting Srivastava Committee can be memorized by:
> **ROME:** Reorientation of medical education in accordance with national needs.

Objectives

Committee worked to meet following objectives:
- To develop a suitable curriculum for training a cadre of health assistants so that they can serve as a link between the qualified medical practitioners and the multipurpose worker. Thus, forming an effective team to deliver healthcare, family welfare and nutritional services to the people.
- To suggest steps for improving the existing medical educational processes as to provide due emphasis on problems particularly relevant to national requirement.
- To make any other suggestions to realize the above objectives and matters incidental thereto.

Recommendations

The group submitted the report in April 1975 and recommended immediate action for the following:
- Creation of bands of para-professional and semi-professional health workers. The workers should be selected from community itself (e.g., school teachers, Gram Sevaks, postmasters) to provide simple promotive preventive and curative health services needed by the community.
- Establishment of two cadres of health workers, namely multipurpose health workers and health assistants, between the community-level workers and the doctors at PHC.
- Development of a referral system from PHC to hospitals at tehsil district, regional level and medical college hospitals.
- Establishment of a "Medical and Health Education Commission for planning and implementing the reforms needed in health and medical education on the lines of the University Grants Commission".
- An educational commission for health sciences should be developed on the lines of UGC.

Mehta Committee (1983)

Mehta Committee is also known as "Medical Education Review Committee." It was appointed by Government of India under the chairmanship of Shri Mehta in 1983 to review the medical education and manpower projections for doctors, nurses and pharmacists.

Bajaj Committee (1986)

The Government of India appointed an "Expert Committee for Health Manpower Planning and Management" in 1985. This was done under the chairmanship of Professor Dr JS Bajaj to tackle the problems of health manpower planning, production and management.

Recommendations

- Formulation of national medical and health education policy.
- Formulation of health manpower policy.
- Establishment of an educational commission for health sciences on the lines of UGC.
- Establishment of health scheme universities in various states and union territories.
- Vocational courses in paramedical sciences to get more health manpower.

Ramalingaswami Committee (1992)

Ramalingaswami committee was appointed by the Government of India under the chairmanship of Dr V Ramalingaswami.

Recommendations

- Involvement of community for health planning and health program implementation 30-bedded hospital for every 1 lakh population.
- The committee gave its recommendations in 1992 regarding urban healthcare.
- It devised Urban Health Post Scheme for the urban slum area and outlined the services to be provided by the same.
- The structure of National Urban Health Mission takes shapes from the recommendation of this committee.
- Integration of health services at all level.
- Redefined the role of doctor in the community.
- Recommended that the PHC and district health center should be under the control of three-tier Panchayati Raj System.

NATIONAL HEALTH POLICY

The National Health Policy (NHP) was announced and placed in the parliament in 1982 during the sixth Five-Year Plan and it was approved by the parliament in1983.

The National Health Policy (1983)

The National Health Policy was adapted in August 1983. It was evolved after global acceptance of health for all by 2000 AD in 1976–1977 through primary healthcare strategy and on the recommendation of the ICMR – ICSSR joint panel. The policy provided political commitment and support to administration in taking decisions which were essential for attaining HFA through the primary healthcare approach.

Objectives

The main objective of NHP-83 was to attain HFA by 2000 AD by establishing an efficient system of healthcare delivery which is accessible to every individual at every corner of the country, especially the most vulnerable groups like women, children, elderly people and under-privileged classes of the society.

Priorities

- Creation of primary healthcare infrastructure
- Coordination with health-related services
- Active involvement of voluntary organizations
- Provision of essential drugs and vaccines
- Qualitative improvement in health and family planning services
- Immunization
- Nutrition
- Maternal and child health services
- Prevention of food adulteration
- Water supply and sanitation
- Health education

Key Elements of NHP-1983

- Making the community aware of their health problems and means to solve these problems.
- Provision of safe drinking water and sanitation using technology that people can afford.
- Reduction of existing disparity in health services between rural and urban areas.
- Establishing a dynamic health management information system which can support health planning and health program implementation.
- Provision of legislative support to health protection and promotion.
- Combating widespread malnutrition.
- Research in alternative methods of healthcare delivery and low-cost health technology.
- Creating coordination of different systems of medicine.

The most important indicators to be achieved by HFA till 2000 AD of NHP 1983 were:

- To reduce the infant mortality rate from 125 in 1983 to below 60 by 2000 AD
- To raise the life expectancy at birth from 52.6 in 1983 to 64 by 2000 AD
- To reduce crude death rate from 14 in 1983 to 9 by 2000 AD
- To reduce crude birth rate from around 33.5 in 1983 to 21 by 2000 AD
- To achieve a net reproduction rate of one by 2000 AD
- To provide potable water to the entire rural population by 2000 AD

Though many objectives of NHP-1983 were fulfilled but the ultimate aim of Health for All by 2000 AD was not achieved. It was due to a lack of financial resources, infrastructure, trained man power, equipment and materials.

National Health Policy (2002)

The objectives and shortcomings of NHP (1983) were reviewed. The Ministry of Health and Family Welfare, Government of India evolved a Revised National Health Policy in 2002.

Objectives

- The main objective of the policy was to achieve an acceptable standard of good health amongst the general population of the country. The approach was to increase access to a decentralized public health system by establishing new infrastructure in deficient areas and by upgrading the infrastructure in the existing institutions.
- Overriding importance would be given to ensure a more equitable access to health services across the social and geographical expanse of the country.
- Emphasis was given to increase the aggregate public health investment through a substantially increased contribution by the central government. It was expected that this initiative will strengthen the capacity of the public health administrative at the state level to render effective service delivery.
- The contribution of the private sector in providing health services would be much enhanced, particularly for the population group which could afford to pay for the services.
- Primacy was to be given to preventive and first-line curative initiatives at the primary health level through increased sectoral share of allocation.
- Emphasis would be paid on rational use of drugs within the allopathic system.
- Increased access to the tried and tested systems of traditional medicine will be ensured.

To translate the objectives into reality, the Health Policy 2002 laid down specific goals which were to be achieved by the year 2005, 2010 and 2015. These goal are mentioned in Table 3.10.

TABLE 3.10: National Health Policy – 2002, goals achieved till 2015

Eradicate polio and yaws	2005
Eliminate leprosy	2005
Establish an integrated system of surveillance, National Health Accounts and health statistics	2005
Increase state sector health spending from 5.5 to 7% of the budget	2005
Achieve zero levels growth of HIV/AIDS	2007
Eliminate kala-azar	2010
Reduce mortality by 50% on account of TB, Malaria and other vector and water-borne diseases	2010
Reduce prevalence of blindness to 0.5%	2010
Reduce IMR to 30/1000 and MMR to 100/lakh	2010
Increase utilization of public health facilities from current level of <20 to >75%	2010
Increase health expenditure by government as a % of GDP from existing 0.9% to 2%	2010
Increase share of central grants to constitute at least 25% of total health spending	2010
Further increase to 8% of the budget	2010
Eliminate lymphatic filariasis	2015

National Health Policy (2015)

Aims

The primary aim of NHP (2015) was to inform, clarify, strengthen and prioritize the role of government in shaping health system in all its dimensions such as:
- Investment in health
- Organization and financing healthcare services
- Prevention of diseases and promotion of good health through cross-sectoral action
- Accessing technologies
- Developing human resources
- Encouraging medical pluralism
- Building the knowledge base required for better health
- Financial protection strategies
- Regulation and legislation for health.

Goal

The goal of NHP (2015) had been to attain highest possible levels of good health and wellbeing through a preventive and promotive healthcare orientation in all development policies.

Objectives

- Universal access to good quality of healthcare services without anyone having to face financial hardship as a consequence.
- Improve population health status through concerted policy action in all sectors and expand preventive, promotive, curative, palliative and rehabilitative services provided by the public health sector.
- Achieve a significant reduction in Out-of-Pocket expenditure due to healthcare costs and reduction in proportion of household experiencing catastrophic health expenditure and consequent impoverishment.
- Assure universal availability of free comprehensive primary healthcare services as an entitlement, for all aspects of reproductive, maternal, child and adolescent health and for the most prevalent communicable and noncommunicable diseases in population.
- Enable universal access to free essential drugs, diagnostics emergency, ambulance services and emergency medical and surgical care services in public health facilities so as to enhance the financial protection, role of public facilities for all sections of the population.
- Ensure improved access and affordability of secondary and tertiary care services through a combination of public hospital and strategic purchasing of services from the private health sector.
- Influence the growth of the private healthcare industry and medical technologies to ensure alignment with public health goals and enable the contribution to making healthcare system more effective, efficient, rational, safe, affordable and ethical.

National Health Policy (2017)

The specific quantitative goals and objective of the policy are:
- Health status and program impact
- Health system strengthening
- Health system performance

Health Status and Program Impact

Life expectancy and Healthy Life

- Increase the life expectancy at birth from 67.5 to 70 by 2025
- Establish regular tracking of disability-adjusted life years (DALY) index as a measure of burden of disease and its trends by major categories by 2022
- Reduce of TFR to 2.1 at national and subnational levels by 2025

Mortality by Age or Cause

- Reduce under-five mortality to 23 by 2025 and MMR from current levels to 100 by 2020
- Reduce infant mortality rate to 28 by 2019
- Reduce neonatal mortality to 16 and stillbirth rate to 'single digit' by 2025

Reduction of Disease Prevalence Incidence

- Achieve global target of 2020, also termed as the target of 90:90:90 for HIV/AIDS:
  - 90% of all people living with HIV know their HIV status
  - 90% of all people diagnosed with HIV infection receive sustained antiretroviral therapy (ART)
  - 90% of all people receiving antiretroviral therapy will have viral suppression.
- Achieve and maintain elimination status of leprosy by 2018, Kala-azar by 2017 and lymphatic filariasis in endemic pockets by 2017
- Achieve and maintain a cure rate of >85% (>85%) in new sputum positive patients for tuberculosis and reduce incidence of new cases to reach elimination status by 2025.
- Reduce the prevalence of blindness to 0.25/1000 by 2025 and disease burden by one third from current level.
- Reduce premature mortality from cardiovascular diseases, cancer, diabetes or chromic respiratory diseases by 25% by 2025.

Health System Performance

Coverage of Health Services

- Increase utilization of public health facilities by 50% from current levels by 2025.
- Antenatal care coverage to be sustained above 90% and skilled attendance at birth above 90% by 2025.
- More than 90% of the newborn are fully immunized by one year of age by 2025.
- Meet need of family planning above 90% at national and subnational levels by 2025.
- 80% of known hypertensive and diabetics individuals at household level maintain, "controlled disease status" by 2025.

Cross-sectoral Goals Related to Health

- Relative reduction in prevalence of current tobacco use by 15% by 2020 and 30% by 2025.
- Reduction of 40% in prevalence of stunting of under-five children by 2025.
- Access to safe water and sanitation to all by 2020 (Swachh Bharat Mission).
- Reduction of occupational injury by 50% from current levels (334/lakh agricultural workers) by 2020.
- National/state level tracking of selected health behavior.

Health System Strengthening

Health Finance

- Increase health expenditure by Government from the existing 1.15% of GDP to 2.5% of GDP by 2025.
- Increase state sector health spending to >8% of their budget by 2020.
- Decrease in proportion of households facing catastrophic health expenditure from the current levels by 25% by 2025.

Health Infrastructure and Human Resource

- Ensure availability of paramedics and doctors as per Indian Public Health Standard (IPHS) norm in high priority districts by 2020.
- Increase community health volunteers to population ratio as per IPHS norms, in high priority districts by 2025.
- Establish primary and secondary care facility as per norms in high priority districts by 2025.

Health Management Information

- Ensure district-level electronic databases of information on health system components by 2020.
- Strengthen the health surveillance system and establish registers for diseases of public health importance by 2020.
- Establish federated integrated health information architecture, Health Information Exchanges and National Health Information Network by 2025.

Summary

- Planning is an organized, conscious and continued attempt to select the best available alternatives to achieve specific goals.
- National Health Planning has been defined by WHO, an orderly process of defining community health problems, identifying unmet needs and surveying the resources to meet them, establishing priority goals that are realistic and feasible.
- The objective of 20-point Program included eradication of poverty, raising productivity, reducing inequalities removing social and economic disparities and improving the quality of life. At least 8 of the 20 points are related directly or indirectly to health.
- National health planning is an integral part of general social and economic planning. The expansion of health services depends upon the states and their resources.
- The Five-Year Plans were planned to rebuild rural India after independence and to lay out industrial program and to secure the balanced development of all parts of the country.
- The National Planning Commission (NPC) was set up in 1950. Major contributions were made by Bhore Committee, (development of primary health centers); Mudaliar Committee (strengthening of existing PHC); Chadha Committee (strict monitoring and implementation of national malaria eradication program); Mukherjee Committee (strengthening of administrative set up at different level from PHC to state health services)
- Other committees which helped to strengthen the healthcare system include Jungalwalla Committee; Kartar Singh Committee; Srivastava Committee; Bajaj Committee; Mehta Committee; Ramalingaswami Committee; and National Health Policies in 1983, 2002.

STUDENT ASSIGNMENT

LONG ANSWER TYPE QUESTIONS

1. Describe national health planning.
2. Discuss the objectives of 20-point Program.
3. Describe characteristic features of the 9th and 10th Five-Year Plans.
4. Explain the major achievements of the third Five-Year Plan.
5. Discuss the purpose of appointing health committees. Enlist various health committee appointed from time to time.
6. Describe the objectives and goals of National Health Policy 2002.
7. Describe the purpose and recommendations of any three of the following health committees.
   a. Bhore Committee (1946)
   b. Mudaliar Committee (1962)
   c. Chadha Committee (1963)
   d. Mukherjee Committee (1966)
   e. Jungalwalla Committee (1967)

SHORT ANSWER TYPE QUESTIONS

1. Enlist the 8-point out of 20-point Program that are related to health
2. Enlist the significant events of 9th Five-Year Plan.
3. Enlist monitorable of 10th Five-Year Plan.
4. Give an account of various health committees appointed by Government of India.
5. Write short note on the following:
   a. Planning Commission
   b. National Development Council
   c. National Health Policy
   d. Kartar Singh Committee 1973
   e. Srivastava Committee 1975–76
6. What are the priorities and major development of First Five-Year Plan?

MULTIPLE CHOICE QUESTIONS

1. **Which one of the following is required for health planning?**
   a. Laws and regulations to facilitate planning
   b. Planning organization for overall socioeconomics planning at policy level
   c. Administrative capacity
   d. All of the above

2. **The basic information for national health planning can be generated from:**
   a. Policy data, demographic data, economic data,
   b. Health status data, environmental health data, data on health services resources and facilities
   c. Health manpower data and unit cost data
   d. All of the above

3. **The Planning Commission was set up by the Government of India in the year of:**
    a. 1952   b. 1950
    c. 1946   d. 1957

4. **Which of the following major division does the planning commission's work through?**
    a. Program advisor   b. General secretariat
    c. Technical division   d. All of these

5. **Which of the following was not the priority of the first Five-Year Plan?**
    a. Safe water supply and sanitation   b. Control of malaria
    c. Control of communicable diseases   d. Healthcare of the rural population

6. **Which of the following major development does not match with its year under the first Five-Year Plan?**
    a. 1951 – BCG Vaccination Program
    b. 1952 – Central Council of Health was constituted
    c. 1953 – National Malaria Control Program was started
    d. 1954 – National Filaria Control Program was started

7. **In which year of the second Five-Year Plan the Mudaliar Committee was appointed by the government of India?**
    a. 1956   b. 1959
    c. 1958   d. 1957

8. **Which of the following is not the major development of the 3rd Five-Year Plan?**
    a. Applied Nutrition program
    b. MTP Act
    c. School Health program
    d. Established of National Institute of Health Administration

9. **Which of the following major development occurred during the year 1977?**
    a. Rural Health Scheme was launched on the basis of Kartar Singh and Srivastava Committee
    b. Reorientation of Medical Education Scheme
    c. The goal of Health for All was adopted by WHO
    d. All of the above

10. **Which of the following major development did not occur during the sixth Five-Year Plan (1980–1985)?**
    a. The National Health Policy was announced and placed in the parliament
    b. Universal Immunization Program was launched on 19th November
    c. National Guinea Worm Eradication Program was started
    d. The Prevention and Control of Air Pollution Act of 1981 was enacted

11. **Which of the following major development does not belong to the 8th Five-Year Plan (1992–1997)?**
    a. Nationwide Pulse Polio Immunization
    b. Community based TB Treatment DOTS as a new strategy
    c. The high power committee on nursing and nursing profession published its report
    d. The ICDS scheme was changed to Integrated Mother and Child Development (IMCD) services scheme

12. **Which of the following is the major development of 9th Five-Year Plan (1997–2002):**
   a. NMEP was renamed as antimalarial program
   b. National Family Health Survey-2 was undertaken and phase-II of National AIDS Control Program was started
   c. Government of India announced National Population Policy
   d. All of the above

13. **Which one is not the important indication of NHP 1983?**
   a. To reduce of infant mortality rate from 125 in 1983 to below 60 by 2000 AD
   b. To reduce crude death rate from 14 in 1983 to 9 by 2000 AD
   c. To provide potable water to entire population by 2000 AD
   d. To increase utilization of public health facilities by 2010

14. **Family Pension Scheme for industrial workers was introduced in the year of:**
   a. 1971
   b. 1975
   c. 1983
   d. 1984

15. **Which one is not the major development during the 4th Five-Year Plan (1969–1974)?**
   a. The Drugs (Price Control) Order was promulgated
   b. Medical Termination of Pregnancy Bill was passed by the parliament
   c. The National Program of Minimum Needs Program (MNP) was formulated
   d. The ROME scheme was started.

16. **Which of the following is called Health Survey and Planning Committee?**
   a. Mudaliar Committee
   b. Chadha Committee
   c. Bhore Committee
   d. Kartar Singh Committee

17. **Which one of the following is known as "Medical Education Review Committee":**
   a. Bajaj Committee
   b. Mehta Committee
   c. Srivastava Committee
   d. Kartar Singh Committee

18. **Which committee is known as "Expert Committee for Health Manpower Planning, Production and Management"?**
   a. Chadha Committee
   b. Jungalwalla Committee
   c. Bajaj Committee
   d. Bhore Committee

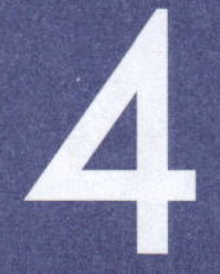

4

Specialized Community Health Services and Nurses' Role

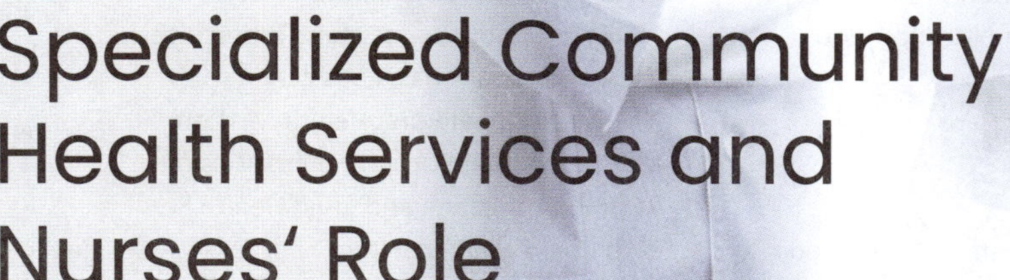

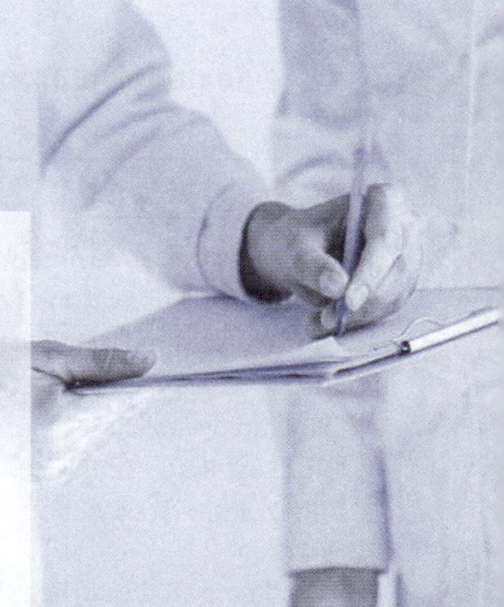

LEARNING OBJECTIVES

After the completion of the unit, the readers will be able to:
- Describe different specialized community health services.
- Discuss the role of nurse in various community health services.

UNIT OUTLINE

- Introduction
- Specialized Community Health Services
- Reproductive and Child Health program
- National Health Mission
- Janani Shishu Suraksha Karyakram
- Emergency Ambulance Services
- Government Health Insurance Schemes
- School Health Services
- Occupational Health Nursing or Industrial Nursing
- Geriatric Nursing
- Physically and Mentally Challenged People
- Rehabilitation Nursing

KEY TERMS

Aging: It is a process of becoming older, a process that is genetically determined and environment modulated.

Emergency obstetric care: It refers to the care of women and newborns during pregnancy, delivery and the time after delivery.

Empowered action group: Eight states—Rajasthan, Uttar Pradesh, Uttarakhand, Bihar, Jharkhand, Madhya Pradesh, Chhattisgarh and Odisha are called 'Empowered Action Group' (EAG). The reason is their development that determines the development of the nation.

Ergonomics: Study of work and working conditions in order to improve people's efficiency.

Gerontological nursing: It involves the care of aging people and emphasizes the promotion of highest possible quality of life and wellness.

Gerontology: Study of aging process and its effects on older persons is known as gerontology.

Intelligent quotient: A total score derived from a set of standardized tests or subtests designed to assess human intelligency.

National health mission: To improve the availability of and access to quality healthcare by people, especially for those residing in rural areas, the poor, women and children.

Reproductive and child health services: Extended maternal child health and family welfare or safe motherhood and child survival program.

Abbreviations

CGHS: Central Government Health Services
CSSM: Child Survival and Safe Motherhood
EAG: Empowered Action Group
EmOC: Emergency Obstetric Care
ESI: Employees' State Insurance
FRU: First Referral Unit
IAPPD: Integrated Action Plan for Pneumonia and Diarrhea
IDCF: Integrated Diarrhea Control Fortnight
ILO: International Labor Organization
IQ: Intelligence Quotient
JSSK: Janani Shishu Suraksha Karyakram
JSY: Janani Suraksha Yojana
MAS: Mahila Arogya Samiti
MDRTB: Multidrug-resistant Tuberculosis
NHM: National Health Mission
NRHM: National Rural Health Mission
NUHM: National Urban Health Mission
RCH: Reproductive and Child Health Services
RKS: Rogi Kalyan Samiti
RMNCH+A: Reproductive, Maternal, Newborn Child and Adolescent Health
RTI: Reproductive Tract Infections
STD: Sexually Transmitted Diseases
VHSNC: Village Health Sanitation and Nutrition Committee

INTRODUCTION

Community health nursing is a combination of nursing practice and public health practice which is applied in order to promote and preserve the health of population. Health promotion, health maintenance, health education and management and coordination and continuity of care, all of these are used as holistic approach in order to manage the healthcare of individuals, families and groups in a community.

SPECIALIZED COMMUNITY HEALTH SERVICES

Specialized community health services include the following:
- Reproductive and Child Health Services
- National Health Mission, i.e., urban and rural
- Janani Shishu Suraksha Karyakram
- Emergency Ambulance Services
- Government Health Insurance Schemes
- School health services
- Occupational health nursing
- Geriatric nursing
- Care of differently abled—physically and mentally ill people
- Rehabilitation nursing.

Nurses play multifaceted role in the aforementioned health services as a direct caregiver, supervisor, administrator, educator, collaborator, advocator and counselor.

REPRODUCTIVE AND CHILD HEALTH PROGRAM

Reproductive and Child Health (RCH) Program was launched on October 15, 1997 with a view to integrate all the services provided to promote maternal and child health services. It includes Family Welfare Program, Universal Immunization Program, oral rehydration therapy, child survival and safe motherhood and acute respiratory infections control, etc. All of these factors are taken care of in order to reduce the cost of inputs on various overlapping programs and bring these programs under one umbrella.

Definition

Reproductive and child health can be defined as a state in which, "people have the ability to reproduce and regulate their fertility, women are able to go through pregnancy and child birth safely, the outcome of pregnancies is successful in terms of maternal and infant survival and well-being, and couples are able to have sexual relations, free of fear of pregnancy and contracting disease."

Objectives

- To reduce the cases of unwanted pregnancies safely and fulfil the reproductive needs of people by providing good quality services
- Safe childhood and healthy children
- Stabilization of population

Main Points

The main points of reproductive and child health are as follows:
- Control of infections and diseases of reproductive system (leukorrhea, menstrual cycle difficulties, cancer of reproductive tract and prolapsed uterus, etc.).
- Safe abortion services
- Treatment of fertility
- Control and treatment of sexually transmitted diseases or infections
- Contraception
- Information and education on protection from human immunodeficiency virus (HIV)/acquired immunodeficiency syndrome (AIDS)
- Child welfare and child health
- Improving the social status of women
- Effective control on maternal mortality and maternal morbidity

Components

Following are the main components:
- Family planning services
- Child survival and safe motherhood (CSSM)
- Prevention and management of reproductive tract infections (STD and AIDS)
- Client-centered approach to healthcare

Other activities include:
- Providing counseling, information and communication services on health, sexuality and gender difference.
- Referral services for all aforementioned intervention
- Growth monitoring, nutrition, education, reproductive health services for adolescent, etc.

RCH–Phase I

Interventions at District Level in All Districts

- Child survival intervention, i.e., provision for immunization, vitamin A (to prevent blindness) oral rehydration therapy and prevention of deaths due to pneumonia
- Safe motherhood intervention, i.e., antenatal check-ups, immunization against tetanus, safe delivery, Anemia Control Program
- Implementation of target free approach
- High quality training at all levels
- Information, education and communication (IEC) activities
- Specially designed RCH package for urban slums and tribal areas
- Districts subprojects under local capacity enhancement
- RTI/STD clinics at district hospital (wherever not available)
- Facility for safe abortions at PHC by providing equipment, contractual doctors, etc.
- Enhanced community participation through Panchayats, women's groups and NGOs
- Adolescent health and reproductive hygiene

Interventions in Selected States/Districts

- Screening and treatment of RTI/STD at subdivisional level
- Emergency obstetric care at selected first referral units (FRUs) by providing drugs
- Essential obstetric care by providing drugs and PHN/staff nurse at PHC
- Additional ANM at subcenters in the weak districts for ensuring MCH care
- Improved delivery services and emergency care by providing equipment kits, IUD insertions and ANM kits at subcenters
- Facility of referral transport for pregnant women during emergency to the nearest referral center through Panchayat in weak districts

Major Interventions under RCH-1

Essential Obstetric Care

It includes:
- Early registration of all pregnant women within 12–16 weeks of gestation
- Provision of minimum 3 antenatal check-ups by ANM or medical officer for screening high risk cases
- Two doses of injection tetanus toxoid to all pregnant women after first trimester of pregnancy at interval of 4 weeks
- Administration of iron and folic acid tablets after 3 months of pregnancy to prevent and treat anemia
- Provision of safe delivery at home or institution
- Provision of 3 postnatal check-ups to monitor the postnatal recovery and to detect any maternal and neonatal complication

Emergency Obstetric Care

Emergency obstetric care is an important intervention to prevent maternal morbidity and mortality. Under the RCH program, the FRUs were strengthened through supply of emergency obstetric kit, equipment kit and provision of skilled manpower on contract basis.

24 Hours Delivery Services at PHCs/CHCs

To promote institutional deliveries, provision has been made to give additional honorarium to the staff in order to encourage round the clock delivery facilities at health centers.

Medical Termination of Pregnancy and IUD Insertion

The aim of MTP services is to reduce maternal morbidity and mortality from unsafe abortions. The services of MTP and IUD insertion are improved at PHC level.

Control of Reproductive Tract Infections (RTI) and Sexually Transmitted Diseases (STD)

The laboratory investigations and specialist services are available at all district hospitals.

Immunization

Immunization of infants, children and pregnant mothers is one of the important activities under RCH-I to reduce the infant mortality due to vaccine preventable diseases.

Essential Newborn Care

The primary goal of essential newborn care is to reduce prenatal and neonatal mortality. It includes resuscitation of newborn with asphyxia, prevention of hypothermia, prevention of infection and exclusive breastfeeding. The strategies are to train medical officer and other health personnel in essential newborn care, provide basic facilities for the care of low birthweight and sick newborn in FRU and district hospitals, etc.

Diarrheal Disease Control

India is the first country in the world to introduce low osmolarity oral rehydration solution (ORS). Zinc is to be used as an adjunct to ORS for the management of diarrhea. Zinc would result in the reduction of the number and severity of episodes of diarrhea. Incidence of diarrhea is reduced by provision of safe drinking water.

Prevention and Control of Vitamin A Deficiency in Children

Under this program, vitamin A is given to all children under the age of 5 years. 1st dose requires 1 lakh units which is given at 9 months of age along with measles vaccination. 2nd dose consists of 2 lakh units given after 9 months. Subsequent doses of 2 lakh units are given at 6-month interval up to 5 years. Every case of malnutrition should be given an additional dose of vitamin A.

Prevention and Control of Anemia

Anemia is most common in young children. Infants after 6 months of age up to 5 years are given elementary iron 20 mg and folic acid 100 mcg in liquid formation up to 100 days in a year. Children under 6–10 years are given 30 mg elementary iron and 200 mcg of folic acid in liquid formation for 100 days in a year. Children above 10 years of age are given iron supplements of adult dose.

Training of Dai

This scheme was initiated during 2001–2002 and implemented in 156 districts in 18 states/UTs of country. The districts have been selected on the basis of safe delivery rate <30%. Scheme has been extended to EAG states. The aim was to train one Dai for 1000 population with the objective of making delivery safe.

Empowered Action Group

The 55% increase in population of India is anticipated in the states of Uttar Pradesh, Bihar, Madhya Pradesh, Rajasthan, Odisha, Chhattisgarh, Jharkhand and Uttarakhand. This comes under empowered action group as constituted by the Ministry of Health and Family Welfare with union Minister of Health and Family Welfare. These states are most deficient in critical socio-demographic indices. Through Empowered Action Group (EAG), these states will be focused and attention on different health and family program would be given.

District Survey

There is no regular source of data to indicate the reproductive health status of women. RCH program conducts district-based rapid household survey to assess the reproductive health status of women. The main indicators are as follows:

- Percentage of women with full ANC
- Percentage of institution deliveries and home deliveries
- Percentage of home delivery by trained birth attendants
- Current contraceptive prevalent rate
- Percentage of children fully immunized
- Percentage of unmet needs for family planning
- Percentage of household reported visits by health worker in previous 3 months

RCH–Phase II

RCH–Phase II was initiated on April 1, 2005.

Objectives

- To reduce total fertility rate
- To reduce infant-mortality rate
- To reduce maternal mortality rate

Main Strategies

The main strategies under second phase of RCH are as follows:
- **Essential obstetric care:**
    - Institutional deliveries
    - Skilled attendants at delivery
- **Emergency obstetric care:**
    - Operationalizing first referral unit.
    - Operationalizing PHCs and CHCs for round the clock delivery services.
- **Strengthening referral system:** The initiatives which have been planned by the Government of India to achieve reduction in maternal mortality and infant mortality rate are as follows:

- **Institutional delivery:** To reduce maternal and fetal mortality rate, institutional deliveries are essential. The envisaged PHCs and all CHCs are to be made operational as 24 hours delivery centers to provide basic emergency obstetric care and essential newborn care and resuscitation.
- **Skilled attendant at birth:** Skilled attendant at birth is a global requirement to reduce maternal and fetal mortality, guide lines for normal delivery and management of obstetric complications for all skilled birth attendants have been formulated and circulated to all states .
- **The policy decision:** In special emergency situations, the staff nurses, LHVs and ANMs have been permitted to use drugs and intervene certain emergencies when the life of the mother is in danger.

- **Emergency obstetric care:** It has been decided that under the RCH–Phase-II, all the first referral units to be made operational for providing emergency and essential obstetric care. The minimum services provided by fully functional FRU are as follows:
  - 24 hours delivery services including normal and assisted delivery
  - Emergency obstetric care including surgical intervention like cesarean sections
  - Newborn care
  - Emergency care of sick children
  - Full range of family planning services including laparoscopic services
  - Safe abortion services
  - Treatment of STI/RTI
  - Blood storage facility
  - Essential laboratory services
  - Referral (transport) services

Nursing Considerations

For fully functioning FRU, there are three determinants on 24-hour basis:
1. Availability of surgical intervention
2. Newborn care
3. Blood storage facility

To perform full range of FRU function, the health facility must have the following facilities:
- Minimum bed strength 20–30, EAG states are relaxed to have 10–12 initially
- Fully functional operation theater
- Fully functional labor room
- An area earmarked and equipped for newborn care in the labor room and in the ward
- A full functional laboratory
- Blood storage facility
- 24 hours water supply and electricity
- Arrangement for waste disposal
- Ambulance facility

- **Strengthening referral system:** During RCH–Phase I, funds were given to Panchayat for providing assistance to poor people in care of obstetric emergencies. But the feedback from states indicated that there was no active involvement of Panchayat in running the schemes.

New Initiatives

- Training of MBBS doctors in life saving anesthetic skills for emergency obstetric care. The timely intervention is most important in saving life of pregnant women during the obstetric emergency to prevent life-threatening maternal and fetal complications. To make FRU operational at subdistrict/CHC level for providing emergency obstetric care (EmOC) to pregnant women who need focused attention. The training of MBBS doctors will be undertaken only in such numbers which is required for functioning of FRUs and CHCs. This is limited to the requirement of tackling emergency situation.
- Government of India has introduced training of MBBS doctors in obstetric management skill but they will not be the replacement of specialist anesthetist.
- Setting up of blood storage centers of FRU according to Government of India guidelines.

Safe Abortion Services

In India, abortions are major causes of maternal morbidity and mortality and account 8–9% of all maternal deaths. Majority of abortions are performed by unskilled and unauthorized persons without observing asepsis. Under RCH–Phase II, the facilities provided are as follows:

- **Medical method of abortions:** Pregnancy can be terminated with the help of two drugs—mifepristone (RU 486) followed by misoprostol. These are safe drugs and their use is recommended up to 7 weeks of amenorrhea in a facility with safe provision of abortion services and blood transfusion. The termination of pregnancy with aforementioned drugs is offered to woman under the provision of MTP Act 1971.
- **Manual vacuum aspiration (MVA):** It is a safe and simple technique. It can be performed in primary health center or in similar settings.

Village Health and Nutrition Day

Village health and nutrition day is organized once a month at Anganwadi center to provide antenatal and postnatal care to pregnant women and to promote institutional delivery.
- To provide immunization, health education, etc.
- To provide family planning services, nutrition services, etc.

Tracking Pregnancy

RCH–Phase II stresses the need for universal screening of pregnant women and providing essential obstetric care:
- Focused antenatal care
- Birth preparation and complication readiness
- Skilled attendant at the time of birth
- Care within first 7 days

All these factors can reduce maternal mortality.

Janani Suraksha Yojana

This scheme was launched on April 12, 2005.

Objectives

To reduce maternal and infant mortality rate through encouraging institutional delivery of women in below poverty line families

Main Features

- Encouraging small family norms
- Encouraging sterilization after completing family
- Provision of cesarean section
- ASHA to be effective link between field level health functionary and women of BPL category
- Payment of incentive to ASHA
- Funds to be released through state department of family welfare

Beneficiaries

- The scheme is applicable for women who lives in low performing states, women of BPL up to all births delivered in the hospital/government sector for cash benefits including cesarean operations
- Scheme is applicable to women of BPL of high performing states up to 2 live births
- **Cash packages** to mothers and ASHA as shown as a table for BPL women from rural area of high and low performing states (HPS and LPS):

Category	Rural Area			Category	Urban Area		
	Mother's Package	ASHA's Package	Total		Mother's Package	ASHA's Package	Total
LPS	1400	600	2000	LPS	1000	400	1400
HPS	700	600	1300	HPS	600	400	1000

- ASHA's incentive in rural areas is ₹600 out of that ₹300 for antenatal component and ₹300 for accompanying pregnant woman for institutional delivery.
- In urban area, it is ₹400 out of that ₹200 for antenatal component and ₹200 for accompanying pregnant woman for institutional delivery.
- In low performing and high performing states, all below poverty line pregnant women preferring to deliver at home are entitled to cash assistance of ₹500 per delivery regardless of age and number of children.

Vande Mataram Scheme

Vande Mataram Scheme is a voluntary scheme launched on February 9, 2004 in all districts of the country.

Aim

To reduce maternal and infant mortality rate and morbidity of the pregnant and expectant mothers by involving and utilizing the specialist/trained work force available in the private sector

Main Features

- It is a voluntary scheme in which any OBG specialist, maternity home, nursing home can volunteer in joining the scheme
- Any lady doctor/MBBS doctor providing safe motherhood services can also join the scheme
- The enrolled Vande Mataram doctors display "Vande Mataram logo" in their clinics
- Iron and folic acid tablets, oral pills and tetanus toxoid injections are provided free of cost to Vande Mataram doctors/clinics by respective district medical officer/CMOs for free distribution
- The cases needing special care and treatment can be referred to government hospital and institutions. For this a Vande Mataram card is given to the referred woman

Activities

- Free antenatal and postnatal check-ups
- Counseling on nutrition
- Encouraging breastfeeding
- Counseling on spacing of birth
- Distribution of iron and folic acid tablets and TT immunization
- Referral services

Child Health Components

The strategy of child health aims to reduce mortality through intervention at every level of service delivery with the help of improved child care practices and child nutrition.

Nutritional Rehabilitation Centers (NRCs)

Severe malnutrition is most common cause of death of children suffering from diarrhea and pneumonia. Deaths among these children are preventable if appropriate and timely action is taken. NRCs are facility-based units which provide medical and nutritional services to severe acute malnourished children, who are under 5 years of age. Feeding skills of mothers are also being focused so that nutritional status can be improved. Also, it is ensured that babies are being breastfed till the age of 1 year.

Activities

The services provided at NRCs are as follows:

- 24 hours of care and monitoring of the child
- Treatment of medical complications
- Therapeutic feeding
- Sensory stimulation and emotional care
- Counseling on appropriate feed
- Demonstration and practice of preparing energy dense food which is available locally, culturally acceptable and affordable food items
- Social assessment of the family to identify and address contributory factors
- Follow-up of children discharged from NRCs

Management of Medical Complication in a Child with Severe Acute Malnutrition

Most deaths occur within 24 hours of admission of such children which can be prevented by prompt treatment on priority basis after screening according to the condition of the child.

Triage

It includes quick examination of the child for emergency signs and provides emergency treatment as necessary. This is done by keeping in mind ABCD steps, i.e., airway, breathing, circulation, coma, convulsions and dehydration.

Assessment of Child on Admission

Child's height, length, weight, mid-arm circumference, edema, pulse, temperature, respiration, signs of dehydration, shock/pallor, eye examination, also signs for vitamin A deficiency, dry conjunctiva, Bitot's spot, corneal ulceration, keratitis, any localized infection, mouth and skin are first inspected.

Principles of Hospital-Based Management

Hospital-based management includes three phases—stabilization, transition and rehabilitation phase.

Stabilization Phase

Child is admitted in hospital and put on starter's diet with high protein and high energy foods. If child cannot eat, tube feeding is given. Treatment of medical complication along with diet is provided. Therapy helps to tide over this phase (after 2 days). Starter diet promotes recovery of normal metabolic function and maintains electrolytes balance. Signs of overfeeding should be monitored.

Transition Phase

Transition phase lasts for 2–3 days. This phase ensures that child is clinically stable and can tolerate an increased energy and protein intake. Child is said to be in transition phase when the following signs are noted:
- Edema starts reducing
- Appetite returns
- No medical problems
- Child is taking oral feeds, no nasogastric feed or infusion
- Child is alert

Rehabilitation Phase

Once the child has recovered appetite and received treatment for medical complication, it enters the rehabilitation phase. The aim of rehabilitation phase is to promote rapid gain in weight, physical development and prepare for normal feeding at home. Child is said to be in rehabilitation phase when:
- Edema has almost disappeared
- No medical complications are there
- Reasonable appetite, child finishes >90% of feed given without a pause.
- Follow-up of children discharged from NRCs. There is a close collaboration between NRCs and community-based care (at PHC, subcenter and AWC) are essential. The list of severe acute malnutrition children discharged from NRS is shared with ANM and ICDS supervisor of the

area. Children should be enrolled in Anganwadi list so that food supplements are provided to them. AWW should prioritize such children for home visit every week for first 4 weeks and once in 2 weeks till the child is discharged from the program.

- Immunization of the children is as per schedule

Integrated Management of Neonatal and Childhood Illness (IMNCI)

Integrated management of childhood illness or IMCI was developed by WHO in collaboration with United Nations Children's Fund (UNICEF) and many other agencies working in the field of child care. IMCI aims to prevent and manage five major childhood diseases, i.e., ARI, diarrhea, measles, malaria and malnutrition. The main focus of IMCI is on preventive, promotive and curative aspects. IMCI strategy is implemented on >100 countries in the world.

IMNCI is the Indian version of IMCI. To introduce IMCI in India a core group was constituted. This group developed Indian version of IMCI guideline and renamed as IMNCI.

The IMCI includes case management charts from 1 week to 2 months, from 2 months to 5 years of age. But in IMNCI, it includes 0–7 days care of newborn neonate along with childhood illness.

Concepts and Needs

Every year >10 million children die in developing countries before the age of 5 years. Most of the deaths are due to ARI, diarrhea, measles, malaria, malnutrition. So, an integrated approach was required to manage the sick children and reduce the child mortality rate. So, WHO responded to the challenge and developed a strategy like IMCI and in India IMNCI. The major reason for developing IMNCI was curative care but it also covers nutrition, immunization and other important aspects of disease prevention and health promotion.

Objectives

- To reduce the mortality rate in children
- To bring down the frequency of illness
- To reduce the severity of illness and disability
- To contribute in improvement of growth and development of children.

Components

The main components of strategy are as follows:
- To strengthen the skill of the healthcare workers
- To strengthen the healthcare infrastructure
- To involve the community

Principles of IMNCI Guidelines

- All sick young infants up to 2 months of age must be assessed for possible bacterial infection and jaundice. They must be assessed for major symptoms of diarrhea.
- All sick children from the age of 2 months up to 5 years must be examined for dangerous signs which indicate immediate referral or admission to hospital. They must be routinely assessed for cough, difficulty in breathing, diarrhea, fever or ear problems.

- All sick young infants and children from age of 2 months up to 5 years must be routinely assessed for nutritional and immunization status, feeding and other potential problem.
- Only a limited number of carefully selected signs are used based on evidence of their sensitivity and specificity to detect disease.
- **Classification**: The diagnosed children are classified for the specific action as:
  - They should be urgently referred to a higher level of care.
  - They require specific treatment such as antibiotic or antimalarial may be safely managed at home.

  The classification is based on color coding:
  - Pink   – Indicates urgent referral or hospital admission
  - Yellow   – Indicates initiation of specific treatment
  - Green   – Calls for home management
- IMNCI guidelines do not describe the management of trauma or other acute emergencies due to accidental injuries.
- IMNCI management uses a limited number of procedures and encourages active participation of caretaker.
- An essential component of IMNCI guidelines is the counseling of caretakers about homecare feeding, fluids and when to return to a health facility.

Nursing Considerations

Elements of Case Management

The case management of a sick child brought to the first level health facility includes the following steps:

1. **Outpatient health facility (OPD cases)**
   - Assessment
   - Classification and identification of treatment
   - Referral, treatment or counseling of child's caretaker
   - Follow-up care
2. **Referrals health facility**
   - Emergency triage assessment and treatment
   - Diagnosis, treatment and monitoring the patient's progress
3. **Appropriate home management:** Teaching mothers how to give oral drugs or treat local infection at home. Counsel mothers and other caretaker regarding feeding, fluids and when to return to health facility

---

Navjaat Shishu Suraksha Karyakram

Navjaat Shishu Suraksha Karyakram (NSSK) is aimed to train health personnel in basic newborn resuscitation, i.e., care at birth—prevention of hypothermia, prevention of infection and early initiation of breastfeeding and basic newborn resuscitation.

Home-based Newborn Care

The strategy of universal access to home-based newborn care following institutional/home delivery aims at reducing neonatal mortality or morbidity. The providers of care include ANMs, Anganwadi and ASHA.

Objectives

The main objective is to reduce neonatal mortality and morbidity which can be achieved through:
- Essential newborn care to all newborn and prevention of complications
- Early detection and special care of preterm and care of babies having low birth weight at the time of birth
- Early detection of illness in the newborn and provision of appropriate care and referral
- Support the family to adopt healthy practices and build confidence and skill of mother to safeguard her health and of newborn

Responsibility of ASHA for Home-based Newborn Care

- Mobilize all antenatal mothers and ensure that they receive full package of antenatal care
- Discuss and plan about choice of delivery (home/institutional) and prepare the lady for labor and care of newborn
- Encourage for institutional delivery
- Provide newborn care through a series of home visits which includes the following:
    - Taking daily weight of newborn
    - Recording temperature of newborn
    - Ensuring warmth
    - Supporting exclusive breastfeed and teaching mother proper positioning and attachment for initiating and maintaining breastfeeding
    - In case any problem is noted in breastfeeding, diagnose the cause and counsel the mother
    - Promoting hand wash
    - Providing skin, cord and eye care
- Health promotion and counseling of mother and families on newborn care and discouraging unhealthy practices like early bathing and bottle feeding
- Increasing number of home visits
- Monitoring weight gain
- Inspecting umbilical cord and eyes for any infection. Inspecting baby's mouth for thrush
- Inspecting mother's breast for engorgement
- Checking involution of uterus
- Inspecting lochia
- Detecting any sign of infection in newborn, provide first level care and refer baby to an appropriate center
- Recognize postpartum complication of mother and refer her appropriately, if needed
- Counsel couple for family planning
- Minimum visits for institution delivery on day 3, 7, 14, 21, 28 and 42, i.e., total—6 visits
- Visits for home delivery—day 1, 3, 7, 14, 21, 28 and 42, i.e., total—7 visits

Incentives Paid to ASHA

The incentive money paid to ASHA on 45th day is subjected to the following:
- Record of birthweight of newborn
- Immunization
- Registration of birth
- Both mother and newborn are safe until 42nd day of delivery

Capacity Building of Healthcare Providers

- Under this, various training programs are conducted for doctors, nurses, ANMs for essential newborn care, early diagnosis and case management of common ailments of children
- The training programs are on Navjaat Shishu Suraksha Karyakram (NSSK), integrated management of neonatal and childhood illness (IMNCI), facility-based newborn care (FBNC), infant and young child feeding practices (IYCF) and others
- Newer interventions are introduced to reduce newborn mortality, vitamin K injection at birth, antenatal corticosteroids for preterm labor, kangaroo mother care and injection gentamycin to young infant in cases of suspected sepsis
- Other interventions initiated are as follows:
    - Home-based newborn care through ASHA
    - Intensified diarrhea control fortnight (IDCF) to be observed in July–August focusing on ORS and zinc distribution for diarrhea management
    - Integrated action plan for pneumonia and diarrhea (APPD)
    - Management of malnutrition through nutritional rehabilitation centers
    - Universal immunization program
    - Mission "Indradhanush" to immunize children who are partially immunized or not immunized
    - Rashtriya Bal Swasthya Karyakram (RBSK) for health screening and early intervention of comprehensive health services under the age of 0–18 years

NATIONAL HEALTH MISSION

The National Health Mission was approved on May 2013. It has got two submissions, i.e., National Urban Health Mission and National Rural Health Mission. The main components of program include health system strengthening in rural and urban areas. This includes reproductive, maternal, newborn child and adolescent health (RMNCH + A). It also involves control of communicable and noncommunicable diseases. Under NHM, the strategies are regularly reviewed, designed and implemented to meet the healthcare needs of the country.

Plans Implemented Under NHM

The plans which are currently implemented under NHM to reduce infant-mortality and maternal mortality rate are mentioned as under:

- Promotion of institutional deliveries through Janani Suraksha Yojana
- Strengthening the training of healthcare personnel in basic and comprehensive obstetric care
- Providing round the clock basic and comprehensive obstetric services in all subcenters, primary health centers, community health centers and district hospitals with adequate manpower, equipment and material
- Antenatal, intranatal and postnatal care including iron and folic acid supplementation to pregnant and lactating women for prevention and treatment of anemia
- Name-based web enabled tracking of pregnant women to ensure antenatal, intranatal and postnatal care
- Mother and child protection card in collaboration with the ministry of women and child development to monitor service delivery for mother and children

- Village health and nutrition day in rural areas as an outreach activity, for provision of maternal and child health services
- Health and nutritional education to promote balanced diet including iron and foliate rich foods as well as food items that promote iron absorption
- Janani Shishu Suraksha Karyakram (JSSK) entitles all pregnant women to deliver in public health institutions absolutely free with no expense including cesarean, free diet, drugs and hospitalization including care of newborn up to 20 days
- Emphasis on facility-based care of newborn at different level to reduce child morbidity and mortality

National Urban Health Mission

National Urban Health Mission (NUHM) was approved by the Ministry of Health and Family Welfare, Government of India in May 2013 as a submission of National Health Mission. The aim of National Urban Health Mission is to improve the health status of urban population, particularly the urban poor and slum dwellers and other vulnerable section of the society. This is done by facilitating equitable access to healthcare. NUHM would cover all state capitals, district headquarters and about 779 other cities/towns with a population of 50,000 and above. Below 50,000 population will be covered by NRHM.

Strategies of NUHM

NUHM focuses on:
- Urban poor population living in listed and unlisted slums
- All other vulnerable population such as homeless, rag pickers, street children, rickshaw pullers, construction and brick and lime-kiln workers, sex workers and other temporary migrants
- Public health thrust on sanitation, clean drinking water, vector control, etc.
- Strengthening public health in urban local bodies
- Ensuring quality healthcare service through Indian Public Health Standard (IPHS)
- Enhanced role of community in planning, management and monitoring of healthcare services through community-based Mahila Arogya Samitis (MASs) and ASHA and Rogi Kalyan Samitis (RKSs)
- Strengthening public health through innovative actions

Essential Services Rendered by ASHA

- Actively promote good health practices and enjoy community support. Provide awareness on RCH services—sexuality, gender equality, age at marriage/pregnancy, motivation on contraception, Medical Termination of Pregnancy (MTP), spacing and sterilization. It also includes early registration of pregnancy and care till delivery, nutritional care during pregnancy, danger signs during pregnancy, immunization, acts as a depot holder on essential drugs, ORS and contraceptives, iron and folic acid tablets.
- ASHA will also create health awareness among the people about health related services at Anganwadi/primary urban health center.
- ASHA will accompany pregnant women and children requiring treatment to urban primary health center.
- ASHA will contribute her services in preventive and promotive health activities along with Anganwadi worker (AWW) and Auxiliary Nurse Midwifery (ANM).

- ASHA will be responsible for maintaining important records of births, deaths, ANC and PNC services including immunization in her area assigned to her
- ASHA will report to ANM about any an unusual event or health problem in her area

Urban Primary Health Center

One UPHC for 50,000–60,000 population located preferably near slum area or within half a kilometer radius, catering to a slum population about 25,000–30,000 with provision of OPD. The cities based upon the population may establish UPHC for 75,000 population for areas with very high density and can also establish one for around 5000–10,000 slum population for isolated slum clusters.

Services provided at UPHC are listed as under:
- OPD consultation
- Basic laboratory diagnosis
- Drugs/contraceptive dispensing
- Health education material delivering RCH services
- Counseling for all communicable and noncommunicable diseases

Referral Unit

One urban community health center (UCHC) for every 4–5 UPHCs for a population of 2,50,000 people.
- In patient services involves 30–50 bed facilities
- For metro cities the UCHS for 5 lakh population with 100 beds

The essential health services provided under NUHM have been mentioned:
- MCH services
- Immunization services
- Family welfare
- Child health and nutrition
- Treatment and prevention of nutritional deficiency diseases
- RTI/STI/HIV/AIDS
- Vector-borne diseases
- Chest infection
- Cardiovascular diseases
- Diabetes mellitus
- Cancer
- Trauma care
- Surgical interventions in surgical cases
- Oral health
- Hearing impairment/deafness
- Eye care primary and secondary

National Rural Health Mission

National Rural Health Mission (NRHM) was launched on April 5, 2005 for a period of 7 years (2005–2012) and then extended up to 2017. It was further extended in March 2018 to continue till March 2020 under the submission of National Health Mission. The mission seeks to improve rural healthcare delivery system. It is operative in every part of the country with special focus on 18 states, i.e., 8 empowered action group states (Bihar, Jharkhand, Madhya Pradesh, Chhattisgarh, Uttar Pradesh, Uttarakhand, Odisha and Rajasthan) 8 Northeastern states (Assam, Arunachal Pradesh, Manipur, Meghalaya, Mizoram, Nagaland, Sikkim and Tripura) and other states like Himachal Pradesh and Jammu and Kashmir.

Aims

- To provide accessible, affordable, accountable, effective and reliable primary healthcare and bridging the gap in rural healthcare through creation of a cadre of accredited social health activist (ASHA)
- The mission is also an instrument to integrate multiple vertical programs along with their funds at the district level

Programs Integrated to NRHM

The programs integrated to NRHM are as follows:
- Health and family welfare including RCH-II
- National Vector-Borne Disease Control Program against malaria, filaria, Kala-azar, dengue fever and Japanese encephalitis
- National Leprosy Eradication Program
- Revised National Tuberculosis Control Program
- National Program for control of blindness, iodine deficiency disorder control program and integrated disease surveillance project.

Core Strategies

- Creation of a cadre of accredited social health activists (ASHA)
- Strengthening subcenters, primary health centers and community health center to match the normative Indian public health standards defining personnel, equipment and management standards
- Promoting synergism through implementation of intersectoral district health plan prepared by the district health mission including drinking water, sanitation, nutrition and hygiene
- Integration of vertical programs operating at national, state, block and district level
- Capacity building and support for data collection, assessment and review for evidence- based planning, monitoring and supervision
- Transport policies for career development of human resources for health

Major Initiatives Under NHRM

- **Introducing ASHA to promote healthcare utilization:** One ASHA for 1000 population. In hilly and tribal area one ASHA for one establishment.
- **Rogi Kalyan Samiti (Patient's Welfare Committee/Hospital Management Society):** This committee is registered society whose members act as trustees to manage the affairs of the hospital and are responsible to keep the facilities up to the mark in the hospital.
- **Untied grants to subcenters:** Subcenters are equipped with essential requirement to provide quality care to the clients.

- **Village Health Sanitation and Nutrition Committee (VHSNC):** It is an important tool of community empowerment and participation. VHSNC reflects the aspiration of local community especially the poor household and children.
- **Janani Suraksha Yojana (JSY):** This aims to reduce maternal mortality. All pregnant women are encouraged to deliver in government health institutions. Under this scheme cash assistance is provided to eligible pregnant women who deliver in government hospital.
- **Janani Shishu Suraksha Karyakram (JSSK):** Under this scheme, all pregnant women are entitled to free delivery/cesarean including free drugs, diet and hospitalization with free transport from home to institution. Free care of the newborn baby up to 30 days after delivery. This scheme was launched on June 1, 2011.
- **National mobile medical unit:** To increase visibility awareness and accountability, all mobile medical units have been repositioned as "National Mobile Medical Unit Service" with universal color and design.
- **National Ambulance Service:** NRHM has supported free ambulance service to provide patients transport in every nook and corner of the country connected with a toll free number from home to public health facilities and back.
- **Web enabled Mother and Child Tracking System (MCTS):** The name-based tracking of pregnant women and children has been initiated under NRHM with an intention to track every pregnant woman, infant and child up to the age of 3 years by name for ensuring delivery of services like timely antenatal care, institutional delivery and postnatal care for the mother. This also ensures child immunization and other related services.

New Initiatives Under NRHS

- Home delivery of contraceptives by ASHA
- Conducting district level household survey-4 in 26 states/UTs where annual health survey is not possible.
- Modification in the scheme for promotion of menstrual hygiene covering 1.5 crore of adolescent girls in 20 states.
- Differential financial approach for comprehensive healthcare by which allocation of untied fund and RKS grants will be made based on the case load and services provided by the health facility.
- Involving ASHA in home-based newborn care
- Revision in the criterion of allocation of funds to the states under NRHM based on the performance of the state against the targets which can be monitored and implemented, taking into consideration the specific reform agenda in the health sector.
- Expansion of village health and sanitation committee to include nutrition as a mandatory requirement and renaming it as village health sanitation and nutrition committee.
- Partial modification of centrally sponsored scheme for development of AYUSH hospitals and dispensaries for maintaining AYUSH under NRHM
- **Rashtriya Bal Swasthya Karyakram (RBSK):** This program was launched on February 2013 and provides child health screening and early intervention services through early detection and management of 4 diseases, i.e., defects of birth, diseases, deficiencies, developmental delays including disability.
- **Rashtriya Kishor Swasthya Karyakram (RKSK):** This scheme was launched in January 2014. It introduces peer-led intervention at the community level, supported by augmentation

of facility-based services. This initiative broadens the focus of the adolescent health program beyond reproductive and sexual health and focuses on life skills, nutrition, injuries and violence (including gender-based violence). This also involves considering noncommunicable diseases, mental health and substance abuse.

- **Maternal and child health wings:** 100/50/30 bedded maternal and child health wings have been sanctioned in public health facilities to cater the increasing demand for services.
- **National iron-plus:** A new initiative launched in February 2013 to prevent anemia in pregnant and lactating women, adolescent girls and also women of reproductive age group to prevent and control iron deficiency anemia by providing iron and folic acid supplementation.
- **Reproductive, maternal, newborn child and adolescent health services (RMNCH + A):** This approach brings focus on adolescent as a critical life stage and focuses on linkages between child survival, maternal health and family planning efforts. It aims to strengthen the referral linkages between community and facility-based health services and between the various levels of health system.
- **Delivery points:** Funds have been allocated to strengthen delivery points in terms of infrastructure, human resource, drugs, equipment, etc. Health facilities that have high demand for services and performance above a certain benchmark are identified as 'delivery points' with the objective of providing comprehensive health services (RHNCH-A) at these facilities.
- **Universal health coverage:** It is a key goal of 12th Five-Year Plan. The National Health Mission is the primary vehicle to move toward this goal.
- **Comprehensive primary healthcare:** Nine areas are proposed to make primary healthcare comprehensive and universal.
  1. Strengthening institutional structures and organization of primary healthcare services.
  2. Improving access to technologies, drugs and diagnostic for comprehensive primary healthcare.
  3. Increasing utilization of information, communication and technology empowering patients and providers.
  4. Promoting continuity of care. Making care patient centered.
  5. Enhancing quality of care.
  6. Focusing of social determinants of health.
  7. Emphasizing community participation and addressing equity concerns in health.
  8. Developing a human resource policy to support primary healthcare.
  9. Strengthening governance including financing, partnerships and accountability.
- **Launch of national anti TB drug resistance survey:** It was launched for 13 anti-tuberculosis drugs to estimate the burden of MDR-TB within the community.
- **Kala-azar elimination plan:** It was launched for Uttar Pradesh, Bihar, West Bengal and Jharkhand to eliminate kala-azar. It includes active search, new drug regimen, coordinated indoor residual spray and use of noninvasive diagnostic kit.

JANANI SHISHU SURAKSHA KARYAKRAM

Janani Shishu Suraksha Karyakram (JSSK) Scheme was launched on June 1, 2011 under the RCH-Phase II program by Ministry of Health and Family Welfare, Government of India to provide better health facilities to the pregnant women and their child. It is an initiative to provide completely free and cashless services to pregnant women and includes normal deliveries, cesarean operation and sick newborn (up to 30 days after birth). These are availed in government health institutions in both rural and urban areas.

Objectives

- To eliminate Out-of-Pocket expenses for families of pregnant women and sick newborn babies in government health facilities
- To reach to the pregnant women who are unable to reach the health institutions (nearly 75 lakh a year who still deliver at home)
- To provide timely access of care for sick newborn

Concept

The scheme is estimated to benefit 12 million pregnant women who access government health facilities for their delivery. This scheme will also motivate those women who still choose to deliver at home to opt for institutional deliveries. It is an initiative with a hope that state would come forward and ensure that the benefits of JSSK would reach every needy pregnant woman coming to government institutional facility. All the states and UTs have initiated implementation of this scheme.

Benefits to the Pregnant Women

- Free and cashless delivery
- Free and cashless cesarean section
- Free diet up to 3 days during normal delivery
- Free diet up to 7 days following cesarean section
- Free drugs and consumables
- Free diagnosis
- Free blood wherever required
- Exemption from user charges
- Free transport from home to health institution
- Free transport between facilities in case of referral
- Free drop back from institution to home after 48 hours stay

Benefits to the Sick Newborn

These benefits are provided up to 30 days after birth, such as:
- Free treatment
- Free drugs and consumables
- Free diagnosis
- Free provision of blood transfusion if required
- No user charges
- Free transport from home to institution
- Free transport between facilities in case of referral
- Free drop back from institutions to home

EMERGENCY AMBULANCE SERVICES

An ambulance is a vehicle which provides mobility from or between places of treatment and in some instances, will also provide out of hospital, medical care to the patient. Emergency ambulance services as a means of transportation of the patient to the healthcare unit are available in India both in private as well as in government sector.

- In government sector, the ambulance with toll free number 108 is available at every nook and corner of the country and round the clock service is provided. In emergency, anyone can dial 108 either from mobile or landline telephone, the ambulance will reach and shift the patient to nearest medical unit free of cost. Recently there is a plan to provide emergency treatment at home to deal with emergency.
- However, in private sector, the emergency ambulance services are equipped with all emergency drugs and required equipment to deal with emergency along with medical team specially trained for such situations. There are specialized and general emergency ambulance services available in the private health sectors.

Medical Team Dealing Emergency Ambulance Services

The medical team for dealing emergency ambulance services consists of a specialist doctor, nurse, laboratory technician and a medical assistant. There are cardiac, respiratory and general emergency services operating in India. The medical team treats the emergency at home till the patient is in a condition to shift to the hospital for further management. In developed countries, there are maternity emergency psychiatric, pediatric, cardiac, respiratory and other general emergency ambulance services are available round the clock.

GOVERNMENT HEALTH INSURANCE SCHEMES

Health Insurance

Health insurance is insurance against risk of incurring medical expenses. By estimating the overall risk of healthcare expenses, an insurer can develop a routine finance structure, such as a monthly premium or payroll tax, to ensure that money is available to pay for the healthcare benefits specified in the insurance agreement. The benefits are administered by a central organization such as government agency, private business or other not for profit entity.

Definition

Protection scheme, process of protecting a person from contingent risk of losses through financial means, in return for a relatively small, regular payment to insurance company. This is considered a hedging instrument against future contingent losses. These instruments help in managing the possible risk. It also guarantees payment to the person in the event of sickness or injury.

Benefits

- Provides financial protection
- Improves the quality of care
- Controls costs
- Increases access

Health Insurance Schemes

The Ministry of Health and Family Welfare (MoHFM) has set up a task force to explore new health financing mechanisms. The ministry has advised to state/UT governments to prepare health insurance models as per their local needs. Government of India will provide support to state governments for health insurance schemes/projects under NRHM. The role of health insurance is very limited in India as compared to foreign countries. Privatization of insurance and the arrival of foreign insurance companies as a result of globalization have brought out lot of improvement in health insurance sector.

The government health insurance schemes in India are as follows:
- Employees State Insurance Scheme
- Rajiv Gandhi Shramik Kalyan Yojana
- Family Planning Insurance Scheme
- Central Government Health Scheme

Employees State Insurance Act, 1948

The ESI Act passed in 1948 (and was amended in 1975, 1984, 1989 and 2010) is an important measure of social security and health insurance in this country. It provides certain cash and medical benefits to the industrial employees in case of sickness, due to employment injury and maternity benefits.

Scope: The Act extends to the whole of India. It has covered all power using factories wherein 10 or more persons are employed excluding mines, railways and defense establishment.

The provision of ESI (Amendment) Act of 1975 were extended to the following new classes of establishment:
- Small factories employed 10 or more persons whether power is used in the process of manufacturing or not.
- Shops
- Hotels and restaurants
- Cinema and theaters
- Road-motor-transport establishments
- Newspaper establishments
- The scheme has been extended to private medical and educational institutions employing 20 or more persons in some states.

W.e.f. May 1, 2010, the Act covers all employees, i.e., manual, clerical, supervisory and technical getting up to ₹15000 per month. This has been further revised to ₹21,000/- per month as per notification of ESIC on September 6, 2016 to any other agricultural or commercial establishment.

Administration: The ESI Corporation has the chairman who is the Union Minister of Labor.

Secretary to the Government of India Ministry of Labor is the vice-chairman. It consists of members representing central and state government's employer and employees' organizations, medical profession and parliament. There is a standing committee constituted from the members of the corporation, which acts as an executive body for the administration of the scheme. The chief executive officer of the corporation is the director general who is assisted by four principal officers.

1. Insurance commissioner
2. Medical commissioner
3. Financial commissioner
4. Actuary

Finance of the ESI corporation: The scheme is run by the contribution of the employees, employers and grants from central and state governments. The employer contributes 4.75% of total wage bill and employees contribute 1.75% of wages (revised rates w.e.f. 1-1-1997). Employees getting daily wages of ₹100 are exempted from payment of contribution. The state government share of expenditure on medical care is 1/8 of total cost of medical care. The ESI corporations share is 7/8 of total cost of medical care.

Benefits to employees:

- **Medical benefit:** It consists of full medical care including hospitalization, lab investigation and all radiological investigation, immunization, all specialists' services, free drugs, family planning services, health education and in-patient's treatment. In complicated cases, where specialized treatment is required, patients are sent to institutional treatment outside the state at the expense of ESI Corporation. Medical treatment extends to the workers, their dependents and families also.

- **Sickness benefit:** As per the ESI Act, an ensured person is entitled for sickness benefit if the sickness is certified by the insurance medical officer or insurance medical practitioner. Sickness benefit is payable for maximum period of 91 days in any continuous period of 365 days in the form of cash. The rate of cash payment is 50% of the daily wages. The person receiving sickness benefit has to remain under medical treatment provided under the act.

  - **Extended sickness benefit:** If the ensured person is suffering from long term disease, then according to the Act, he/she is entitled for extended sickness benefit for maximum period of two years in addition to 91 days sickness benefit. There are 34 diseases for which the extended benefit can be paid to ensured person who has been in continuous employment for 2 years.

  - **Enhanced sickness benefit:** An ensured woman is entitled for 14 days of enhanced sickness benefit after undergoing tubectomy and 7 days for ensured male who has undergone vasectomy.

- **Maternity benefit:** It is payable to an insured woman for confinements/miscarriage or sickness arising out of pregnancy, confinement or premature birth of a child or miscarriage. For confinement the duration of benefit is 26 weeks, for miscarriage 6 weeks, and for sickness arising out of confinement 30 days. The benefit is allowed at about full wages. The rate of confinement expenses has been increased from ₹5000 to ₹7500 per confinement if medical facilities are not available under ESI.

- **Disablement benefit:**

  - **Temporary disablement benefit (TDB):** Payable from day one of entering insurable employment and irrespective of having paid any contribution in case of employment injury at the rate of 90% of the wage is payable as long as disability continues.

  - **Permanent disablement benefit:** It is paid at the rate of 90% of wage in the form of monthly payment depending upon the extent of loss of earning capacity as certified by a medical board.

- **Dependent benefits:** These are paid at the rate of 90% of the wage in the form of monthly payment to the dependents of a deceased, injured person in case where death occurs due to employment injury or occupational hazard.

- **Funeral expenses:** It is a cash payment payable on the death of an insured person toward the expenses on his funeral. The amount not exceeding ₹10,000 w.e.f. 1st April 2011.

Rehabilitation allowance: On monthly payment of ₹10, the insured person and his/her family members continue to get medical treatment after permanent disablement or retirement.

Benefits to the employer:
- Employer is exempted from the applicability of workman's compensation Act, 1923
- Exemption from Maternity Benefit Act, 1961
- Exemption from payment of medical allowance to employees and their dependents or arranging for their medical care
- Rebate under the Income Tax Act on contribution deposited in the ESI account

Rajiv Gandhi Shramik Kalyan Yojana

This scheme was launched on April 1, 2005 by the ESI Corporation. This scheme provides an employment allowance for the employees covered under ESI scheme who are rendered unemployed involuntarily due to closure of factory, etc. An employee can avail the benefit of this yojana only after fulfilling certain eligibility conditions.

As per this scheme, an insured person going out of insurable employment involuntarily on account of closure of a factory or establishment, retrenchment or permanent invalidity arising out of nonemployment injury after rendering insurable employment and having contributed under the scheme for five or more years is entitled to claim unemployment allowance for maximum period of 6 months during his/her entire service. The allowance can be availed in one spell or different spells of not less than one month.

The daily rate of employment allowance is the "standard benefit rate" as specified in the table of standard benefit rate under Rule 54 of ESI (Central) Rule 1950 corresponding to the average daily wage drawn by the insured person. During this period for which the insured person is entitled for employment allowance, he/she is also entitled to utilize medical benefits for himself/herself and the entire family members from ESI hospitals to which he/she was attached.

Central Government Health Scheme (CGHS)

The CGHS was introduced in 1954 in New Delhi to provide comprehensive medical care to the central government employees, pensioners and their dependents residing in CGHS covered cities. The scheme is based on the principle of cooperative effort by the employee and the employer, to the mutual advantage of both.

Beneficiaries: The scheme is applicable to the following category of people residing in CGHS covered cities:
- All central government servants paid from civil estimates (other than employed in railway services and those employed under Delhi administration except members of Delhi Police Force)
- Pensioners drawing pension from civil estimates and their family members (Pensioners residing in non-CGHS area may also obtain CGHS card from nearest CGHS covered city).
- Honorable members of parliament of autonomous bodies covered under CGHS (Delhi).
- Ex-governors and Ex-vice presidents
- Former judges of honorable Supreme Court of India and honorable High Courts
- Widows receiving family pension
- Freedom fighters

Services rendered: CGHS provides services through the following categories of systems:
- Allopathic

- Homeopathic
- Indian System of Medicine, i.e., AYUSH

Components:
- Dispensary services including domiciliary care
- Family welfare and MCH services
- Specialists consultations at dispensaries, polyclinics and hospital level
- Hospitalization
- Organization for the purchase, storage, distribution and supply of medicines and other requirement
- X-rays, ECG and laboratory examination

Facilities:
- Outpatient care through a network of dispensaries
- Supply of necessary drugs
- Laboratory and X-ray investigations
- Domiciliary visits
- Hospitalization facilities at government as well as private hospitals recognized for the purpose
- Specialist consultations
- Pediatric services including immunization
- Antenatal and postnatal services
- Emergency treatment
- Supply of optical and dental aids at reasonable rate
- Family welfare services
- Services of Ayurvedic, Unani, Siddha and homeopathy system of medicine

Family Planning Insurance Scheme

Government of India has launched family planning insurance scheme w.e.f. November 29, 2005 for acceptors of sterilization and indemnity insurance cover for doctor performing sterilization procedures both in government and accredited private/NGO/corporate health facilities. MoHFW is also implementing a central sponsored family welfare linked to health insurance scheme. This has been done since 1981 to compensate the acceptors of the sterilization for the loss of wages for the days on which he/she attended the medical facility for undergoing sterilization.

SCHOOL HEALTH SERVICES

School health is an important branch of preventive and social medicine. The Government of India has given an important place to school health services in Five-Year Plan and in 20-point Program. The health of the school children is vital for the future of the country as today's children will be tomorrow's leader and administrator of the nation. School Health Program aims at providing a package of preventive, promotional and curative health services directed toward improving the current health status of the school age children.

Historical Development

The beginning of school health services dates back to 1909, when for the first-time medical examination of school children was carried out at Baroda city. The Bhore Committee (1946) reported that school health services are nonexistent in India and where they existed, they were poorly conducted. In 1953, the secondary education committee emphasized the need for medical examination of pupils and School Feeding Program.

During the second Five-Year Plan, many state governments provided school feeding program. In 1960, Government of India constituted a School Health Committee to assess the present standards of health and nutrition in school children and suggest ways and means to improve them. The committee recommended certain measures for the improvement of school health services. Government of India emphasized the importance of the medical check-up of primary and secondary class students. Keeping in view the importance of medical check-up programs for school going children, the program was launched all over the state with the available existing medical and paramedical staff at PHCs and CHCs since 1993–1994.

Definition

The school health is defined as "the school procedures that contribute to the maintenance and improvement of the health of the pupils and school personnel including health services, healthful living and health education."

Features

- **Large number of groups:** The children between the age group of five and fourteen, i.e., school going children comprises 25% of India's population. The social and economic development of the country is possible only through care and development of this group. The school health services should be improved.
- **Stage of growth and development:** The school age is the period of growth and development of the child so it is very important to check up the health and give appropriate guidance.
- **Group life:** School is a social group that child gets after home. Contribution of the school is vital in socialization of children. Child can spread or get any infection owing to this group life.
- **Easy implementation:** School age is learning stage. School children are very receptive for anything taught to them like health education and importance of good health. If health services are implemented at this age they will follow it throughout their life.
- **Early detection of diseases:** Many health problems which remain undetected like eye problem, hearing problem, mental retardation, nutritional deficiency disease and dental problem can be detected at early stage and treated. Infectious diseases can also be prevented by detecting it at the earliest.
- **Adaptability:** School children have ability to quickly adopt and acquire new knowledge. School can be used for giving effective healthy habits in them.

Objectives

- The promotion of positive health
- Early detection of health-related problem and their treatment through referral services
- Awakening health consciousness in children
- Provision of healthy environment
- To advise the school authority on safe drinking water supply, good environmental sanitation, cleanliness and good ventilation and lighting in the classroom
- Impart knowledge to the class teachers for early detection of eye, skin, ear and dental problems in children

- Health education to the school children and teachers
- To reduce morbidity among the school children by preventing them from diseases and thus reducing the dropout rate among the school children

Common Problems of School Children

Health Problems

- Malnutrition—anemia, PEM, vitamin A deficiency, etc.
- Skin problems—scabies, lice, acnes, dermatitis rash, etc.
- Eye disorders—refractory defects, trachoma, conjunctivitis
- Respiratory diseases—asthma, TB, pneumonia, etc.
- Infectious diseases—diarrheal diseases and intestinal parasites, etc.

Behavioral Problems

Behavioral problems may be due to various conditions like mental deficiencies, organic disease or failure to adjust in internal and external environment. These problems include:
- Antisocial problem
- Habit disorder
- Personality disorder
- Educational problems—school fear, absenteeism and lack of interest in study

Aspects of School Health Services

The school health services are multifaceted and vary according to the local priorities, special school health services may be developed if the resources are enough. The aspects of school health service are as follows:
- Health appraisal of school children and school personnel
- Remedial measures and follow-up
- Prevention of communicable diseases
- Healthy school environment
- Nutritional services
- First aid and emergency care
- Mental health
- Dental health
- Eye health
- Health education
- Education of handicapped children
- Proper maintenance and use of school health records

Health Appraisal

The health appraisal should cover not only the students but also the teachers and other school personnel. The School Health Committee (1961) in India recommended medical examination of children at the time of entry and thereafter every four years. The initial examination should be thorough. It includes:

- Thorough careful history of the child
- Physical examination
- Tests for vision, hearing and speech
- Laboratory test—blood, urine and stool examination

Parents should be present at the time of entrance medical examination. Teacher should help in medical examination by taking height, weight, testing of vision and preparing children for medical examination.

- **School personnel:** The medical examination should be given to the teachers and other school personnel as they form the school environment to which the child is exposed.
- **Daily morning inspection:** Teacher should do daily inspection to detect changes in appearance and behavior of the students which suggests illness or improper growth and development. The following points will help the teacher to identify which student needs medical treatment:
  - Unusually flushed face
  - Any rash or spots on the skin
  - Coughing and sneezing
  - Sore throat
  - Rigid neck
  - Nausea and vomiting
  - Red or watery eyes
  - Headache
  - Chills or fever
  - Restlessness or sleepiness
  - Disinclination to play
  - Diarrhea
  - Pain in the body
  - Skin conditions, i.e., excessive itching to detect scabies, ringworm or pediculosis

Children showing any of the aforementioned signs should be referred to school medical officer. Teacher's observation of school children is very important to detect any health problem as in India the limited number of trained personnel monitoring school health are available. So the teachers should be adequately trained about medical examination of children during teacher's training course.

Remedial Measures and Follow-up

After medical examination, if any health problem is detected, it should be followed by appropriate treatment and follow-up care. There should be exclusively separate clinic for children at primary health center in the rural area in one of the selected school or dispensaries for a group of 5000 children in the urban area. Clinics days and time should be intimated to all concerned schools. There is a high prevalence of eye, ear, dental, nose and throat defects in school children in India. Special clinics should be provided for school children for treatment.

Prevention of Communicable Diseases

Communicable diseases are controlled by timely immunization. A well-planned immunization program should be drawn up against the communicable diseases. A record should be maintained as a part of school health records. Health record should be given to the child at the time of leaving the school.

Healthy School Environment

The school should serve as a good demonstration center of good sanitation to the community. The school building, site and equipment are part of environment in which the child grows and develops. Healthy environment is necessary for the best emotional, social and personal health of the child. Minimum standard for sanitation of school and its environment have been suggested in India are as follows:

- **Location:** School should be located at far distance from noisy places like railway roads, cinema, factories and market. The premises of the school should be properly fenced and kept free from all hazards.
- **Site:** School should be located on suitable high land and should not be subjected to dampness and shall be properly drained. The School Health Committee recommended 10 acres of land for higher elementary school and 5 acres of land area for primary schools with an additional one acre per 100 students.
- **Structure:** Nursery and secondary school should be single storey. The exterior wall should be heat resistant.
- **Classroom:** Varandha should be attached to classroom. Minimum 40 students should be allowed in each classroom.
- **Furniture:** It should suit the age group. There should be single desk and chair. The chair should have proper back rest.
- **Floor:** It should not be slippery
- **Lighting:** Sufficient natural light should be available from the left side and not from the front.
- **Water supply:** An independent source of safe and potable water should be there and it must be distributed from clean taps.
- **Doors and windows:** Windows should be broad with a height 2″–6″ from the floor area. Combined windows and doors area should be 25% of floor space. Windows should be placed on different walls for cross ventilation. The ventilators should not be <2% of floor area.
- **Color:** Inside color of classroom should be white and should be periodically whitewashed.
- **Toilets:** For 100 students there should be 2 urinals and 1 toilet.
- **Eating facilities:** The vendors should not be permitted inside school premises other than approved by school authorities.

Nutritional Services

The diet of school child is very important. A child who is physically weak, will be mentally weak as well and cannot be expected to take full advantage of schooling. Diet should have adequate nutrients and calories for proper development of the child. Nutritional deficiency diseases are more prevalent in India among the children, particularly related to protein, vitamins A, C, thiamine, riboflavin, iron and calcium elements. To ensure proper diet, the Government of India is providing one whole some meal to school children in government and aided school, under the scheme of "Midday Meal".

- **Midday meal:** It was started in 1995 by the Government of India to ensure adequate nutrition. The meal should provide one-third of daily calories requirement and half the protein requirement.

This meal is in addition to meals which the child gets at home. The meal is prepared at school and served to the children in lunch.

- **Applied Nutrition Program:** The Applied Nutrition Program was started by the Indian government in 1963. It began through an agreement with FAO, WHO and UNICEF. UNICEF is assisting in the form of implementing policies, providing seeds, manure and water supply equipment. Wherever land is available, the facilities provided by UNICEF should be utilized in developing school gardens. The products should be utilized in school feeding program as well as nutrition education.

First Aid and Emergency Care

All teachers should have sufficient knowledge of providing first aid and emergency treatment. Their knowledge should be updated through "In Service Training Program" to prepare them to carry out their responsibilities. The emergencies usually met within the school are as follows:

- Accidents or injuries which can be either minor or serious injuries.
- Medical emergencies such as fever, gastroenteritis, colic pain, fits and fainting, etc. Every school should have an equipped first aid kit. Nowadays, most of the schools employ school health nurse who is capable of tackling all emergencies.

Mental Health

The school is the best tool to shape child's behavior and promote their health. The school routine should be planned in such a way that there should be enough time for relaxation between the periods of intense work to relieve the tension of classroom. The school teacher has a positive and preventive role in mental health of the child. Many problems like juvenile delinquency, maladjustment and drug addiction can be prevented by keeping extracurricular activities sports and competitions in the school. Many schools have counselor and clinical psychologist to counsel and provide career guidance to the students so that they can opt for career which is best suited for them.

Dental Health

The dental examination should be conducted periodically. Dental caries and periodontal diseases are more common in India. Health education on oral hygiene can prevent many diseases of the oral cavity. Early detection and treatment of dental caries and gum diseases prevents the spread of infection.

Eye Health Services

The teachers can detect early signs of refractive errors, poor eye sight, squint and amblyopia condition. These conditions should be treated at the earliest. Eye infections like conjunctivitis and trachoma should be detected and treated. Administration of vitamin A can prevent Xerophthalmia and night blindness. Children should be provided education on primary eye care.

Health Education

The goal of health education is to bring a desirable change in health knowledge, attitude and in practice. Health education is the responsibility of school teacher. The health officers, public health nurse and health assistant may assist the school teacher by providing teaching material and aids. It should be provided on:

- **Personal hygiene:** The need of hygiene of skin, hair, teeth, clothing and good posture.
- **Environmental hygiene:** Children should take part in health activities and keep their environment clean. Visits should be planned to observe community health program where they can observe and learn, measure to control flies and rodents, sanitary wells, sanitary latrines.
- **Nutrition:** Education on balanced diet and regular meals and its importance in health.
- **Sports and physical activities:** It promotes not only physical health of children but also inculcates team spirit.
- **Family life education:** Healthy attitude toward human reproduction is an important aspect of health education. Family life education includes premarriage education, married life education and responsible parenthood.

Education of Handicapped Children

The main aim of education is to assist the handicapped child and his/her family to help the child become independent and lead a normal life as much as possible. It requires the cooperation of health, welfare, social and educational agencies.

School Health Administration

The health of the schoolchild is the joint responsibility of parents, teachers and health administration. The success and efficiency depend upon the effective coordination of the participating agencies.

Primary health centers are charged with responsibility of school health services within their jurisdiction. It requires a whole-time medical officer to examine 5,000–6,000 children in a year.

School Health Committee

The Government of India recommended a School Health Committee in 1961 at the village level, block level, district level, state level and national level. This committee should mobilize the community resources and make school health program continuous and self-supporting. The national school health council will be an advisory and coordinating body.

School Health Records

A cumulative health record of each child should be maintained. It should have name of the child, date of birth, parent's name and address, etc. The record must also contain past history, records of findings of physical examination and screening test, etc. and services provided. The purpose of records is to have cumulative information on the health aspects of child in order to provide continuing intelligent health supervision.

Role of School Health Nurse

School health nurse acts as a direct care provider, advocate, coordinator, manager and educator. She collaborates with the parents, teachers and community health professional to provide quality healthcare to the students in the school community.

Functions of School Health Nurse

- **Direct care provider:** Provides first aid and emergency treatment as per the standing order.
- **Advocate:** Takes an active part in implementation of school health services. Takes permission from school administration before implementing school health services, collects information about school environment and facilities available and number of students and teachers.
- **Coordinator:** She fixes up the appointment with medical officer about student's health check-up and informs the other department related to health. Informs the teachers involved in health checkup of the students.
- **Educator:** She is health educator and counselor. Takes the responsibility of training the teachers about daily checkup including first aid and emergency care.
- **School health records:** She is responsible for maintaining school health records of the students.
- Identifies the children at risk and takes appropriate action
- Assists the medical officer during the health checkup days of the students
- Provides treatment as per the advice of the medical officer
- Provides follow-up services
- Conducts and directs the immunization program of the students
- Conducts health clinics related to children's health
- Assists the administration in maintaining healthful environment at school

OCCUPATIONAL HEALTH NURSING OR INDUSTRIAL NURSING

Occupational Environment

Occupational environment is the sum total of external conditions and the influence which exists in work place and which may affect the health of people in that environment. The external conditions which may affect the health of workers include the following:

- **External conditions:**
  - **Physical agents:** Physical agents which have adverse effect on health of workers are heat, cold, humidity, air moments, radiation, light, noise, vibrations and ionizing radiation, breathing and work space, toilet, hand washing and bathing facilities.
  - **Chemical agents:** These consist of number of toxic chemicals, toxic dust and gases, vapors, fumes, etc., which are potential hazards to the health of workers. Some chemical agents may cause disabling respiratory illness; some can cause injury to the skins. Some may have deleterious effect on blood and other organs.
  - **Biological agents:** The work environment may be a source of infectious agents such as virus, rickettsia, bacteria and parasites. Workers may contact infections while coming in contact with the source.
- **Man and machines:** In industries, there are machines driven by power with emphasis on mass production. The unguarded machine, protruding and moving parts of poor installation of the plant, lack of safety measures are the causes of accidents which are the major problem in industry. Working for long hours in unphysiological posture is the cause of fatigue, backache diseases of joints and muscles and impairment of the workers' health.

- **Man and psychosocial factors in work place:** The numerous psychosocial factors also operate in the work place. The human relationship among the workers on one side and with the authority and administrators on the other side. The psychosocial factors also include the type and rhythm of work, work stability, service conditions, job satisfaction, security, welfare conditions, degree of responsible leadership style and incentive, etc., and lies under the field of human relationship.

Occupation environment cannot be separated from domestic environment. If a worker is having stress at work place it may affect his physical and mental health reducing his efficiency at work. Similarly, workers can take such problems at home which would create a disturbing environment at home. If they have home problems, it may also effect on his work performance.

There should be equilibrium between the industrial worker and his occupational environment.

Occupational Hazards

An industrial worker may be exposed to the following hazards (Fig. 4.1):
- Physical hazards
- Chemical hazards
- Biological hazards
- Mechanical hazards
- Psychosocial hazards

Physical Hazards

Exposure to conditions such as heat and cold. Workers may be exposed to high temperature by working in the sun such as

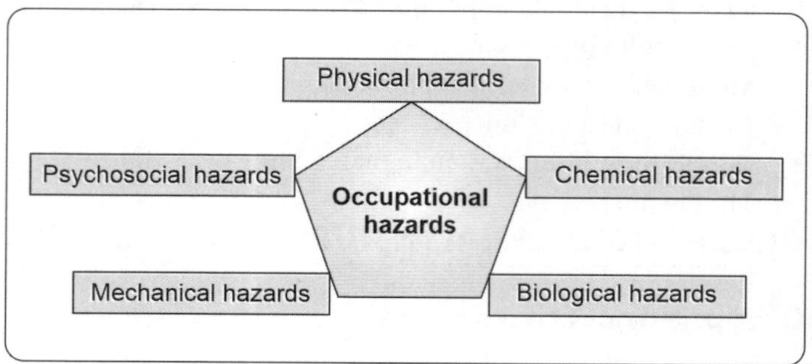

Figure 4.1: Occupational hazards

farmers, builders and laborers. High temperature also found in the mines, e.g., Kolar Gold Mine of Mysore, some industries will have local 'hot spots' ovens and furnaces which radiate heat like in bakeries, metal works, asbestos factory engine room, etc. The effect of high temperature includes prickly heat, heat allergy, heat exhaustions, muscle cramp, etc.

Many workers are exposed to low temperature such as ice factories, high altitude, cold storage, cold laboratories, etc., these workers may develop chilblains, erythron cyanosis and respiratory problems.

- **High humidity:** It along with exposure to extreme temperature in many industries such as textiles, paper and ice factories, aggravates the effect of heat and cold.
- **Noise:** Loud noise is produced in steel, oil, textile and automobile factories. Noise is injurious to health. Its effect depends upon the intensity and duration of exposure leading to fatigue, nervousness, irritation and partial or complete hearing loss.
- **Light:** Workers may be exposed to poor or glaring and bright light. Poor light causes eye strain and pain, eye fatigue, headache. Blaring and bright light causes discomfort, blurring of vision, annoyance and visual fatigue.
- **Vibration:** It occurs while working on machines like grinding, cutting, drilling boring machines, etc. Vibrations may cause fatigue, nervousness and local effects such as injury of hands and joints, etc.

- **Radiations:** Exposure to radiation from X-rays and radioactive isotopes can cause skin and blood cancer. It can result in genetic changes, malformations, sterility, etc. Persons working in radiology department, watch factories, ammunition factories are exposed to ionizing radiation. Ultraviolet (UV) radiation such as during welding causes conjunctivitis and keratitis. Ultraviolet radiation may cause sunburns. Road builders, sailors, shepherds and farmers can be affected with ultraviolet radiation.

Chemical Hazards

Almost all factories make use of some or other chemicals. The chemicals act in three ways.
1. **Local action:** Some chemical causes dermatitis, eczema, etc.
2. **Inhalation:** Gases and vapors are inhaled cause respiratory diseases
3. **Ingestion:** Mercury, lead, arsenic, zinc, chromium and cadmium, phosphorous, etc., cause various diseases

Types of chemicals which are hazardous:
- Gases like carbon monoxide, ozone, carbon dioxide, hydrogen and cyanide, etc.
- Fumes and vapor from various types of acids, mercury vapors, etc.
- **Mists:** Mists in electroplating industries
- **Dusts:** Solid particles liberated as a result of crushing and grinding rock, ores, metals, coal wood, etc.
- The chemical agents are harmful to skin, respiratory system and gastrointestinal system.
- Skin problems include dermatitis, eczema, urticaria, ulcers and cancer, etc.
- Respiratory problems include different types of pneumoconiosis, e.g., silicosis due to quartz dust, anthracosis due to coal dust, byssinosis due to cotton dust, asbestosis due to asbestos dust, asphyxia due to carbon monoxide, hydrogen sulfide and hydrogen cyanide. Throat irritation can occur due to various pungent gases like chlorine, ozone, nitrogen oxide, sulfur dioxide. Lung cancer can result due to asbestos, beryllium, coal tar, mineral oil.
- Gastrointestinal problems are diarrheal problems due to irritation and toxic effects of various chemical ingested along with water and food.

Biological Hazards

Biological hazards are due to infective and parasitic agents like virus, rickettsia, bacteria and parasites. These may cause hookworm infestations in farmers. Leptospirosis in miners. Workers working in tanning factory, veterinary hospital and dispensaries, zoo, circus, farming butchering houses, etc., are exposed to various zoonotic diseases such as brucellosis, mycotic infections, parasitic infections and anthrax, etc.

Health personnel working in hospitals/dispensaries may contact infections from patients, such as tuberculosis, HIV and serum hepatitis, etc.

Mechanical Hazards

Variety of accidents and injuries may result due to unprotected machines, their protruding moving parts and lack of safety measures. The injuries and accident caused due to mechanical hazards may result in partial or permanent disabilities.

Psychosocial Hazards

These may result due to various maladjustment problems either with the coworkers or due to employers conditions of employment like lack of job satisfaction, insecurity, frustration and emotional tension or may not be able to adjust. All these conditions cause physical health problems of high or low blood pressure, indigestion, insomnia loss of appetite and hurt burn, etc.

Occupational Diseases

Occupational diseases are usually defined as diseases arising out of or in the course of employment. These are given in Tables 4.1 and 4.2:

- **Diseases due to biological agents:** These include brucellosis, leptospirosis, anthrax, actinomycosis, hydatidosis, psittacosis, tetanus, encephalitis, fungal infections, etc.
- **Occupational cancers:** Cancer of skin, lungs and bladder.
- **Occupational dermatosis:** Dermatitis, eczema.
- **Diseases of psychological origin:** These include industrial neurosis, hypertension, peptic ulcer, etc.

TABLE 4.1: Diseases due to physical agents

Heat	Heat hyperpyrexia, heat exhaustion, heat syncope, heat cramps, burns and local effects like prickly heat
Cold	Trench foot, frost bite, chilblains
Light	Occupational cataract, miners' nystagmus
Pressure	Air embolism, caisson disease, blast, etc.
Noise	Occupational deafness
Radiation	Cancer, leukemia, aplastic anemia, pancytopenia
Mechanical factors	Injuries and accidents
Electricity	Electric burns

TABLE 4.2: Diseases due to chemical agents

Gases:	Carbon dioxide, carbon monoxide, chlorine, hydrogen sulfide, hydrogen cyanide cause gas poisoning			
	Inorganic dust		**Organic dust**	
	Inorganic dust	**Diseases**	**Organic dust**	**Diseases**
Dusts:	Silica	Silicosis	Cane fiber	Bagassosis
	Coal dust	Anthracosis	Cotton dust	Byssinosis
	Asbestos	Asbestosis	Tobacco	Tobaccosis
	Iron	Siderosis	Hay or grain dust	Farmers disease
Metals and their compounds	Toxic hazards from lead, mercury, cadmium, manganese, beryllium, arsenic and chromium, etc., various diseases of GIT, kidneys, lungs and skin			
Chemicals	Acids, alkalis and pesticides, etc., cause dermatitis			
Solvents	Toxic hazards from carbon bisulfide, benzene trichloroethylene chloroform, etc., cause liver and kidney diseases			

Occupational Health Services

The joint ILO/WHO committee on occupational health, in the course of first session in 1950, gave the following general aims:

Aims

- Promotion and maintenance of the highest degree of physical, mental and social well-being of workers in all occupations
- Protection of workers in their employment from risks resulting from factors adverse to health
- Placing and maintenance of the workers in an occupational environment adopted to his physiological and psychological equipment

Objectives

- Identify the hazardous conditions which might be there in work place.
- Plan and implement protective and control measures to deal with identified hazardous conditions in work place.
- Ensure that the physical and psychological demands imposed on workers by their respective jobs are properly matched with their individual anatomical, physical and psychological needs, capabilities and limitations.
- Provide effective services to protect those who are especially vulnerable to adverse working conditions.
- Provide effective services to workers who are incapacitated for any reason to rehabilitate them as soon as possible.

Health Aspects Under Occupational Health Services

As per the definitions of occupational health nursing, the healthcare of the workers includes the following health aspects:

- Health promotion measures
- Health protection measures
- Early diagnosis and treatment
- Disability limitations and rehabilitation

The occupational health nurse plays an active role in all the aspects of health of the workers:

Health Promotion Measures

To promote the health of workers the following health promotive measures have been recommended:

- **Pre-employment examination for preplacement:** Occupational health nurse helps in the preplacement examination. The purpose of this is to detect any physical or medical problem so that healthy employees are recruited.
- **Job training and continuing education:** Workers are given adequate training and education about their work environment to improve their abilities and get acclimatized to the work environment efficiently.
- **Periodical health check-up:** Routine periodical health check-up is done for screening of health problems due to occupational exposure and take early action to promote health and efficiency of the worker. Periodic examination of workers those who are exposed to radiation noise, food handler and drivers is a must.

- **Health education and counseling:** The occupational health nurse provides health education to the workers on aspects of healthy living and on occupational hazards. Counseling of workers and their family members done to help them to deal with these problems related to their occupations.
- **Provision of wholesome environment:** It includes physical, biological and psychosocial aspects of environment. The occupational health nurse helps the administrators to provide adequate lighting, well-ventilated work place, adequate temperature and humidity, washing and toilet facilities. Environment should be clean, free from harmful organisms. Healthy working relations between the workers and the authority should be encouraged.
- **Provision of welfare facilities:** It includes first aid services, place for meals, rest, change of clothes, etc., insurance against loss of job, illness and disablement, MCH and family welfare services.
- **Suitable working hours:** Working hours should be as per the laws of workers. Weekly holidays and earned leave, etc., should be provided as per the organization policy. Workers should not be exposed to continuous noise or long-standing work. In such cases, they should be frequently changed.
- Provision of housing facilities, recreation ground and clubs, etc., should be there

Health Protection Measures

The protective measures include:
- Immunization against BCG, tuberculosis, hepatitis B, etc.
- Use of shoes against hookworm
- Protection against noise using ear plugs, ear muffs above 85 decibels and frequency above 150 Hz.
- Use of goggles in bright light
- Shielding when exposed to ionizing radiation
- Protection against chemicals by using face mask to prevent inhalation of chemical substances
- Suitable clothes, gloves, shoes, aprons, barrier creams for skin protection
- Proper designing of construction of work place to ensure wholesome physical environment
- Proper designing and layout of machines to minimize their hazards
- Health education for workers for specific health protection measures which need to be implemented by the workers themselves but to be supervised by occupational health nurse

Early Diagnosis and Treatment

The occupational health team should identify the health problems in early stage and early diagnosis and treatment should be done to prevent disabilities. The occupational disease identified to be notified as per Factory Act, 1976. The purpose of notification is to plan and implement preventive and protective measures effectively. The medical services are provided by ESI corporation for the workers as well as for the family members.

Disability Limitation and Rehabilitation

Disability limitation requires early diagnosis and prompt treatment, rectification of conditions responsible for occupational health problems. If a worker develops any health problem due to occupational hazard, he/she should be immediately assigned other suitable job and proper care of disability. In case, the worker is handicapped, he/she should be assigned alternative job and other benefits permissible under the ACT, i.e., ESI Act, 1948.

Occupational Healthcare Team

The aim of occupational health service is to provide primary, secondary and tertiary preventive facilities to the workers. Several people working inside and outside of the commercial institutions are included in the team which includes the following members:

- Occupational health nurse
- Physiotherapist
- Specialist doctor
- Industrial manager
- Supervisor
- Shift in charge
- Rehabilitation specialist
- Labor welfare officer
- Labor union representative
- Representative of voluntary organization
- Other invited members as per the need

Occupational Health Nursing

In the past, it was customary to think occupational health entirely in relation to factories and mines, hence, the term industrial hygiene, industrial health, industrial nursing was in vogue. But the modern concepts of occupational health embrace all types of employment including factories, mines, industries, transport, newspaper, hotels and restaurants, farming, forestry, cinema, theaters, building construction and shops, etc. Hence, the term occupational health nursing is used and industrial nursing is a part of it.

Occupational health like health of people in general deals with promotion and protection of health of workers, control of diseases by early diagnosis and rehabilitation of the disabled workers. Occupational health services thus include primary, secondary and tertiary level preventive and control measure.

History

In 1888, in America, a group of coal-mine company had appointed an occupational health nurse on contract to take care of injured coal-mine workers and their families. Gradually occupational health nursing started taking place of doctors in factories so the first occupational health nurse has become the root pillar of modern occupational health nursing.

Occupational health nursing is a specialized branch of nursing by which the health of workers engaged in different occupations is taken care of and the disorders are treated.

Definitions

- The American association of occupational health nurse defined occupational health nursing as, "the application of nursing principles in conserving the health of workers in all occupations. It involves prevention, recognition and treatment of illness and injury, and required special skill and knowledge in the fields of health, education, counseling, environmental health, rehabilitation and human relations."

- Similar definition is given by Killer, "Occupational health nursing is the application of nursing and public health philosophy and skills to the relationship of people to their occupations for the purpose of prevention of disease and injury and the promotion of optimal health, productivity and social adjustment." This definition is based on the statements given by Brown and Page.
- The joint committee of ILO/WHO on Occupational Health, held in 1950, for the first time gave the following definition about occupational health. It is defined as "The general aim of occupational health should be the promotion and maintenance of highest degree of physical, mental and social well-being of workers in all occupations, the protection of workers in their respective employment from risks resulting from factors adverse to health, the placing and maintenance of the workers in an occupational environment adopted to their physiological and psychological needs". In order to summarize, it is the adoption of work to man and each man to his job.

The occupational health thus implies the application of principles of prevention and control of health problems in workers at various levels to promote, protect and preserve their health and to rehabilitate when required. So, the health personnel working in occupational health setting, require special education and training in occupational health in addition to their basic professional education.

Educational Preparation of an Occupational Health Nursing

In addition to basic professional education the following subjects are included in the occupational health nursing:
- Epidemiology and toxicology
- Occupational health problems
- Occupational hazards and diseases
- Industrial hygiene
- Industrial security
- Different labor law and labor welfare programs
- Industrial health program
- Preparation of industrial budget
- Occupational rehabilitation
- Occupational psychology
- Work evaluation technique
- Occupational health management.

Ergonomics

The term means adaptation of work to man and man to work for the improvement of human efficiency and well-being. The science of ergonomics deals with layout designs of work place, work environment, methods of work, designing of equipment, machines, etc. It aims to prevent and control accidents, disabilities, etc., and to improve the efficiency and well-being of the workers. The application of the science of ergonomics resulted in improvement in working conditions by detecting existing health hazards and by designing the work place and activities according to workers physical and psychological ability and requirement.

> **Must Know**
>
> Ergonomics is an integral part of any advanced occupational health service. The term ergonomics is derived from the Greek word, Ergonomics: Ergon + Nomos
> - Ergon means—work
> - Nomos means—law

Roles and Responsibilities of Occupational Health Nurse in Occupational Health

The occupational health nurse has her primary responsibility to promote, protect and preserve the health of the workers. She has also the accountability to protect the employer from adverse effects of work processes and hazardous substances on worker. She is an important member of the occupational health team. She has got independent role as a care provider within the goals and objectives of the team work. She coordinates the services of all members of the team. She identifies health and nursing needs of workers by making assessment and plans and implements nursing care within her capabilities and limitations. The functions of nursing personnel are stated by WHO Technical Report (Series 24) and also by second joint ILO/WHO committee on occupational health convened in Geneva 1952.

Functions of Nursing Personnel in Occupational Health

The functions of nursing personnel as stated by WHO Technical Report, Series 24 are as follows:
- Carrying out the therapeutic program designed by the physician for sick patients including personal services aimed at hygiene and comfort.
- Maintenance of the physical and psychological environment conductive to recovery and health.
- Engaging the patient and his/her family in his/her recovery and rehabilitation.
- Carrying out measures for the prevention of diseases.
- Interacting people sick or well, in measures promoting total health (physical and mental) in a positive sense.
- Coordinating nursing efforts with other members of community groups.

Functions of Nursing Personnel in Occupational Health

The functions of nursing personnel as Stated by Joint ILO/WHO Committee in 1952, are as follows:
- Assistance in general administration, maintenance and arrangement of health facilities in the plant.
- Emergency and primary treatment of accidents and illness based on standing orders from physicians.
- Assistance with preplacement and medical examination.
- Arranging follow-up treatment where indicated, including health supervision of employees returning to work after illness.
- Health education and counseling.
- Assistance in supervision of factory hygiene and accident prevention.
- Advice on specific health question to management and workers.
- Maintenance of records and statistics.
- Cooperation with referral of workers to general community agencies for help as and when necessary.

GERIATRIC NURSING

Geriatric nursing refers to the care of sick aged when he/she is not well. Geriatric is the branch of health science concerned with the study and treatment of problems and diseases associated with aging.

Definition

Geriatrics is defined as "the study of the medicine aspects of old age and the application of knowledge related to the biological, behavior, biomedical and social aspect of aging to prevention, diagnosis, treatment and the care of old persons."   —**Butler, 1987**

Population Aging

Population aging is one of the most significant emerging problems in all developing and developed countries. Government of India in its national policy on older persons in January 1999, defines "Senior citizen" or "elderly" as a person who is of 60 years age and above.

According to United Nations Population Fund (UNFPA) data, the global elderly population aged 65 years and above nearly doubled from 5.5% in 1974 to 10.5% in 2024. This figure is projected to reach 20.7% by 2074. In India, according to new UN report, there is sharp growth of elderly population from 2010 onward along with a decline in the age group of those below 15 years in the country (which is currently the largest cohort of the young). Going by projection in 2046 India's elderly population will be higher than the population size of children between 0 and 14 years and there will be dip in number of those between 15 and 49 years. The UNFPA report 2023, highlighted that undoubtedly, relatively young India will turn into a rapidly aging society in the coming decades. The report highlighted that there are 14.9 crore persons aged 60 years and above in 2022 (as on 1st July 2022) comprising around 10.5% of the country's population and estimated to increase 15% (around 27 crore) by 2036.

Causes of Increase in Elderly Population

This increase in elderly population is due to:
- Increased awareness on healthy lifestyle
- Access to healthcare
- Improvement in nutrition and sanitation
- Decline in premature mortality from infections and chronic diseases due to discovery of antibiotics and improved medical technology.

Aging Process and the Change

The life cycle has got four stages:
1. Childhood
2. Youth
3. Adulthood
4. Old age

Aging is not a health problem but it is gradual lifelong biological process affecting irreversible changes. The natural aging process is known as senescence. The change takes place in the body as time goes by in the absence of recognized disease. This natural aging refers to inexorable and universal physiological changes that occur with age. These changes are genetically programed.

These changes are inevitable but it can be delayed, controlled or prevented by modifying lifestyle, habits, diet exercise and by retaining autonomy and social support. The concept of prevention and control of changes by modifying lifestyle gave origin to successful aging. Successful aging refers to modification of behavioral process to achieve the best possible outcome of aging. The aging population is to be encouraged to adopt healthy lifestyle and safe environment to live long and have quality life. In 1999, WHO had chosen the theme for World Health Day: "Active Aging makes the difference". Health is vital to maintain well-being and quality of life. Active aging refers to active and disability free life. Healthy and active aging means:

- Retention of physical, physiological, mental and social fitness of its maximum and to lead a normal life as possible like earlier years
- Being mobile, coping well with physical, mental, social and spiritual activities of daily life
- Enjoying sound and fulfilling life
- Being productive and contribute to family and community

"Healthy and active aging can be defined in terms of ability to function autonomously within a given social setting"

The older persons can be healthy and active in spite of some chronic problems. Healthy and active aging is influenced by:

- Life time habits
- Environment
- Social support system and
- Emotional outlook

Changes that Occur in the Body due to Aging

Physical Changes

All the body system and organs undergo changes.

Nervous System

Enlargement of ventricles, as the people get older, the volume of ventricles get increased. Cells surrounding ventricles are lost. Reduced brain weight and volume probably caused by loss of neurons. Gradual mental dysfunction due to gradual decline in intelligence, memory, sensory changes resulting in inaccurate communication, disruption of sleep.

Eye and ENT Changes

The richness of human experience is perceived through the sense especially through vision and hearing. As people's age increases, their ability to perceive the information received from their senses is impaired and distorted.

- **Vision:** Visual acuity decreases and night vision also decreases. Sclera becomes yellow and less elastic. Lacrimal secretion is reduced giving rise to dry eye.
- **Hearing:** There is a 25% of hearing loss at the age of 60–74 and 50% above the age of 75 and above. Impaired hearing results in incomplete perception of information.
- **Smell and taste:** Sense of smell and taste is reduced.

Digestive System

- **Oral cavity:** As a person ages, there is atrophy of oral mucosa. Increased infection of teeth and gums has been observed. Recession of gingiva and increased sensitivity is present. Less production of saliva leading to dry mouth and falling of teeth in old aged people.

- **Esophagus:** Smooth muscles weaken resulting in delayed emptying and possible dilatation. It gives an unpleasant feeling of fullness in their chest under sternum.
- **Stomach:** Decreased gastric secretions, presence of atrophic gastritis with diminished level of hydrochloric acid, mucus and pepsin are observed. Impaired digestion and absorption of iron, vitamin B_{12} and protein has been seen.
- **Small intestine:** Decrease in function due to poor peristaltic movement of intestine. Atrophy of small intestine may affect protein, fat and carbohydrate metabolism and absorption and malabsorption of other nutrients like calcium and vitamin D, constipation are common.
- **Liver:** Metabolic decreases as there is decreased number of hepatic cells and marked decrease in alcohol intolerance.

Cardiovascular System

The blood vessels become less distensible with aging. Thickening of the walls of arteries leads to hypertension. Cardiac muscles fibers and other structures get calcified and thickened. Increase in the deposition of collagen and lipids contribute to stiffening of the heart muscles. The valves of heart become thickened and more rigid. The rate of blood circulation by the heart decreases.

Respiratory System

Age-related changes in the structures can influence comfort and functioning. Connective tissue changes can cause columella (lower edge of septum) to have reduced flow of air through nasal cavity. This can lead to mouth breathing. Lung's capacity gets reduced ineffective gas exchange, osteoporosis of the ribs and vertebrae, calcification of the cartilage causes increased stiffness or rigidity decreased mobility and reduced compliance of chest wall. Muscles involved in respiration weakens with age. Vital capacity decreases by 25%.

Integumentary System

Due to systemic decrease in circulation, there is loss of cells and loss of elastic collagen fibers and muscle mass resulting in decreased elasticity of skin. Light touch and pressure sensations decrease with age. It predisposes to mechanical and chemical injuries, subcutaneous atrophy of face and hands. Decreased production of sweat, sebum and vitamin D, wrinkles appear, age spots appear. There is loss of hair from scalp, axilla and pubic region.

Musculoskeletal System

Normal age-related changes include decreased height up to 2 inches, muscle atrophy, stiffening of joints, kyphosis, swelling in joints.

Bones become weak leading to osteoporosis and degenerative changes in joints and bones. Mobility decreases if proper exercises not done.

Genitourinary System

Age-related changes include urinary incontinence due to impaired sphincter control. Loss of nephrons and renal mass, diminished blood flow, decreased creatinine clearance, decline in endocrine functions of the kidney. Decrease in bladder capacity due to smooth muscle and elastic tissue replacement with fibrous connective tissue. Fluid and electrolyte imbalance. Enlargement of prostate gland in males. Atrophy of reproductive organs in females. Vaginal secretion decreases.

Endocrine System

Thyroid gland becomes less active. Alertness decreases. More susceptible to cold. Secretions of testosterone, estrogen and progesterone decreases. Less secretions of insulin by pancreas.

Sociological Changes

There is reduced income due to retirement or reduced capacity to work and earn, change in lifestyle, widowhood, loss of other family members and friends, failed relationship, social isolation, isolation from service and other activities, person feels the sense of 'uselessness'.

Spiritual Changes

The religious attitude and feelings tend to increase while attendance of religious services tend to decrease with age for many reasons such as functional disability, lack of company, shortage of funds and related means and facilities. All these changes may cause feeling of rejection, loneliness, anxiety and insecurity.

Factors Affecting Changes

Hereditary Factors

Hereditary diseases, the capacity for longevity and physical capacities influence the aging process

Environmental Factors

Three types of factors affect aging:
1. **Abiotic factors:** Factors like climate, radiation, chemical and physical elements of pollution, etc.
2. **Biotic factors:** Living organisms in the environment like pathogens, parasites, the availability and quality of food. etc., all these influence the aging process
3. **Socioeconomic factors:** Several socioeconomic factors responsible are adverse living or working condition increase the "wear and tear" of life. Such tensions make people grow old early.

Life Events of Older Adulthood

- **Widowhood:** It is inevitable for one of the two partners and chances are greater of males dying first and female windows are more than male widows.
- **Relocation:** Another area of psychosocial adjustment for older adults is the decision to move from family home. Relocation to the nursing home or old age home is a common and significant life event of the older adult. It leads to:
  - Loss of space
  - Change of neighborhood
  - Move away from friends
- **Cognitive and intellectual:**
  - Cognitive speed and memory performance decline with age. Poor health, lower activity high BP predict faster cognitive decline.
  - Intellectual process such as reasoning and abstract thinking remain the same throughout the life unless they are affected by physical or mental degeneration. Intellectual does not decline with age.

- **Death of friends or family member:** The loss of family members and friends becomes more inevitable with each advancing years of age. Loneliness and social isolation are two consequences of these two losses. It can also be a threat on anxiety.

Problems of Old Age

- **Physiological problems:** It is estimated that 95% of the elderly have chronic disabilities. Most common diseases in this segment are hypertension, cataract, diabetes mellitus, osteoporosis, coronary artery disease, chronic obstructive pulmonary disease (COPD), constipation and urinary incontinence.
- **Psychological problems:** Include delirium, dementia, depression, anxiety and stress.

Elderly Abuse

Elderly abuse (Fig. 4.2) is an act that causes harm. Abuse of elderly especially disturbing them as they are helpless to fight back and often unable to call help because they love family so much.

Forms of Elderly Abuse

Elderly abuse includes the following:

- **Physical abuse:** It includes the behavior of the care giver toward the elderly person which results in bodily harm such as

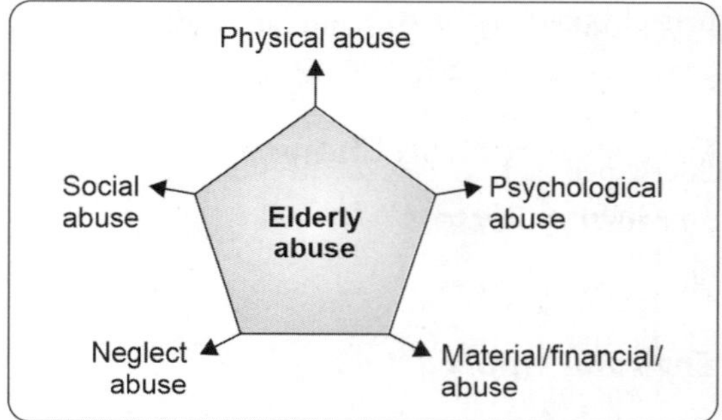

Figure 4.2: Elderly abuse

slapping, dragging, kicking, throwing, bites, cuts burns and injuries locking them in the house, physical punishment or restraining, etc. It may also include sexual harassment.
- **Psychological abuse:** The care giver threats to the elderly person which provoke the fear of violence or isolation. It may result in mental tension, anxiety and depression. Examples of psychological abuse is calling name, insulting, frightening, yelling, screaming and using ridiculous language.
- **Material/financial abuse:** This form of abuse includes owning the property of the elderly person by illegal means without his/her consent. It may include unethical use of his/her money. Not providing necessities such as good food, clothing, wheel chair, hearing aid, dentures and spectacles, etc., or it may be unusual bank activity.
- **Neglect:** It can be active neglect or passive neglect
  - **Active neglect:** Includes the willful deprivation of the services which are necessary to maintain physical or mental health. Examples of active neglect are not giving adequate food, medicine on time. Not changing clothes or giving bath on time or not attending to his/her needs on time.
  - **Passive neglect:** Deleting the care and needs of the elderly or failing to recognize the needs of the elderly person. It may be due to ignorance also.
- **Social abuse:** Not providing proper respect or proper place in the family, neglecting his/her advice. Not including him or her in decision-making in family activities.

General Considerations in Assessing Health Needs of Elderly

- Elderly people may have multiple health problems and needs which they may not explore, so they should be encouraged to speak out so that attention may be given to their difficulties
- They may have difficulties in communicating their problems so careful attention should be given to their needs
- They may under report or may have multiple nonspecific complaints which require interrogation
- They may show a typical signs and symptoms
- They may show decreased tolerance to stress. They may require longer time to readjust
- Normal effects of aging must be differentiated from pathology
- Normal effects of aging must be constantly redefined

Elderly people have an increased vulnerability to diseases due to decreased physiological reserves less flexible hemostatic of the body, so their care should be efficiently planned to meet their physiological needs.

Health Needs of the Elderly

Elderly people have specific health needs which demand extra attention. These include:
- **Good nutrition**: To maintain optimal weight and good digestion, the food should have low fat, moderate carbohydrate and high protein. Food should be cooked properly and served at frequent intervals in small quantities as their reserves are poor and they feel hungry soon. Ideally the meals should be divided into five times. They should avoid laxatives. Diet should have sufficient amount of fibers. More fluids should be given during early hours of the day and restricted fluid during late hours of the day.
- **Exercise**: Physical activity contributes flexibility of the joints and muscles. It also prevents the stiffness of the joints and adds to the quality of intellectual and physical performance.
- **Economic security**: It is another major need of older adults. Often financial worries are the cause of debilitation. Fear of the cost of major illness leads to cut short on expenses for good food, full and active life, etc. There is a need for economic security and appropriate healthcare services.
- **Need for independence:** Elderly people like to make their decision and manage their own life even if they are having, disabilities and limitations as it makes them to feel independent and have self-respect and dignity.
- **Need for companionship**: Older people need company and social interaction for expression and response. It adds meaning to their life.
- **Meaningful activity**: Meaningful activities add purpose to life and are good for mental health. It may be hobbies or part-time or full-time employment.
- **Need for dignified death**: Dignified death means death which is free from pains as far as possible, humiliation, discomfort or financial concerns, etc. People need to consider for their choice for place, spiritual counseling for presence of family members, etc.

Role of Geriatric Nurse in Management of Geriatric People

The family members should be counseled and involved in the care of the elderly whether the person is in hospital or at home.

Nursing Management of Physiological Problems

They should be taught about the care of the person with physiological problems at home. Care of some disorders are as follows:

- **Hypertension**: If the person is hospitalized see that he/she is taking proper medicine. If he/she cannot afford, refer him/her to appropriate social services. Blood pressure should be monitored. Health education to the patient and family regarding his/her diet and exercise.
- **Stroke**: After strokes, many people become dependent on others in daily activities and self-care.
  - Improve patient's quality of life, pay attention to both physical and psychological aspects.
  - Enhance patient's self-care ability and minimize dependency. This can slow down the aging process.
  - Maintain limb and body function to avoid pressure sores, chest complications, aspirations and frozen shoulders, etc.
- **Urinary incontinence**: It is a common problem in elderly because of weakened pelvic floor muscles and sphincter muscles. Assess the family's behavior toward problem
  - An indwelling catheter should be passed and released intermittently
  - Avoid coffee or more fluid at night
  - Use of absorbent pad
- **Osteoporosis:** In this there is a gradual loss of bone density. The affected bone becomes thinner and can be fractured easily which result in loss of independence. This condition can be taken care by:
  - Preventing fall
  - Doing exercise
  - Ensuring adequate calcium intake
- **Accidents:** Due to sensory deficit like vision, altered perception, poor hearing and slower response elderly people are prone to accidents and falls. Older people are encouraged to take safety measures.
- **Malnutrition:** It is common due to decreased appetite, poor food choices, physical limitations of chewing, loss of teeth and social isolation. They should be given soft, easily digestible, palatable food with adequate calories and nutrients.
- **Immobility:** Physical activity is the key point for healthy aging. A planned exercise is important for adults.
- **Self-care deficit:** Family is educated to assist in self-care needs as with advancing age; ability to perform self-care is impaired.

Nursing Management of Neurological and Psychological Problems

- **Delirium:** It is a condition in which cerebral circulation is affected and can cause disturbance in cognitive function. The onset may be rapid and can include disturbed intellectual functions, disorientation to time and place, worsened memory, poor adjustment can alter the level of consciousness.
- **Dementia:** Chance of dementia increases after the age of 60. Estimated 4 million of people suffer from dementia. Most common is Alzheimer's disease. This has been noticed as the patient does not remember when asked about things. He/she needs special attention toward nutrition and personal hygiene and medicine, etc.

- **Depression:** Depression is referred to as "Common cold of elderly". It is most frequent problem that psychiatrists treat in elderly and its incidence is on the increase. Severity of depression is also higher in older adults.

Management of 3Ds includes:

- Prompt detection. Treating the condition as a medical emergency can prevent permanent damage.
- Monitoring level of consciousness.

Anxiety

Anxiety is common in elder population. Overseas research found that anxiety symptoms are present in 20% of the old community. Main areas associated with anxiety are as follows:

- Health
- Finance
- Life stressors

Coping with Anxiety

In order to cope with anxiety, one needs to be optimistic and should have positive thinking.

Stress

Common source of stress in elderly includes:

- Changes of lifestyle and financial status after retirement.
- Caring of grand children
- Caring of sick spouse
- Chronic illness
- Dependency

High Yield Point

Myths and Truths related to senior citizens

Myths related to senior citizens	Truths about senior citizens
Older people are mentally and physically weak	They help us deal with our disappointment, grief and illness
We cannot expect any creativity or contribution from older people	They have creative ideas learnt from the years of experience which they can teach others
All older people have alike needs	We can gain practical experience
Older people are not worth	They can be helpful in guiding us on how to conduct us of self-esteem, self-respect and self-discipline
Expense on older people is a waste	They are valuable for a family as they know the traditions which young generation do not
Older people take away resources from young people	They have learnt the lessons of humanity
Older people want to live in isolation	They are fun companions
Older people are not suited to modern work place—you cannot teach old dogs' new tricks	They know things we would never guess unless we ask
Older people experiences cannot make wonders in modern society	They will teach us through experience
Old people want to be quiet and calm	They make our environment joyful

Management of Stress

An active social life. The modern philosophy is that the old people must continue to participate in the responsibilities and have enjoyment of privileges, which are essential features to remain active. The community must assist the old aged people to fight from triple evils—poverty, loneliness and ill health. The following things should be considered management:

- Engaging in voluntary work
- Positive thinking
- Seek help from professionals

Welfare Programs for Senior Citizens

Ministry of social justice and empowerment is the nodal ministry responsible for welfare of the senior citizens. It has announced the national policy on older persons covering all concerns pertaining to the welfare of older persons.

Maintenance and Welfare of Parent's and Senior Citizens Act, 2007

The Maintenance and Welfare of Parents and Senior Citizens Act, 2007, was introduced in December 2007 to promote need-based maintenance for parents and senior citizens.

The act provides for the following:

- Maintenance of parents/senior citizens by children/relatives made obligatory
- Justice through court reversal or transfer of property by senior citizen in case of negligence by relatives
- Penalization in case of abandonment of senior citizens
- Establishment of old age home for senior citizens
- Facilitate adequate medical facilities and security for senior citizen
- NGOs and voluntary organizations

National Program for Healthcare for Elderly

National Program for Healthcare for Elderly (NPHCE) was implemented by the Ministry of Health and Family Welfare in the year 2010–2011 with an approval amount of ₹288 crore for the period of 11th Five-Year Plan.

The Ministry also considers the following provisions for senior citizens:

- Separate queues for older persons in government hospitals
- Geriatric clinic in several hospitals
- Separate registration and medicine counter
- Indira Gandhi National old age scheme was launched on November 19, 2007 to provide monthly pension to people above 65 years living below poverty line.
- More interest on saving in banks/post office
- **Travel:**
    - Reservation of two seats for senior citizens on front row of buses of the state road transport under takings
    - Some states are giving fare concession
    - Indian railway provides 30% fare concession in all mail/express for senior citizens aged 60 years and above

- Indian Railway also has the facility for separate counter for senior citizens for purchase/booking/cancellation of tickets.
- Wheel chairs for use of older persons are available at all junctions.
- Ramps for wheel chair are available in some important stations.
- Air India is offering discount to senior citizens who are above 60 years of age, on flights to USA, UK and Europe.
- Under the Antyodaya Scheme—the below poverty line (BPL) families that have older persons are issued food grains 35 kg/family/month. The food grains are issued at the rate of ₹3/- per kg for rice ₹2/- per kg for wheat.
- **Income tax exemption:** Tax exemption is provided to the senior citizens by the Ministry of Finance. The senior citizens of 60 years and above are exempted from ₹3 lakh/annum, and 80 years and above are exempted ₹5 lakh per annum.

Responsibilities of Community Health Nurse in Geriatric Care

The main objective of gerontological nursing is to improve the quality of life of old people, i.e., "Add life to the years but not years to the life." She has to fulfil the following roles in gerontological nursing:

- Caregiver
- Health educator
- Coordinator of health services
- Counselor or guardian

Nurse has to perform different functions in relation to aforementioned roles:

Health Assessment

A detailed examination of the old person to assess the entire needs, i.e., physical, mental, social and economic resources. The following assessment is made:

- Daily activities of living, i.e., bathing, clothing, eating, excretion, urinary control, etc.
- Activities related to the use of equipment or procedures (telephone, bank account, food, preparation, etc.) and his/her ability in these activities
- Health screening, ability to see, hear, dental problems, blood pressure, examination of breast, and uterus, cancer testing, examination of skin
- In laboratory tests, blood examination, urine analysis, blood sugar, cholesterol, thyroid function test, etc.

Arranging/Promoting Good Nutrition

Proper assessment of nutritional requirement needs to be done if an elderly is living alone. Proper assessment should be done in order to know whether the person is able to prepare the food, ensure availability of food stuff and finance to purchase. Complete assessment of nutrition is done to protect from under nutrition. If living in a family, the family is educated about nutrition aspect, i.e., soft and easily digestible food with adequate calorie and nutrients according to preference. Small and frequent meals should be provided to prevent malnutrition.

Activities and Exercises

Physical activity and exercises apart from keeping physically fit, also protect from anxiety, depression and other mental problems. Physical activities prevent stiffening of joints, arthritis, hypertension, constipation and insomnia. They should be encouraged to take part in games, cultural, artistic and educational activities in addition to morning and evening walk.

Preventive Care of Elderly

The physical and mental safety of elders is very important. The care given should pay special attention to the following safety measures:
- Protection from unhealthy environment
- Protection from mental tension
- Protection from physical and mental injuries, threats and fatigues
- Providing rehabilitation services

Providing Psychological Support

The mental health of old people depends largely on the mental status in their entire life. Loneliness, neglect, sense of uneasiness of being a burden and social inactivity may create imbalance in mind. The family members should be educated to encourage them in taking part in social, religious and cultural activities. Different program should be organized for old people to keep them occupied.

PHYSICALLY AND MENTALLY CHALLENGED PEOPLE

Care of Differently Abled—Physically and Mentally Challenged People

Physically or mentally challenged or disabled handicapped means weakening or damage of the normal body structure or mental activities. There may be defects in anatomical structure or having problems with mental function.

Definition

According to WHO International Classification of Impairment, Disabilities and Handicaps (ICIDH), these terms can be defined as:
- **Impairment:** "Any loss or abnormality of psychological, physiological or anatomical structure or function", e.g., missing limb, paralysis after polio, mental retardation, etc.

   Impairment may cause functional limitations which may be partial or total visible or invisible, temporary or permanent.
- **Disability:** It is defined as, "Any restriction or lack (resulting from an impairment) of ability to perform an activity in a manner within the range considered normal for a human being."

   Or disability is the inability to carry out certain activities due to impairment.
- **Handicap:** "A disadvantage for a given individual resulting from an impairment or disability that limits or prevents the fulfilment of a role that is normal (depending on age, sex, social and cultural factors) for that individual."

- **Incidence:** It is very difficult to know the exact incidence of disability because no such comprehensive surveys are possible at global level. It has been estimated by WHO that approximately 10% of the population suffers from disability. In India, some sample surveys indicate that 2–5% of Indian population is suffering from some kind of disability.

Management

It includes prevention, early detection, treatment and rehabilitation.

- **Primary prevention:** Most of the condition can be prevented through adequate prenatal, natal, postnatal services and genetic counseling.
- **Secondary prevention:** It includes early diagnosis and prompt treatment. The congenital conditions like hare-lip, cleft palate and talipes are diagnosed at birth and treated by surgical intervention. The hearing and visual disability should be diagnosed from the milestone of the child and early intervention is sought.

Nursing Considerations

Management of locomotors, disabilities resulting from accidents, polio or cerebral palsy and burns, etc.:
- Prevention at all levels
- Maximum elimination of the disability by medical or surgical intervention
- Training in daily activities of living and making the disabled to be independent as much as possible
- Prevention from contractures and other complications
- Keen observation on any signs of pressure sore
- Regulation of bladder and bowel activities
- Provision of self-help devices and aids like wheelchair, walker, walking stick and commode or urinal, etc.

- **Rehabilitation:** It includes psychological and vocational rehabilitation. In India, the Ministry of Social Welfare operates through five major schemes of assistance to voluntary organization providing services to disabled persons. These include:
  1. Assistance to voluntary organization for the disabled, 90% in the urban and 95% in rural areas is given to NGOs for education, training and rehabilitation of the disabled. For rehabilitation of people recovering from mental illness, emphasis is on vocational guidance and training, liaison with nearest psychiatric center or hospital.
  2. Assistance for aids and appliances.
     - Aids and assistance are provided free to the disabled if up to ₹3600/-
     - At 50% cost if the income of the disabled is ₹1201–2500/- per month
  3. Assistance to voluntary organization for rehabilitation of leprosy cured persons. Assistance to voluntary organization given up to 90% for public education and awareness, early intervention, educational and vocational training, economic rehabilitation and social integration.
  4. Development in the field of cerebral palsy and mental retardation. For manpower training of professionals and developing organizational infrastructure such as class room/library/hostel in the field of cerebral palsy and mental retardation.
  5. Assistance to voluntary organization for establishing special schools. 90% grant to NGOs opening new schools in new districts and upgrading the existing one.

> **Must Know**
>
> **Pension for People with Disabilities**
>
> On August 26, 1995, Ministry of Social Welfare, Government of India introduced a comprehensive bill in the Parliament known as "Pensions with Disabilities (Equal Opportunities, Protection of Right and Full Participation) Bill, 1995." It deals with preventive and promotional aspect of rehabilitation. The scheme is known as Subsistence Allowance/Financial Allowance to person with special need. The grant is ₹2500 per month.
>
> **Eligibility Criteria:**
> 1. Age of disabled persons should not be >60 years (0 to 60 years)
> 2. Family income should not be more than ₹75,000/annum from all sources
> 3. A resident of the National Capital Territory of Delhi for at least 5 years preceding the date of submission of application
> 4. Disability of the applicant should not be <40%. The Medical Board of Government Hospital should issue the disability certificate
> 5. Should have a 'single-operated' account in any Bank or Post Office for receiving the payment through electronic clearing system

Classification of Disability

Handicapped/disabled are classified into the following categories:
- Physically handicapped
- Mentally handicapped
- Socially handicapped

Physically Handicapped

In this category, the persons/children who are blind, deaf and mute, those with harelip, cleft palate, talipes and the "crippled" resulting from polio, cerebral palsy, congenital heart disease, road accidents, burns, injuries, etc.

Causes

The causes of physically disabled are as follows:
- Birth defects
- Infections
- Accidents

Hearing and Speech Disability

Hearing disability: Hearing impairment or disability indicates deafness. Deafness is a condition in which a child/adult suffers from hearing difficulties. The degree of deafness depends upon the impairment. Deafness at childhood has greater impact on normal living than that which comes at later stage.

Definition: According to the Persons with disabilities (Equal Opportunities, Protection of Rights and Full Participation) Act 1995, hearing impairment means "loss of 60 decibels or more in the better ear in the conversational range of frequencies."

Incidence: Exact data of hearing impairment is not possible to detect as large number of people retain usable hearing. According to one survey (NSSO, 1991), India has about 3–5 million deaf people.

Deafness leads to lack of speech development in those who cannot hear from early childhood where others learn words. The deaf child does not speak as he/she cannot hear and so cannot learn speaking.

Classification of hearing loss:
- **On the basis of onset of loss**
  - Congenital
  - Acquired
- **On the basis of site of lesion**
  - **Conductive hearing loss:** Outer ear/middle ear is affected
  - **Sensory neural hearing loss:** Acoustic nerve is damaged
  - **Mixed hearing loss:** Combination of conductive and sensory neural loss
  - **Central auditory disorder:** Problems with the auditory system

Causes:
- **Prenatal causes:** Use of drugs in early pregnancy and Rubella infections during first trimester of pregnancy
- **Natal causes:** Low-birth weight, traumatic delivery, asphyxia, hypoxia, respiratory distress
- **Postnatal causes:** Genetic, inflammatory conditions, otitis media, foreign bodies in ear, trauma to the ear, infection of mumps, measles and meningitis

Detection of deafness:
- Child using excessive gestures to communicate.
- Child not responding to his/her name when called from a distance
- Child has defective speech or even unable to speak a word
- Child does not respond to various soft and loud sounds

If a child is having any of the aforementioned conditions, it should be taken seriously and child should be investigated.

Management:
- **Prevention:** All measures to control the occurrence of disease should be taken, such as:
  - Improving the MCH services
  - MTP facilities should be enhanced to control illegal abortion or taking toxic drugs to induce abortions, which can lead to deafness
  - Avoid putting pin, pens, pencil or cleaning ear with sharp things
  - Avoid bathing in stagnant water
  - Ear protector should be used while diving in water
  - Avoid entering noisy places
  - Marriage in a history of deafness and consanguineous marriages should be avoided
  - Sound pollution should be controlled
    - Proper immunization
    - Proper ear hygiene
    - Health education on safety of the hearing capabilities and ears
- **Early diagnosis and intervention:**
  - Hearing problems of the child should be assessed from the very beginning
  - Appropriate assessment for the type and degree of hearing loss
  - Careful history, from the mother regarding antenatal, natal and postnatal and any infection of the child after birth

- Medical and surgical intervention
- Providing hearing aids
- **Rehabilitation:** Special education can be given as there are many institutions providing communication training to the child with hearing disability. These are as follows:
  - Home-based training program
  - Residential school
  - Day school
  - Vocational rehabilitation
  - Psychological support
  - National Program for Prevention and Control of Deafness was launched on January 1, 2007. According to this program, manpower training and development, capacity building, service provision including rehabilitation, awareness through IEC and monitoring and evaluation of the program to prevent and control deafness.

Speech and Language Disability

Speech impairment does not interfere with the normal activities of a person. But the person is unable to communicate verbally by speaking. Speech handicapped may be associated with deafness.

Classification of speech disorders:

- Articulation (speech sound) disorder includes substitutions, distortions, omissions and additions, etc.
- Fluency disorders (stuttering)
- Voice disorders, i.e., alteration in pitch, quality and loudness.
- People with speech and language disorders suffer with the following problems:
  - Hearing impairment
  - Cleft palate
  - Cerebral palsy
  - Neurogenic disorders
  - Aphasia

Detection of speech disability:

Usually, a child at the age of 10–12 months can speak 3–5 meaningful words and at the age of 2–3 years can speak well. Mother should note when the child is not able to repeat the words taught to him at the age of 10–12 months. Also, the following points must be observed:

- Child struggles to speak, may repeat a sound, prolong a sound or hesitate or nod head
- Male has female voice and female has male voice
- Child has horse, nasal or whispered voice
- Child does not speak or speaks only few words at the age of 3 years or above
- Child's speech is not clear and sound is produced wrongly

Causes of speech impairment:

- Congenital defects
- Deformities of mouth
- Injury to tongue, mouth, vocal cords, larynx, etc.
- Paralysis of vocal cords
- Deafness
- Lack of speech training

- Cleft palate, cerebral palsy, laryngeal tumors
- Neurogenic, genetic or psychological

Management:
- Early detection of speech impairment
- Appropriate preventive measures should be taken to prevent speech impairment
- Elimination of hearing impairment
- Medical and surgical intervention as and when needed
- Consulting speech pathologist
- Speech therapy
- Providing good model of speech to child
- Psychological support to the child and parents
- Positive attitude of society toward speech handicaps, avoid making fun of their speech as it hurts them

Visual Disability and Blindness

According to WHO, "Blindness is a visual acuity of <3/60 (Snellen) or its equivalent. The current WHO International classification of disease describes the level of visual impairment as follows:

WHO International classification of level of visual impairment

Category	Presenting distance visual acuity	
	Worse than	Equal to or better than
Mild or no visual impairment 0		6/18
Moderate visual impairment 1	6/18	6/60
Severe visual impairment 2	6/18	3/60
Blindness 3	3/60	1/60*
Blindness 4	1/60*	Light perception
Blindness 5 9	No light perception Unspecified	–

* Counts finger at 1 meter

Definition of blindness: According to persons with disabilities Act 1995, blindness refers to a condition where a person suffers from any of the following conditions.
- Total absence of sight
- Visual acuity not exceeding 6/60 or 20/200 (Snellen) in the better eye with correcting lenses.
- Limitation of the field of vision subtending an angle of 20 degree or worse

The problem:

World: In 2010, an estimated 285 million people worldwide were visually disabled of whom 39 million were blind and 246 million were with low vision. About 90% of them living in developing countries. About 80% of the blindness is avoidable.

India: The estimated prevalence of blindness in India in 2004 was about 11.2/1000 population. According to rapid national survey 2006–2007, the prevalence reduced from 1.1 to 1.0%.

Causes of blindness:

- **Eye diseases:** Cataract is the main cause of blindness in India and responsible for 81% of the blind.
  - Trachoma
  - Glaucoma
  - Corneal opacity
- **Congenital disorder** of the eye like refraction errors, glaucoma, eye malformations.
- **Malnutrition:** Vitamin A deficiency causing diseases like xerophthalmia, night blindness, keratomalacia. But nowadays with the routine distribution of vitamin A along with immunization, these diseases are under control.
- **Injury or accidents** may cause blindness
- **Systemic diseases:** Diseases like diabetes, hypertension, tumors, and neurological disorders are also responsible for loss of vision.
- **Premature retinopathy** is another emerging cause of blindness. The survival of premature babies has improved but due to administration of oxygen, babies are at risk of retinopathy.
- **Socioeconomic and environmental factors**—occupation, dust, dirt, airborne infections, poverty, poor eye hygiene, illiteracy and unemployment are the contributory factors of blindness.

Management:

- Prevention
- Early detection of the defects
- Medical or surgical intervention
- Rehabilitation

Prevention: Includes primary, secondary and tertiary eye care and correction of malnutrition in children.

- **Primary eye care:** The objective of primary eye care is to prevent the various infections and conditions at the grass root level. The ultimate goal of intervention is protection and promotion of eye health. Primary care includes:
  - Training of the health workers providing primary level of care at village, subcenter and primary health center level, i.e., multipurpose health workers, VHG
  - Anganwadi workers to teach about the eye-hygiene
  - Supply of essential drugs to aforementioned workers for first aid treatment of eye infection
  - Providing vitamin A solution or capsule for distribution to eliminate vitamin A deficiency diseases among the population
  - Referring the ophthalmic cases to the CHC/district hospital for treatment and correction of refractive error
  - Enhancing the knowledge of village level health workers about eye safety, personal hygiene, nutrition, etc., for eye health promotion
- **Secondary level care (Early detection):** Early detection of eye diseases and prompt treatment, i.e., medical or surgical intervention. Surgery for cataract, glaucoma, entropion, etc.
  - By organizing eye camps for operation
  - Providing services of eye specialist through eye clinics/eye care mobile units

- Follow-up after eye surgery
- Mass education for eye care
- **Tertiary care (Medical or surgical intervention):** This includes specialized eye care like corneal grafting, retinal detachment surgery provided through specialized or teaching hospitals.
- **Rehabilitation:** Rehabilitation services for visually handicapped include vocational training, better job orientation, employment, reservation facilities and psychological rehabilitation.

Management of visually handicapped:
- Assessment of visual impairment to control and reduce the severity of blindness
- Preventive and therapeutic eye care at all levels of care
- Conducting specific programs, e.g.:
  - Vitamin A prophylactic program
  - School eye health services for early detection and management
  - Occupational eye health services
  - National program for control of blindness
- Involving all concepts of eye care:
  - **Epidemiological concept:** Measurement of incidence and to identify risk factors
  - **Team concept:** Working as a team member to fulfil the gap between patient and eye specialist
  - **Primary care concept:** Including eye care in the primary healthcare
- Evaluating intervention and prevention program periodically, this includes:
  - Creating community awareness through IEC about eye care and safety
  - Providing help and aids for blind handicapped
- **Providing educational services:** There are about 300 special schools in India providing education to 30,000 visually handicapped children. Along with Braille system schools, these children can be educated in general schools. This is called integrated education.
- Counseling for better adjustment.

Mental Retardation and Mentally Handicapped

Mental retardation is not a medical problem, but it is an educational, psychological and social problem. It is not mental illness also but it may influence all aspects of human functioning such as speech, language development, hearing, visual and as well as muscular coordination.

Definition

- It is a condition of subaverage intellectual function combined with deficit in adaptive behavior.
- According to Persons with Disabilities Act 1995, "Mental retardation means a condition of arrested or incomplete development of mind of a person which is specially, characterized by subnormal intelligence." The terms like idiot, imbecile, moron, etc., are not used to describe mental retardation.

Recent Updates

According to one survey (NSSO, 1991), about 3% of our child population below the age of 16 years have the problem of mental retardation.
Another study indicates that about 21 million adults are mentally handicaped.

Categories of Mental Retardation

Psychologist has used the concept of IQ to classify the degree of mental retardation. WHO gave the following classification for mental retardation:

Mild mental retardation (Intelligent quotient): IQ 50–70

Moderate mental retardation: IQ 35–49

Severe mental retardation: IQ 20–34

Profound mental retardation: IQ under 20

Causes of Mental Retardation

- Genetic causes (or endogenous)
- Environmental causes (or exogenous)

Genetic causes:

- Chromosomal abnormalities, e.g., Down's syndrome and Klinefelter syndrome
- Cretinism—impaired deficiency of thyroid gland
- Phenylketonuria, i.e., defect in amino acid metabolism
- Galactosemia—inborn error of carbohydrate metabolism
- Consanguineous marriages—marriage between blood relations

Environmental causes:

- **Antenatal causes:** Physical trauma, malnutrition, Rh factor incompatibility, exposure to radiation, toxic agents, alcohol, drugs, asphyxia, infection like rubella, cytomegalovirus, toxoplasmosis and syphilis.
- **Perinatal causes:** These include birth injuries, hypoxia and cerebral palsy and prolonged labor.
- **Postnatal factors:** Head injuries to the baby, accidents, postnatal infection, hypopyrexia physical and chemical agents such as mercury and lead.
- **Miscellaneous:** Maternal malnutrition. Protein energy malnutrition. Iodine deficiency late pregnancy (after the age of 40 years)

Prevention of Mental Retardation

Primary prevention:

- Public education through IEC, mass education regarding preventive measures against mental retardation.
- Medical intervention includes:
    - Good standard of MCH services including appropriate care during antenatal, natal and postnatal period
    - Proper immunization to prevent childhood diseases
    - Care about Rh incompatibility
    - Avoid exposure to radiation during pregnancy
- Genetic counseling: Taking careful history of the parents, avoiding pregnancy in late age
- Screening at risk cases
- Improving socioeconomic and nutritional status

Secondary prevention:

- Early diagnosis and prompt care of socially deprived children
- Treatment of hereditary disorders
- Proper handling of handicapped children

Tertiary prevention:

- Special education: With special education, the mentally retarded children can contribute more to the society.
- Checking the deterioration of the personality of handicaps
- Psychotherapeutic intervention to solve emotional problems of mentally retarded

Management of Mentally Handicapped

- Assessing the extent of the problem and informing the parents/relatives accordingly
- Innovative teaching methodology for providing special education to mentally handicapped
- Psychotherapeutic intervention as and when necessary
- Psychological support to the family members and counseling them about the care and training of handicaps
- Taking help of NGOs/Voluntary agencies in the care and management of mentally handicapped along with government measures
- Creating positive attitude in the society toward mentally handicaps
- Loving, tender care at all levels of management
- Proper rehabilitation according to individual needs including vocational rehabilitation of the mentally handicaps

Socially Handicapped Children

A "socially handicapped child" may be defined as a child whose opportunities for a healthy personality development and a full unfolding of potentialities are hampered by certain elements in the social environment such as parental inadequacy, environmental deprivation i.e., lack of stimulation of learning process and emotional disturbances. Children included in this category are as follows:

- Orphan children either due to death or loss of parents
- Neglected and destitute children
- Delinquent children
- Mentally handicapped child also meets with social handicaps to the extent to which he/she is subject to social rejection or misunderstanding and cannot make use of normal value of social fulfilment.
- Management includes prevention at the earliest by seeking help of voluntary organization for care and education of the child and vocational training so that they become useful members of the society.

REHABILITATION NURSING

Rehabilitation nursing is an important component of comprehensive nursing. It starts from the moment that the patient enters the healthcare system. The purpose of rehabilitation is to minimize the disabilities which may occur due to diseases, injury or addiction and bring back the individual to its normal functioning level.

Concepts

Rehabilitation has become an integral part of the nursing care of the patient. It has gained wide acceptance since for the last few decades. World Health Organization estimated that 10% of the world's population has some form of disability. In India, statistics from different sources show that at least 3.8% of the population has disabilities like locomotors, visual, communication and mental retardation, etc. WHO in its technical report suggested that rehabilitation services must be considered a natural and essential part of the healthcare system. It was further strengthened by Alma-Ata declaration. Following the UN declaration of 1981 as the international year of disabled persons, many developing countries (including India) formulated policies and priorities in disability and rehabilitation services. The rehabilitation services in India are mainly institutional-based and urban centered. Only 3% of the disabled population can have access to these services. With the promotion of rehabilitation programs by government and NGOs, it had been demonstrated that rehabilitation program can be simplified and carried out by nonprofessionals. Nowadays, there is emphasis on shifting toward universal coverage of services and decentralization of development planning to involve local communities. The institutional services are costing high and many people cannot afford it and as a consequence, the community-based rehabilitation approach is viewed in many developing countries as a possible alternative.

Definitions

- According to WHO, "Rehabilitation is the combined and coordinated use of the medical, social, educational and vocational measures for training and retraining to the individual to the highest possible level of functional ability."

  It includes all measures of reducing the impact of disability and handicapping conditions and enable the disabled and handicapped to achieve social integration. The social integration means active participation of the disabled in the mainstream of the community.
- "Rehabilitation is a process of restoring people to useful functions in physical, mental, social, economic and vocational areas of their lives." It means rehabilitation is a process of restoring patients or persons to their previous level of health, that is to their previous capabilities or to the level that is possible for them.
- Rehabilitation is the restoration of a person to the fullest physical, mental, social, vocational and economic usefulness possible. Rehabilitation actually means a combination of academic, professional and therapeutic training that provides a person maximum possible activity and capabilities.

Rehabilitation includes issues like:
- Physiotherapy
- Occupational therapy
- Speech therapy
- Audiology
- Psychotherapy and
- Educational vocational guidance

Objectives

- To restore affected abilities to the highest possible level of function
- To prevent further disability/handicap
- To protect the person's present abilities
- To assist the patient or person to use his or her abilities

Rehabilitation comes under the tertiary level of prevention when the patients recover from acute illness but are left with some functional disabilities.

Scope

Rehabilitation nursing requires intersectoral or intrasectoral discipline or specialties. There is a wide scope of rehabilitation nursing. The main areas of rehabilitation nursing include the following:

- Physiotherapy
- Occupational therapy
- Speech therapy
- Psychotherapy
- Social work
- Audiology
- Placement services
- Health education

Criteria to be Considered Handicapped

A person is considered to have a disability, when he/she has difficulty in:
- Talking
- Walking
- Hearing
- Climbing stairs
- Seeing
- Lifting or carrying objects
- Performing activities of daily living
- Doing school work/working at a job

Rehabilitation Team

The rehabilitation team consists of the following members:
- Nurse
- Physiotherapist
- Occupational therapist
- Speech pathologist
- Vocational rehabilitation counselor
- Medical social worker
- Psychologist
- Dietician
- Recreational therapist
- Rehabilitation engineer and other auxiliary staff

Activities of Team Members

Rehabilitation is a creative, dynamic process that requires a team of professionals working together with patients and families.
- Team members hold frequent group lessons to collaborate, evaluate program and modify goals as needed to facilitate rehabilitation
- To promote independence, self-respect and acceptable quality of life for the patient
- Patient and the patient's family also incorporated into team
- The nurse develops a therapeutic and supportive relationship with the patient and family

Types of Rehabilitation

Rehabilitation is generally classified into the following types (Fig. 4.3) based on the causes:

- **Medical rehabilitation:** It is related to the increasing potential capabilities and correction of deformities, and restoration of functions.
- **Social rehabilitation:** It implies to the social life, restoration of family, social interaction or relationship.
- **Psychological rehabilitation:** It includes psychological normalization, restoration of personal dignity and confidence of the disabled or handicapped.
- **Vocational rehabilitation:** It is concerned with economic aspects, restoration of the ability to earn the means of livelihood.

Medical	Types of rehabilitation	Social
Vocational		Psychological

Figure 4.3: Types of rehabilitation

Rehabilitation is again described on the basis of providing services. It is of two types:

1. Institutional-based rehabilitation
2. Community-based rehabilitation

Institutional-Based Rehabilitation

Institutional-based rehabilitation (IBR) is performed in an institution, that may be regional rehabilitation or district rehabilitation or research rehabilitation center or in a special educational institute (i.e., deaf and dumb school for mentally retarded children, etc.) or it may be done in a general rehabilitation unit of hospital i.e., physiotherapy center, speech therapy, or vocational training center.

Community-Based Rehabilitation

This is a new strategy, a unique concept of WHO, to provide universal coverage of rehabilitation to all segments of society. Community-based rehabilitation (CBR) involves active role of people with disabilities, their families and communities in the rehabilitation program. In CBR, the knowledge and skills for the training of disabled people are transferred to disabled adults, their families and community members.

Features of CBR

The main features of community-based rehabilitation are as follows:

- Removal of physical and attitudinal barriers in the community toward disabled/handicapped
- Ensuring opportunities for disabled to participate in school work, leisure, social and potential activities within the community
- Caring for the family of disabled persons by community groups
- Providing local job training for disabled adults and facilities for disabled children in school at their own village/community
- Assisting disabled in transportation, getting loans and income generating activities
- Training of community persons, community workers for intervention in the rehabilitation services
- Maximum community participation in the care of disabled/handicapped within the community
- Supporting the referral services

Rehabilitation Services in India

All patients, regardless of age, gender ethnic group, socioeconomic status, have a right to rehabilitation services. There are government departments, NGOs institutions and voluntary agencies which are functioning for the disabled/handicapped for their rehabilitation and care. Some of the organizations are given as follows:

- Ministry of Social Justice and Empowerment
- Ministry of Health and Family Welfare, Human Resource Development, Labor, Information and Broadcasting, etc.
- Regional and District Rehabilitation centers.
- Rehabilitation Council of India
- Occupational therapy schools at Mumbai and Nagpur
- All India Institute of Physical Medicine and Rehabilitation at Mumbai and CMC Vellore.
- Occupational Therapy College Mumbai.
- National Institute of Mentally Handicapped (NIMH) Secunderabad, (Regional branch at Mumbai, New Delhi, Kolkata)
- Ali Yavar Jung National Institute for the Hearing Handicapped, Mumbai (Regional branches at Delhi, Kolkata and Secunderabad)
- National Institute of Visually Handicapped, Dehradun.
- National Institute for the Orthopedically Handicapped (NIOH), Kolkata, etc.

Responsibilities of Nurse in Rehabilitation

The early diagnosis and prompt treatment is the only effective remedy to minimize the disability and to reduce the overload on rehabilitation services. The nurse plays a vital role in coordinating the services of the medical team for early diagnosis and treatment to minimize the disability and also plays a key role in coordinating the efforts of rehabilitation team. The responsibilities of the rehabilitation nurse are as follows:

- Assessing the type and extent of disability
- Determining the nature and type of rehabilitation
- Seeking the advice of specialist according to the needs of rehabilitation
- Organizing the rehabilitation team
- Coordinating among the team members
- Maintaining normal body functions of disabled person as much as possible
- Preventing further complications or disability
- Providing psychological support to the disabled or handicapped along with their family members
- Providing legal, financial and occupational assistance to disabled
- Providing health education to the disabled and family
- Evaluating the rehabilitation program

Summary

- The specialized community health services include RCH, National Health Mission (rural and urban), Janani Shishu Suraksha Karyakram, emergency ambulance services, government health insurance schemes, school health services, occupational health nursing, geriatric nursing, care of differently abled, i.e., physically and mentally disabled and rehabilitation nursing.
- Components of RCH program include birth spacing, immunization, anemia, prophylaxis against vitamin A deficiency, oral rehydration therapy and acute respiratory functions.
- In RCH–phase-I program, the components included are family planning, child survival and safe motherhood, client centered approach and prevention and management of STI/STD and AIDS.
- In RCH–Phase II, the main focus is on emergency obstetric care, essential obstetric care of newborn and strengthening of referral system.
- Role of community health nurse in RCH is direct care provider, communicator, supervisor, educator, manager and evaluator.
- National Health Mission was approved in May 2013. The strategies of NHM are promoting institutional deliveries, strengthening of training of health workers and providing round the clock health services.
- Urban Health Mission started in May 2013. The strategies are strengthening healthcare of urban poor and slums communities.
- Rural Health Mission was launched in 2005 for a period of 7 years, i.e., up to 2012 and extended for another 5 years. The main strategies on strengthening subcenter PHC and CHC to provide effective and round the clock health services.
- Government health insurance schemes include ESI Act 1948, CGHS and family planning insurance schemes.
- The main aim of school health services is health screening at the earliest and prompt intervention to improve the health of the pupils and prevent dropout of students and reduce morbidity and mortality rate. The aspects of school health services include first aid and emergency care, immunization and prevention of communicable diseases, early detection, treatment and follow-up care of common problems of school children.
- Occupational health nursing deals with the work environment and health problems as a result of occupational hazards.
- Geriatric nursing deals with the health problems and care of elderly persons.
- Care of physically and mentally handicapped includes assessment, early diagnosis, prompt treatment and rehabilitation counseling of the parents and family members about the limitations of the affected individual and helping them to cope up with disabilities.
- Rehabilitation comes under tertiary level of care. The main objective of rehabilitation is to restore the affected abilities to the highest possible level of function.

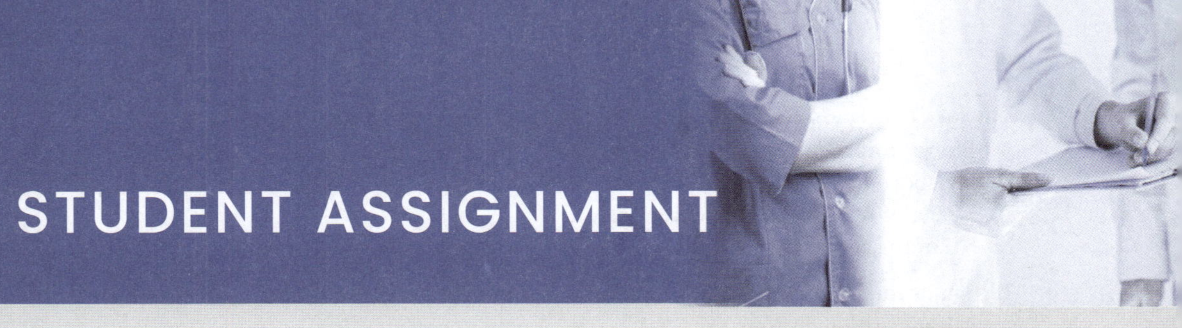

STUDENT ASSIGNMENT

LONG ANSWER TYPE QUESTIONS

1. Enumerate the specialized community health services and describe reproduction and child health services.
2. Describe National Health Mission along with it submissions (rural and urban).
3. Enlist the Government Health Insurance Schemes and describe CGHS.
4. State the facilities available in Employees Health Insurance Scheme.
5. Discuss the role of school health nurse in school health services.
6. What are the hazards of occupational services? As an occupational health nurse, what are your responsibilities toward the health of workers?
7. Define geriatric nursing. State the problem of old age and management of those problems.
8. Write the classification of disabilities. Describe the management of physical disabilities.

SHORT ANSWER TYPE QUESTIONS

1. State the objectives of school health services.
2. Enlist the strategies of RCH–Phase I.
3. Briefly enlist the role of community health nurse in RCH services.
4. Write an account of occupational diseases.
5. State the causes of mental retardation.
6. Define the following terms:
   a. Impairment
   b. Disability
   c. Handicap
   d. Amentia
7. Write short notes on:
   a. Rehabilitation
   b. ESI Act
   c. Janani Shishu Suraksha Karyakram
   d. NHM

MULTIPLE CHOICE QUESTIONS

1. Which of the following has not been included in the reproductive and child health?
   a. Pregnant mothers
   b. Lactating mothers
   c. Infant and children under 5 years of age
   d. Children of 6–10 years

2. Which of the following is not the main focus of RCH–phase II program?
   a. Essential obstetric care
   b. Family planning
   c. Emergency obstetric care
   d. Strengthening referral system

3. **The facilities that FRU have:**
    a. Blood storage facility on a 24 hours basis
    b. Newborn care
    c. Availability of surgical intervention
    d. All of the above

4. **Which of the following is not included in the school health services?**
    a. School administration
    b. Health teaching and health education
    c. Maintenance of health giving environment
    d. Comprehensive healthcare

5. **Which of the following is included in maternal health services?**
    a. Antenatal care
    b. Intranatal care
    c. Postnatal care
    d. All of these

6. **Occupational health deals with:**
    a. Promotion and protection of health of workers
    b. Early diagnosis and prompt treatment of occupational diseases
    c. Rehabilitation in case of disablement
    d. All of the above

7. **What percentage of disabilities the Indian population has?**
    a. 7.7
    b. 5.8
    c. 4.8
    d. 3.8

8. **The cut of age of senior citizens in India is:**
    a. 70 years
    b. 65 years
    c. 60 years
    d. 58 years

9. **Incontinence of urine may occur in old people due to:**
    a. Poor sphincter control due to lack of elasticity of the muscles
    b. Diminished capacity of bladder due to replacement of smooth muscles and elastic tissue with fibrous connective tissue
    c. Enlargement of prostate gland in male
    d. All of the above

10. **Aging can be delayed by:**
    a. Active lifestyle
    b. Good nutrition and social support
    c. Exercise
    d. All of these

11. **The ESI Act was passed in:**
    a. 1948
    b. 1950
    c. 1952
    d. 1962

12. **A child having IQ between 50 and 70 is included in which group of mental retardation?**
    a. Mild
    b. Moderate
    c. Severe
    d. Profound

13. **The disease Byssinosis is caused due to prolonged exposure to:**
    a. Cotton dust
    b. Grain dust
    c. Cane fiber
    d. None of these

14. **Which of the following disease, a factory worker exposed to coal dust is prone to get?**
    a. Siderosis
    b. Silicosis
    c. Anthracosis
    d. Asbestosis

Note

5

National Health Problems

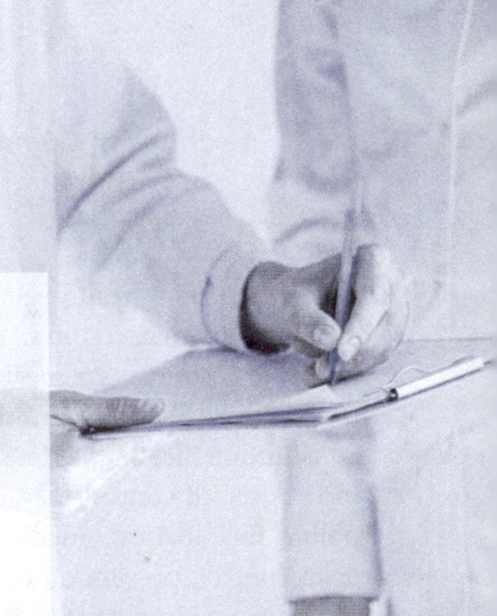

After the completion of the unit, the readers will be able to:
- Identify the health problems in India.
- Discuss major health problems prevalent in India.
- Explain the population explosion problems causing hindrance in development of the country.

UNIT OUTLINE

- Introduction
- Health Problems in India

KEY TERMS

Acute respiratory infections: An infection that may interfere with normal breathing. It can affect just upper respiratory system (starts at sinuses and ends at vocal cords), or just lower respiratory system (which starts at vocal cords and ends at lungs).

GDP: Measures the monetary value of final goods and services—that is, those that are bought by the final user—produced in a country in a given period of time (say a quarter or a year). It counts all of the output generated within the borders of a country.

Health problems: A state in which person is unable to function normally.

Intraocular lens: Clear, artificial lenses that replace the eye's natural lens.

Mass drug administration: Involves giving treatment to an entire population or every person in a geographical area.

Abbreviations

ARI: Acute Respiratory Infections	**NIMH:** National Institute of Mental Health
GDP: Gross Domestic Product	**NIN:** National Institute of Nutrition
IOL: Intraocular Lens	**PF:** *Plasmodium falciparum*
LF: Lymphatic Filaria	**RNTCP:** Revised National Tuberculosis Control Program
MDA: Mass Drug Administration	**STD:** Sexually Transmitted Diseases
NFHS: National Family Health Survey	**STI:** Sexually Transmitted Infections

INTRODUCTION

Before planning health services of any nation, it is the first requisite to know the existing health problems of that country. Based on the health problems, the priorities are set according to the available resources to meet those health needs. After independence of India has been planning its health services according to the priorities of problems through Five-Year Plans. Under the constitution, health is a state subject, central government can intervene to assist the state government in the area of control/eradication of major communicable and noncommunicable diseases. Broad policy formulation, medical and paramedical education combined with regulatory measures, drug control, prevention of food adulteration, child survival and safe motherhood, immunization program, environment and sanitation, all these are the responsibility of the State Government. According to WHO, "Health is a state of complete physical, mental and social well-being and not nearly the absence of disease or infirmity."

HEALTH PROBLEMS IN INDIA

Health problem is a state in which person is unable to function normally (state of ill health and unhealthiness).

Health problems (Fig. 5.1) may be grouped under the following headings:
1. Communicable diseases
2. Noncommunicable diseases
3. Nutritional problems
4. Environmental sanitation problems
5. Medical care problems
6. Population problems

Figure 5.1: Health problems in India

Communicable Diseases

Communicable diseases continue to be one of the major health problems in India. Communicable diseases like malaria, tuberculosis, leprosy, dengue, chikungunya, filaria, Japanese encephalitis, waterborne diseases like cholera, diarrheal diseases, typhoid, viral hepatitis A and E, Zoonotic diseases like rabies, plague, leptospirosis, anthrax, brucellosis, etc., and vaccine preventable diseases like measles, diphtheria, pertussis, poliomyelitis, viral hepatitis B, etc., are endemic in many parts of the country and it would continue to be a major public health problems in India. The diseases considered of great importance today are mentioned as follows:

Malaria

Malaria continues to be a major health problem in India. Although total malaria cases have been declined as compared to the previous years, the proportion of *P. falciparum* has increased. About 36% of the World's population is exposed to the risk of contracting malaria. According to WHO's report, on malaria day on 25th April 2023, there was an estimation of 249 million malaria cases with 608,000 malaria deaths in 85 countries. In India 1,80,000 cases of malaria were reported and 83 deaths were due to malaria. The Government of India has launched the National Framework for Malaria Elimination (NFME), 2016 and 2030 to eliminate malaria by 2030.

Tuberculosis

India is a country with the highest TB burden. It remains a major public health problem. India accounts one-fifth of the world incidence of tuberculosis. Every year about 2.2 million people develop tuberculosis of which 0.62 million are new smear positive highly infections cases and 0.24 million people die of tuberculosis every year. The emergence of HIV-TB co-infection and multidrug resistance of TB has increased the severity and magnitude of the disease. Ministry of Health and Family Welfare released the India TB report 2024, which highlights that mortality rate due to TB had declined from 28 per lakh population in 2015–23 per lakh population in 2022. In March 2006, RNTCP has achieved nationwide coverage.

Leprosy

It is another important health problem in India. Despite India being declared "Leprosy Eliminated" in 2005, the country still accounts for over half (52%) of world's new leprosy patients according to the National Strategic Plan and roadmap for leprosy 2023–2027. The Union Health Minister has devised a strategic roadmap for achieving zero cases of leprosy by 2030. All the states and union territories report cases of leprosy but there is a considerable variation not only between the states but also between one district and another. The prevalence rate of leprosy has come down from 0.69 per 10,000 populations in 2014–15 to 0.45 in 2021–22. Further annual new cases detection rate per 100,000 populations has come down from 9.73 in 2014–15 to 5.2 in 2021–22 according to the data published on 30th June 2023. World Leprosy Day is observed on 30th January every year.

Diarrheal Diseases

The diarrheal diseases are counted as one of the major causes of morbidity and mortality among children less than five years of age. The National Family Health Survey shows that the prevalence of childhood diarrhea has increased from 9% to 9.2% from 2016 to 2020 in India. It is third most common disease responsible for under-five mortalities. Globally, there are nearby 1.7 billion cases of childhood diarrheal disease every year. Diarrhea is a leading cause of malnutrition in children under-five years of age. Each year diarrhea kills around 443,832 children under-five and an additional 50,851 children aged 5–9 years. Outbreaks of diarrheal diseases (including cholera) continue to occur in India due to pool environmental conditions. Diarrhea is preventable with improvement in environmental sanitation and practicing good hygiene. Diarrhea Control Program was started in 1978 and it has reduced the mortality from diarrhea by 50%. To increase awareness about use of ORS and Zinc in diarrhea, an intensified diarrhea control fortnight (IDCF) is being observed during premonsoon/monsoon season with the aim of zero child death due to childhood diarrhea since 2014.

Acute Respiratory Diseases

Acute respiratory diseases/infections (ARDs/ARIs) are one of the major causes of morbidity and mortality in children below 5 years of age. The National Family Health Survey-4 (NFHS-4) estimated the prevalence of ARDs or acute respiratory infections (ARIs) to be 2.7% in 2015–16 in India which is 50% decline from 5.6% reported in 2005–2006 by the NFHS-3. According to WHO, ARI causes 3.9 million deaths globally. The prevalence of ARI is 59.1%. In urban areas, it is 63.7% and in rural population it is 53%. Overcrowding, place of residence and mother's education are significantly associated with ARIs. During COVID-19 pandemic, on 19th February 2021, India reported 1.09 million cases with 1,56111 deaths due to COVID-19.

Filariasis

It is endemic in 256 districts of 17 states and 6 union territories. About 31 million people are estimated to be infected. Approximately 21 million people have symptomatic filariasis and 27 million people are microfilaria carriers. To achieve elimination of filariasis, Government of India has launched nationwide annual Mass Drug Administration (MDA) with annual single recommended dose of diethylcarbamazine citrate tablets, in addition to scaling up home-based foot care and hydrocele operations. In 2014, 250 endemic districts implemented MDA targeting population of about 554 million with coverage rate 87%. The National Filaria Control Program (NFCP) was launched in 1955. National Filaria Day is observed on 11th November, every year.

HIV/AIDS

HIV/AIDS is epidemic in India. The National AIDS Control Organization (NACO) estimated 3.14 million people were living with HIV/AIDS in India in 2023. Despite being home to the HIV/AIDS (as of 2023, South Africa and Nigeria have more prevalence), the AIDS prevalence rate is lower than that of many other countries in India. In 2016, the AIDS prevalence was highest in the world, i.e., 0.30%. According to the latest United Nations Program on HIV/AIDS (UNAIDS) estimate, in India, in 2022, there were 66,000 new HIV cases that is an incidence of 0.05 new infections per 10,000 populations. Government of India estimates in 2024 reports that, about 2.40 million Indians were living with HIV in 2022. India reported an estimate of 39.6 thousand annual AIDS related deaths.

STDs/STIs Infections

There are >1 million people who acquire sexually transmitted infections every day. The most common infections are Chlamydia, gonorrhea, syphilis and trichomoniasis. The STDs/STIs are sexually transmitted and present a huge burden of the diseases, and cause suffering in both males and females. The exact data of these infections in general population is lacking but the disease prevalence is estimated to be 6% in India and total 30 million people may be affected out of 340 million worldwide. Under the umbrella of NRHM, along with RCH-II, the prevention and management of STDs/STIs services are accessible to the public at PHC and CHC.

Noncommunicable Diseases

There is a rapid epidemiological transition with large and rising burden of chronic diseases, which are estimated to account for 74% deaths globally of all noncommunicable diseases (NCDs) deaths 77% are in low-and middle-income countries. These NCDs are diabetes mellitus, CVDs, cancer, strokes and chronic lung diseases which have emerged as a major public health problem due to an aging population and environmentally driven changes in behavior.

Hypertension

As per the 2023, data, about 220 million adults are having high blood pressure. According to the recent report of Indian Council of Medical Research India Diabetes (ICMR-INDIAB), about

300–320 million are having hypertension. National Family Health Survey-5 (2019–21) reported that 21% of women and 24% of men aged 15 and above have hypertension and 39% women and 49% men are prehypertensive. In India, the prevalence of hypertension is 24%–30% and 12%–14% in urban and rural areas, respectively. Worldwide 13.5% of premature deaths and 47% of ischemic heart diseases cases were attributed to hypertension.

Cardiovascular Disorders

Ischemic heart disease (IHD) is the leading cause of death in economically developed countries and cases are rapidly increasing in developing countries. In India, the most common is IHD with 200% increase in cardiac ailments in 20–50 years of age group. Globally about 200 million persons have IHD and the prevalence rate of 3820 cases per 100,000 populations worldwide according to 2023 data and India has highest burden of cardiovascular disease worldwide. Main causes are sedentary lifestyle, obesity, alcohol consumption and excessive tobacco consumption. More than half a billion people around the world continue to be affected by cardiovascular diseases which accounted for 2005 million deaths in 2011 (close to a third of all deaths globally) and an overall increase on the estimate 121 million CVD deaths. In India, 80% CVD deaths are due to IHD and strokes. As per the reports of 24th January 2024, CVD accounted for approximately 19.91 million global deaths in 2021. These diseases tend to develop gradually with age and life style. The risk factors include high blood pressure, smoking, alcohol use, poor diet, lack of physical activities and air pollution. Death rates in many countries have fallen due to improvement in life style, better health facilities and health education. The impact of cardiovascular disease can be reduced much with greater understanding and public health efforts.

Cancer

Cancer has become an important public health problem in India with an estimated 1.1 million cases occurring every year. At any point of time, it is estimated that there are 3.9 million cases of cancer in the country. In 2022, the projected number of new cancer cases in India was 1461427 with a crude incidence rate of 100.4 per 100,000 population. A study projected the number of annual cancer cases to rise from 1.4 million in 2020 to 1.57 million by 2025. WHO reported that breast cancer was the leading cause of death (98,337 or 13.7%), followed by oral cancer 79,979 or 5.6% and cervical cancer (79,906 or 11.2% in India in 2022. Globally, there were an estimated 20 million new cancer cases and 9.7 million deaths in 2022.

Most common cancer among males is oral cancer (11.2%) and 5th common cancer in women (4.3%). Tobacco consumption continues to be the cause of oral cancer.

Diabetes Mellitus

According to the recent reports by the National NCD Monitoring Survey (NNMS), the diabetes prevalence in India stood at 9.3% in 2018. Similar estimate has been given by IDF, where diabetes prevalence was estimated at 9.6% in 2021 and projected to increase to 10.4% by 2030. The lifestyle and sedentary habits are two contributory factors among the others. In India, 77 million people are estimated above the age of 18 years are estimated to be suffering from diabetes (type-2) and nearly 25 million from prediabetes. >50% of people are unaware of their diabetic status which leads to health complications of not treated early.

Mental Disorders

WHO estimated that the mental problems in India are 2443 disability adjusted life years (DALYs) per 10,000 population. The age adjusted suicide rate per 100,000 population is 21.1%. The economic loss due to mental health conditions between 2012 and 2030 is estimated as $1.03 trillion. The Mental Healthcare Act, 2017 provides the legal framework for providing services to protect, promote and fulfil the rights of people with mental illness. The National Mental Health Program, and health and wellness centers are efforts to provide quality care at the primary healthcare level.

Tobacco Consumption

Tobacco use is responsible for approximately 33% of cancer related deaths, worldwide. In India, tobacco related cancer contributed to 27% of the nation's cancer burden in 2020. According to WHO, there will be >8 million tobacco related deaths per year by 2030 accounting for 10% of all yearly fatalities globally. According to the global adult tobacco survey (GATS-2), 28.6% (266.8 million) of adults in India aged 15 years and older now use tobacco in some form. In 2022, an estimated 253 million adults aged 15 and older in India are tobacco product users which is the highest rate of tobacco use in the world. Tobacco drives a large of burden of communicable and noncommunicable diseases. About 42.4% of men and 14.2% of women consume tobacco in one or other form.

Alcoholism

The pattern of alcohol consumption varies with the geographical regions. Highest incidence is in Punjab, Andhra Pradesh, Goa and North Eastern States which have higher proportion of male alcohol consumption than the rest of the country. Women alcoholics are more in the states of Arunachal Pradesh, Assam and Sikkim. About 14.6% of the population in the age group of 10–75 years use alcohol, as per 2019 survey by the government. Use of alcohol is higher among men (27.3%) compared to women (1.6%). The number of alcohol related deaths in India are 38.5 per 100,000 population. According to the recent studies, the number increased sharply for Indian males (63%) as compared to China's (29.6), according to the recent studies.

Accidents

As per the report, a total 4,61312 road accidents have been reported by the states and union territories (UTs) during the calendar year 2022 which claimed 1,68491 lives and caused injuries to 4,43366 persons. The number of road accidents in 2022 increased by 11.9% compared to 2021. Similarly, the number of deaths and injuries on account of road accidents also increased by 9.4% and 15.3%, respectively.

Chronic Lung Disease

India contributes to 15.69% of global chronic respiratory diseases but 30.28% of all global deaths due to chronic respiratory disease occur in India. India has the highest number of chronic obstructive pulmonary disease (COPD) cases in the world. The COPD and asthma cases are increasing at a swift pace. COPD alone causes 64 deaths per 100,000 population. The Government of India in the health sector has critical options. On one hand, disease is increasing for various reasons, on the other hand resources are enormously required for prevention and management. Smoking, air pollution, poor housing and overcrowding and socioeconomic conditions are contributory factors for many lung diseases. The public health perspectives mainly emphasize risk reduction, secondary and tertiary prevention. Target three of 3rd Sustainable Development Goal (SDG) states, "by 2030 reduce premature mortality from noncommunicable diseases by one third through prevention and treatment and promote mental health and well-being". Pollution of air, contamination of water and soil and unhygienic conditions at workplace are important threats to human development.

Cataract

It is a major cause of blindness in India. The incidence is higher in low socioeconomic status communities, largely due to reduced access to cataract surgery. Poor diet, occupational sunlight exposure, and use of biomass fuels may increase the prevalence of cataract in settings with low socioeconomic status. Currently there are 4.95 million blind persons and 70 million are visually impaired persons in India, out of which 0.24 million are blind children. Cataract and refractive errors are the main causes of blindness in India. There is a significant reduction in blindness since the initiative "Vision 2020, the Sight to Sight".

Oral Healthcare

It has not been given significant importance in India. People suffering from oral health problems like caries, gingivitis, mouth ulcers, leukoplakia, oral cancers, etc., have to spend large amount of their budget to seek treatment from private practitioners. National Oral Health Program (NOHP) was launched during 2014–2015 to strengthen the public health facilities of the country for an accessible, affordable and quality oral healthcare delivery.

Strokes

It is the second most leading cause of deaths in India—about 1,85000 strokes every year in India (with nearly one stroke every 40 seconds and one stroke death every 4 minutes). About 34% of all people hospitalized for strokes are younger than 65 years of age. The prevalence of strokes has increased by 50% over the last 17 years, and at present 1 in 4 people are at risk of setting stroke in their life time. The chances of getting stroke at 55 years and above is 1 in 5 among women and 1 in 6 among men. The current prevalence ratio varies from 44.54 to 150 per 100,000 population. A global burden of disease study in India found that stroke was alone responsible for 9.4 million fatalities and 28.5 million DALYS loss. Despite the availability of numerous medical innovations, interventions and therapeutic approaches, it continues to be one of the leading causes of disability, worldwide.

Nutritional Problems

One of the major causes of malnutrition in India is economic inequality. Due to the low economic status of some parts of the population, their diet lacks both quality and quantity. Indian society is a dual society consisting of small group of well-fed and very large group of under nourished children. Under nourished cases are mainly found in rural areas. India's ranking in the Global Hunger Index 2023 is at index 111 (slipped from 2022 index of 107) out of 125 countries. 35.5% of children under the age of five years are stunted, 19.3% are wasted, 32.1% are underweight, 3% are overweight as per the latest data of June 2024. The specific nutritional problems are discussed as follows:

Protein-energy Undernutrition

Protein-energy undernutrition (PEU) previously known as protein-energy malnutrition, (PEM) is an energy deficit due to deficiency of all macronutrients but primarily protein. The insufficiency of food, also called 'food gap' is the main cause of PEU, which is a major health problem. The majority of PEU, 80% of cases are mild and moderate. The incidence of severe PEU is 1–2% in preschool children. The problem exists in all the states either due to poverty or lack of knowledge. The nutritional marasmus is more frequent than kwashiorkor.

Nutritional Anemia

India has the highest prevalence of nutritional anemia among women and children. As per the latest National Family Health Survey-5 (NFHS-5) of 2019–2021, 25% of men (15–49 years), and 57% of women (15–49 years), 50.4% to 52.2% of pregnant women and 53.2% to 57.2% of nonpregnant women are suffering from anemia. Incidence of anemia in children aged 6–35 months is 79.2% with 72.7% urban areas and 81.2% in rural areas. The most frequent cause is iron deficiency and less frequent is folic acid and vitamin B_{12} deficiency.

Low Birthweight Babies

This is also a major public health problem in many developing countries. According to NFHS-4 and NFHS-5, in India, there were 17.6% and 17.4% of babies born with low-birth-weight (<2 kg). The cause of low birth weight babies is maternal malnutrition and anemia in most of the cases. Other associated conditions with pregnancy like preeclampsia and hydramnios are other causes of low birth weight babies.

Xerophthalmia

It is the general term applied to all the ocular manifestations right from night blindness through complete corneal destruction due to vitamin A deficiency. It is the main contributing factor in childhood blindness. Xerophthalmia is due to deficiency of vitamin A that causes childhood blindness. About 0.4% of blindness in India is attributed to vitamin A deficiency. According to latest studies, there is 4.43% prevalence of xerophthalmia in children of 2–6 years of age. According to National Program of Corneal Blindness (NPCB), there are 1,20,000 corneal blindness cases in the country with addition of 25000 to 30000 corneal cases every year. Keratomalacia is major nutritional blindness of children of 1–3 years of age.

Iodine Deficiency Disorders (IDDs)

One third (33%) of the world's population is exposed to the risk of Iodine deficiency disorder. In India, >6.1 crore people are suffering from endemic goiter and 88 Lakh people are suffering from mental and physical disabilities. According to the latest data of June 2021, out of 167 million people are at risk of IDD, 54 million suffer from goiter and two million from cretinism. World Iodine deficiency day is observed on 21st October every year to raise the awareness about importance of iodine consumption and effect on health.

Others

Other nutritional problems of importance are lathyrism and endemic fluorosis in certain parts of the country. This is due to widespread adulteration of foodstuffs.

Environmental Sanitation Problems

Environmental sanitation problems are multifaceted and multifactorial. These problems include:

- **Lack of access to clean water:** Over 163 million people in India lack access to clean water.
- **Lack of sanitation facilities:** In many parts of the country, primitive methods of excreta disposal and open defecation are the big problem in rural area, though it has been reduced, but the practice is not completely vanished.
- **Environmental sanitation:** It includes not only safe drinking water and excreta disposal but also covers arrangements for drainage of rainwater, effluents, collection and disposal of garbage and pure air and clean surroundings. Environmental sanitation is an important indicator of the millennium.
- **Developmental goals:** By 2020, to achieve a significant improvement in the lives of at least 100 million slum dwellers. Forty percent of India's waste remains uncollected and untreated, with human sewage directly flowing into rivers in many cities. According to the World Bank data of 2020, 72% of the Indians have access to the basic sanitation facilities. India has implemented various solutions to solve environmental sanitation problems like Swachh Bharat Abhiyan, Jal Shakti Abhiyan. Community led total sanitation E-toilets, biodigester, rainwater harvesting, mobile toilets. Public-private partnership sanitation, workers' training, behavior change and communication to improve environment sanitation in India.

Medical Care Problems

The healthcare issues are the biggest problem that the country is facing. In spite of various healthcare programs and policies launched by the Government of India and steps taken to improve the healthcare delivery system, it is difficult to meet the health needs of the vast population of India as the financial resources are limited. India has shortage of hospitals, particularly in rural areas and many existing healthcare facilities lack basic equipment and resource. According to the National Health Profile, India has only 0.9 beds per 1000 population and out of which only 30% are in rural areas. The main problem of healthcare in India includes shortage of health professionals, health infrastructure digital healthcare and medical research rising cost of health services and financial challenges for the government. The country ranks 112 out of 191 countries on the World Health Organization's ranking of Global Healthcare System. Rising population of India, emerging of new communicable and noncommunicable diseases are the challenges to the health system. With the launch of 1,50,000 AB-HWCs in India since 2018. Still the rural population is unable to avail these services either due to lack of awareness, education, and nonaccessibility of these services to the periphery. Due to nonaccessibility of health services and low quality of healthcare services, majority of people turn to local private sector as their first choice of care. There is also an inadequate distribution of available health resources between urban and rural areas and lack of penetration of health services to the social periphery. The "Health for All" by 2000 AD slogan and primary healthcare approach lays stern approach on equity, intersectoral coordination and community participation to redress these imbalances.

Population Problems

The population explosion is the serious problem faced by India. The current population of India is 1,441,981,744 as on 9th July 2024, based on worldometer elaboration of the latest United Nations data. About 36.3% of the population is urban. The Government of India sets a goal to achieve population growth rate of 1% by the year 2000 AD which was not achieved. India's population is growing at an unsustainable rate. The population is expected to exceed 1.5 billion by 2030 and 2 billion by 2050. India is the most populous country in the world and is number one in world population. The cause of over population is high birth rate, lack of knowledge about family planning options and access to family planning, services, sociocultural desire for bigger families and advancement is healthcare that lowers the death rate. There is also a variation between male and female population. With the large population of India, the country is facing the consequences on all developmental aspects, i.e., employment, education, housing, healthcare, sanitation, environment and economic development. The population size and structure represent the single most factor is health and manpower planning in India. Today when the law of diminishing returns, among other factors plays an important role in the economic development of the country. There is a strong need to control population to sustain available resources.

Summary

- Planning of healthcare delivery system depends on two major factors; the one is to solving health problems and needs of the people and second is the resources available to meet those needs or solve these problems.
- It is very important to have in depth knowledge of the health problems of the country so that the priorities are set and objectives are planned.
- The major health problems of India are communicable and noncommunicable diseases, environmental sanitation, medical care problems, and population.

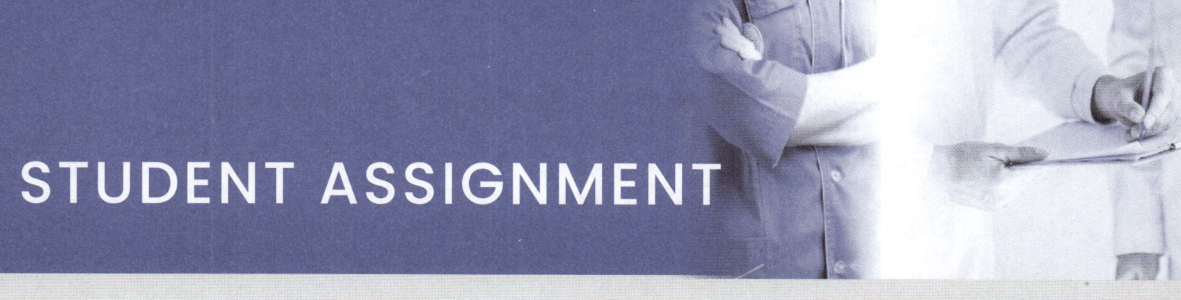

STUDENT ASSIGNMENT

LONG ANSWER TYPE QUESTIONS

1. Explain briefly the major health problems in India.
2. Describe the major communicable disease problems in India.
3. What are the main noncommunicable diseases which contribute to high mortality rate in India?
4. Discuss the nutritional problems of under-five age group.

SHORT ANSWER TYPE QUESTIONS

1. State the causes of poor health services in the rural areas of India.
2. List the communicable diseases causing major health problems in India.
3. Enlist the consequences of population problems in India.
4. Enlist the nutritional problems in India.

MULTIPLE CHOICE QUESTIONS

1. **Which of the following is not a communicable disease?**
   a. Diabetes mellitus
   b. Tuberculosis
   c. Malaria
   d. AIDS

2. **Which of the following is not a noncommunicable disease?**
   a. Cardiovascular accidents
   b. Mental disorders
   c. Cancer
   d. Filaria

3. **Which of the following is not a preventive strategy against diarrheal disease?**
   a. Immunization
   b. Sanitation
   c. Health education
   d. ORS therapy

4. **The followings are the nutritional deficiency diseases; except:**
   a. PEM
   b. Anemia
   c. Xerophthalmia
   d. Down syndrome

5. **The National Filarial Control Program was launched in:**
   a. 1965
   b. 1955
   c. 1986
   d. 1990

6. **The National Health Problems in India are:**
   a. Communicable and noncommunicable diseases
   b. Nutritional problem, medical problem and population problem
   c. a and b
   d. a alone

7. **India spends on healthcare:**
    a. 1% of GDP
    b. 2.5% of GDP
    c. 0.5% of GDP
    d. 3% of GDP

8. **The consequences of population problems in India are:**
    a. Inadequate healthcare facilities
    b. Poor sanitation, housing and environment health
    c. Lack of economic development
    d. All of the above

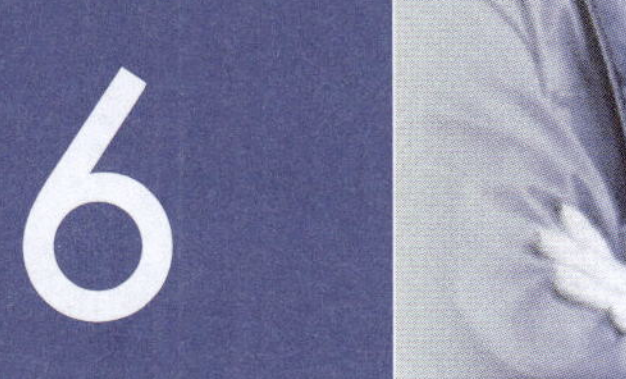

6

National Health Programs

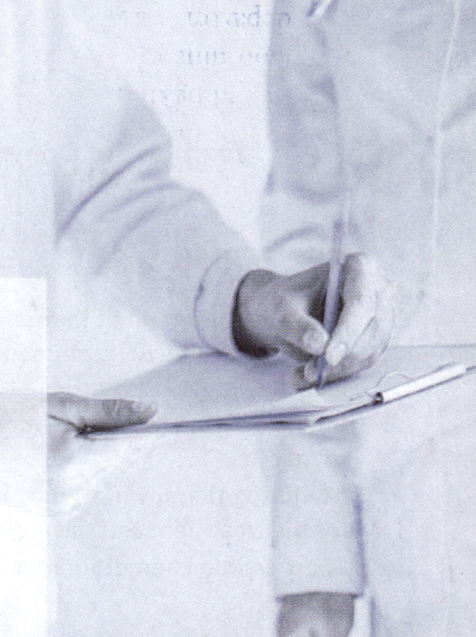

LEARNING OBJECTIVES

After the completion of the unit, the readers will be able to:
- Describe the National Health and Family Welfare Programs in India.
- Understand the role of a nurse in the National Health Programs.

UNIT OUTLINE

- Introduction
- Major Health Problems in India
- National Health Programs
- Acute Respiratory Infection
- Revised National Tuberculosis Control Program
- National Strategic Plan for TB Elimination (2017–2025)
- National Antimalaria Program
- National Filaria Control Program
- National Guinea Worm Eradication Program
- National Leprosy Eradication Program
- National AIDS Control Program
- National Strategic Plan for HIV/AIDS and STI 2017–2024
- National STD Control Program
- National Program for Control of Blindness
- Iodine Deficiency Disorder Control Program
- Expanded Program on Immunization
- National Family Welfare Program
- National Water Supply and Sanitation Program
- Drinking Water Supply Programs and Policies
- Swajaldhara
- National Sanitation Program
- Nirmal Bharat Abhiyan
- Swachh Bharat Mission
- Minimum Needs Program
- Ayushman Bharat Program
- National Diabetes Control Program
- Polio Eradication—Pulse Polio Program
- National Cancer Control Program
- Yaws Eradication Program
- National Nutritional Anemia Prophylaxis Program
- Twenty Point Program
- Integrated Child Development Scheme Program
- Midday Meal Program
- Midday Meal Scheme
- National Mental Health Program
- Mental Health Policy
- Integration of Mental Health with Primary Healthcare
- District Mental Health Program
- Adolescent Health Program
- Tribal Health
- Role of a Nurse in National Health Programs

KEY TERMS

Expanded program of immunization: Established in 1976 to ensure that infants/children and mothers have access to routinely recommended infant/childhood vaccines. Six vaccine-preventable diseases were initially included in the EPI which are tuberculosis, poliomyelitis, diphtheria, tetanus, pertussis and measles.

Iodine deficiency: It is the most common cause of thyroid disease, specifically hypothyroidism (underactive thyroid).

Multidrug therapy: Dapsone, rifampicin and clofazimine are combined. This therapeutic regimen is effective for the treatment and the prevention of drug resistance.

Short course chemotherapy: It has excellent patient acceptance, short duration, fewer doses, and modest toxicity.

Abbreviations

ART: Antiretroviral Therapy

EPI: Expanded Program of Immunization

IDD: Iodine Deficiency Diseases

LEC: Leprosy Eradication Campaign

MDM: Midday Meal

MDR-TB: Multidrug resistant–TB

MDT: Multidrug Therapy

NGCP: National Goiter Control Program

NID: National Immunization Day

NPCB: National Program for Control of Blindness

PLWA: People Living with AIDS

SCC: Short Course Chemotherapy

TPP: Twenty Points Program

UIP: Universal Immunization Program

WHA: World Health Assembly

INTRODUCTION

Since India became independent, several measures have been undertaken by the government to improve the health status of the people. The important program among these measures are National Health Program, which has been launched by the central government for the control and eradication of noncommunicable and communicable diseases, improvement of environmental sanitation, raising the standard of nutrition, control of population and improving the health of rural society. National Health Program should be in consistent with National Health Policies and should contribute toward the achievement of the goals and objectives of the program. Various international agencies like WHO, UNICEF, UNFPA, World Bank along with other agencies such as SIDA, DANIDA and USAID have been providing technical and material assistance in the implementation of these programs.

MAJOR HEALTH PROBLEMS IN INDIA

India is facing a variety of health problems. Detailed analysis of health situation of the country is done and problems related with health along with health needs of the country are identified. The problems identified are ranked according to priority or urgency for allocation of resources. The major health problems of India are malaria, filaria, acute respiratory infections, tuberculosis, guinea worm infestations, leprosy, AIDS/STD, blindness, and iodine deficiency diseases. Other major concerns are control of communicable diseases, family welfare, environmental sanitation, diabetes, cancer, anemia, mental health, adolescent health, etc. These problems have been identified as the major health problems.

Kindly refer the details on this topic which is already discussed in Unit 5.

NATIONAL HEALTH PROGRAMS

The National Health Programs are launched to tackle the aforementioned health problems of the country. These programs have been discussed in this chapter.

ACUTE RESPIRATORY INFECTION

Introduction

Acute respiratory infections (ARI) are the leading causes of mortality among children in most of the developing countries. Poor living standard, malnutrition, air pollution, unavailability of health services or ignorance, poverty or even inappropriate case management at health centers are the main reasons of acute respiratory infection. In mid 1980s, WHO initiated a control program for ARI that focused on cases managed by health workers. Simple case management procedures have been designed for diagnosis and treatment of such infections in situations without any laboratory and radiological facilities. United Nation Children's fund has set a target of 33% reduction in child death due to ARI by 2000.

Problem Statement

WHO, UNICEF and MOHFW estimated in 2013 that around the world 20% of mortality in children under-five is due to ARI which includes pneumonia (including neonatal pneumonia) and 3.5% mortality is caused by ARI. According to recent community-based estimates from prospective study 70% of the childhood morbidities among children aged <5 years are due to ARI. While in developing countries a child is likely to get around 0.3 episodes of pneumonia per year but in developed countries it is 0.03 episodes per child every year. On this basis India is predicated to have over 700 million episodes of ARI and over 52 million episodes of pneumonia every year.

Risk Factors of ARI

- Poor socioeconomic status
- Low level of literacy
- Inadequate breastfeeding
- Malnutrition and poor weaning
- Incomplete immunization
- Smoke due to burning of wood as fuel
- Unavailability of health services

Acute Respiratory Infection Control Program

Acute Respiratory Infection Control Program was launched in India in 1990. The scientific protocol for case management of pneumonia with antibiotic, bronchodilator, antipyretics and adequate fluid intake. Since 1992, the program was implemented as a part of CSSM and later with RCH. Under RCH-II activities, it is implemented in an integrated way with other child health interventions.

Objectives

To reduce mortality rate in children due to acute respiratory infections, 20% by 1995 and 40% by 2000.

Strategies

- To ensure standard case management of ARI under-five by trained health personnel.
- To train peripheral health staff to recognize and treat cases of pneumonia.
- To promote timely referral of severe cases of pneumonia by the peripheral health personnel.
- To educate mothers about home management of cough, cold, fever and recognize early signs of pneumonia for seeking medical help.
- To promote immunization, exclusive breastfeeding in the first 4–6 months. Proper weaning and vitamin A administration.

Prevention and Control of Respiratory Diseases

- **Breastfeeding:** In developing countries, children who are exclusively breastfed for 6 months had 30–42% lower incidence of ARI as compared to children who did not receive for the same duration of breastfeeding. Breastfeeding falls under WHO/UNICEF Global Action Plan to stop pneumonia. It is one of the lifesaving tools in prevention of pneumonia. In addition, hand washing, improved nutrition and reducing of indoor air pollution are the primary strategies to protect children under the age of 5 years from pneumonia.
- **Hand washing:** Simple hand washing reduces the incidence of respiratory infection by 24% (ranging from 6% to 44%).
- **Indoor air pollution from solid biomass:** Exposure to indoor air pollution has increased the risk of respiratory infection by 2.3 times. Use of CNG has proven to be a cost-effective method in order to reduce incidence of indoor air pollution.
- **Proper immunization:** National immunization schedule introduces DPT at 5 years of age instead of DT and raising the upper age limit for DPT vaccine to 7 years.
    - **Measles:** The recent strategic plan is to give an opportunity to Indian children to receive the second dose of measles vaccine. According to this plan immunization or vaccination is to be given to avoid development of measles, mumps and rubella (MMR). This dose has to be given when the child is of 15–18 months.
    - **Vaccine against *H. influenzae*:** 95% influenza infection occurs only among children. According to recent estimate *H. influenza* contributes to annual burden of 8.13 million serious illness and 371,000 deaths worldwide. The vaccine not only protects against severe pneumonia but also prevents the colonization, thereby helping in prevention of the disease transmission.
    - **Pneumococcal vaccines:** The first dose of vaccine is to be given when the infant is of 6 weeks. Total 3 doses are to be prescribed at an interval of 4 weeks and booster dose after 6 months, after last dose as per WHO recommendation in routine immunization for children.
    - **MMR and chicken pox vaccines:** Secondary pneumonia due to exanthematous illness (like measles and chicken pox) is next common causes for ARI among children. For countries like India where second dose of measles is given, it has been proposed recently (MMR at the age of 15–18 months) that special emphasis is to be given on high coverage. Adults who are exposed to varicella are advised to get vaccinated within 48 hours of exposure.

REVISED NATIONAL TUBERCULOSIS CONTROL PROGRAM

Introduction

India accounts for nearly one-fifth of the global TB incidence. In 2007, out of the global annual incidence of 9.23 million TB cases, 1.96 million were estimated to have occurred in India. National Tuberculosis Control Program has been in operation since 1962 and is associated with general health services. The treatment success rate was unacceptably low. The death and default rate remained high. HIV/AIDS epidemics and the spread of multidrug resistance TB mere threatening to further worsen the situation. In 1992, the Government of India along with WHO and SIDA reviewed the TB situation and concluded the barriers of success as follows:

- Technically sound, suffered from managerial weakness.
- Inadequate funding.
- Over reliance on X-rays for diagnosis.
- Frequent interrupted supplies of drugs.
- Low rate of treatment completion.

In 1993, in order to overcome the shortcoming of TB control program, Government of India decided to give new thrust to TB control activities with the assistance of international agencies and thus formulated the Revised National Tuberculosis Control Program (RNTCP). This program adopted the internationally recommended directly observed treatment short-course (DOTS) strategy as the most systematic and cost-effective approval to revitalize TB control program in India. According to recommendation of the review, India adopted the following amendments:

- Introduction of DOTS (short course).
- Ensuring strong political and administrative commitment to achieve success in TB control program.
- Adoption of smear microscopy for reliable diagnosis.
- Strengthening of supply of drugs.

Objectives of RNTCP

- To achieve and maintain cure rate of at least 85% of newly detected infections cases (New sputum smear positive) through DOTS involving peripheral health functionaries.
- To achieve and maintain detection of at least 70% cases through quality sputum microscopy.
- To eliminate TB by 2025.

Organization of RNTCP

The organization of Revised National Tuberculosis Control Program (RNTCP) (Fig. 6.1) operates at five levels:

1. At national level
2. At state level
3. At district level
4. Subdistrict level
5. At peripheral health institutes

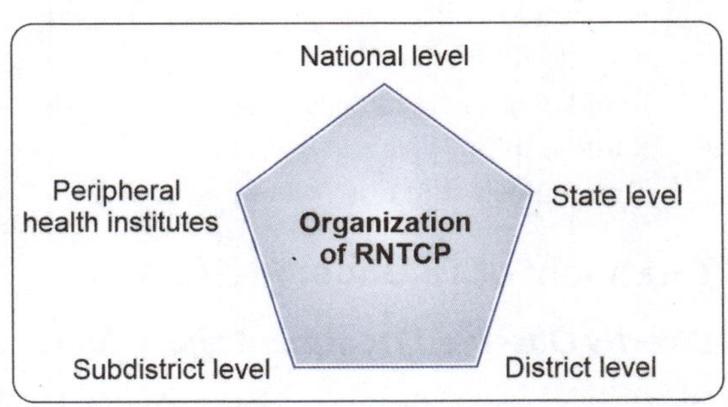

Figure 6.1: Organization of RNTCP

Laboratory Network by RNTCP

RNTCP has established a laboratory network throughout the country having 14,000 designated microscopy centers (DMCs) which are supervised by intermediate reference laboratories (IRL) at state level and national reference laboratories (NRLs) at central TB division at the National level.

National Reference Laboratories (NRLs)

There are six national reference laboratories. These are at Chennai, Bengaluru, Delhi, Agra, Bhubaneswar and Bhopal. The National reference laboratories work closely with intermediate reference laboratories. The NRLs monitor and supervise the IRLs activities.

Intermediate Reference Laboratories (IRLs)

There is one IRL in the state tuberculosis training and demonstration center/public health laboratory medical college of the respective state.

Function of IRLs:

- Supervision and monitoring of external quality assessment activities
- Mycobacterial culture
- Drug sensitivity testing
- Drug resistance surveillance (DRS) in selected states
- To ensure proficiency of the staff in performing smear microscopy activities
- Provide technical training to the district and subdistrict laboratory technicians and senior TB laboratory supervisors
- On site evaluation and panel testing to each district in the state at least once in a year.

Designated Microscopy Center

The Designated Microscopy Center (DMC) is the peripheral laboratory which serves a population of one lakh in plain and fifty thousand in hilly and tribal area.

TB diagnostics under RNTCP include the following:

- Smear microscopy for acid fast bacilli at CHC or PHC:
    - Sputum smear stained with Ziehl-Neelsen staining
    - Fluorescence staining
- Culture:
    - Solid media or
    - Liquid media
- Rapid diagnostic molecular test
- Radiography
- Tuberculosis skin test

Nursing Consideration

Direct observed therapy/direct observed treatment is given by peripheral health staff such as multipurpose health workers or through voluntary workers, e.g., teachers, anganwadi workers or through ex-patients or social workers, etc. They are known as "DOTS" agents and are paid incentive/honorarium of ₹150 per patient on completion of treatment.

Treatment of TB Under RNTCP

Directly Observed Treatment Short Course

Directly Observed Treatment Short Course (DOTS) is the standardized treatment protocol for management of tuberculosis under RNTCP DOTS. It is governed by the principle of "directly observed" treatment system to ensure proper doses and completion of treatment under supervision of the provider.

Components of DOTS Treatment

There are five components of treatment as given ahead:

1. Political and administrative commitment, i.e., continued financial assistance, human resources and administrative support.
2. Good quality diagnosis by sputum smear microscopy at designated RNTCP microscopy center.
3. Uninterrupted supply of quality drugs.
4. Directly observed treatment, an observer or trained community volunteer, i.e., teachers, anganwadi workers, *dais*, ex-patients or social workers or MPW.
5. **Systematic monitoring and accountability:** All patients are provided short course chemotherapy free of charge. During the intensive phase of chemotherapy, all the drugs are administered under direct supervision called direct observed therapy short-term (DOTS).

Benefits of DOTS

- It is a supervised treatment. Patient takes the full medication. No chance of omitting the dose.
- DOTS is a community-based treatment and patient receives community-based care and support.
- High cure rate because of appropriate medical treatment, supervision and motivation by the healthcare workers.
- Monitoring of disease status by the healthcare services.

Must Know

Abbreviations used in treatment regimens of DOTS

Amx/Clv	: Amoxicillin and clavulanic acid	Km	: Kanamycin
Cfz	: Clofazimine	Lzd	: Linezolid
Cm	: Capreomycin	Mfx	: Moxifloxacin
E	: Ethambutol	PAS	: Para-aminosalicylic acid
Eto	: Ethionamide	Pto	: Prothionamide
H(INH)	: Isoniazid	R	: Rifampicin
Hh dose	: High-dose isoniazid	Z	: Pyrazinamide

First Line Regimen for Drug Sensitive TB

- Drugs are given daily.
- Dose of drugs are according to body weight.
- Fixed dose combination (FDC) tablets are used.
- No need for extension of intensive phase.
- Continuation phase may be extended by 12–24 weeks in certain focus of TB like CNS TB, skeletal TB and disseminated TB, etc., based on the clinical decision of the physician.
- Extension beyond 12 weeks should only be on recommendation of experts concerned of the concerned filed.
- No separate regimen for re-treatment cases.

Treatment Plan for Drug Sensitive TB Adults

All new and previously treated patients are given the first line treatment, i.e., in intensive phase isoniazid, rifampicin, pyrazinamide, and ethambutol (HRZE) for two months. During the continuation phase isoniazid and rifampicin with ethambutol (HRE) for four months. The duration of continuation phase may be increased according to the type of TB.

Drugs are given according to the body weight and the fixed dose combination tablets are used. Dose of drugs as per the body weight is given in Table 6.1.

TABLE 6.1: Dose of drugs as per the body weight

Weight category	Fixed dose combination tablets	
	Intensive phase (IP)	Continuation phase (CP)
	HRZE	HRE
	75/150/400/275 mg tablet	75/150/275/275 mg tablet
25–39 kg	2	2
40–54 kg	3	3
55–69 kg	4	4
>70 kg	5	5

Tablet pyridoxine (B_6) should be given to avoid the side effects of isoniazid.

Treatment plan for drug sensitive TB-pediatric cases is given in Table 6.2.

TABLE 6.2: Treatment plan for drug sensitive TB pediatric cases

Weight in kg	Number of fixed dose combination tablets (FDCs) dispersible			
	Intensive phase (IP)		Continuation phase (CP)	
	HRZ	E	HR	E
	50/75/150 mg tablet	100 mg	50/75 mg tablet	100 mg
4–7 kg	1	1	1	1
8–11 kg	2	2	2	2
12–15 kg	3	3	3	3
16–24 kg	4	4	4	4
25–29 kg	3 + 1A[+]	3	3 + 1A[+]	3
30–39 kg	3 + 2A[+]	2	2 + 2A[+]	2

A[+] = Adult FDC (HRZE = 75/150/400/275 tablet) (HRE = 75/150/275 mg tablet)

Treatment plan for multi-drug resistance (MDR-TB)/rifampicin resistance TB (RR-TB) is shown in Table 6.3.

TABLE 6.3: Treatment plan for MDR-TB/RR-TB

Regimen class	Regimen pattern	Intensive phase	Continuation phase	Total duration
Shorter MDR-TB regimen	RR/MDR-TB	(4–6) Mfx[h] km[*][h] Eto Cfz Zhe	(5) Mfx[h] Cfz Z E	9–11 months
Conventional MDR-TB regimen	MDR-TB	(6–9) Lfx km Eto Cs Z E	(18) Lfx Eto Cs E	24–27 months

Follow-up Protocol for Drug Resistance TB

- Sputum culture monthly during the intensive phase and every three months during the continuation phase.
- Intensive phase is extended if culture is positive during intensive phase (IP)
- Drug sensitivity testing (DST) is repeated if culture is positive at the end of IP and extended IP or any time during CP.
- Weight recording monthly.
- X-ray chest at the end of IP, end of treatment or whenever clinically indicated.
- ECG once in a month in IP if moxifloxacin uses.
- Serum creatinine, liver function test, kidney function test monthly for first three months and every three months during the CP.
- Thyroid function test during pretreatment evaluation and whenever indicated.
- Complete blood count and platelet count weekly in first month then monthly to rule out bone marrow suppression and anemia as a side effect of linezolid.

Pregnancy with MDR-TB

- All MDR-TB suspects and patients of child bearing age should be tested for pregnancy as part of pretreatment evaluation and also while on treatment.
- **Family planning methods:** Oral contraceptives are avoided during treatment, barrier methods, intrauterine devices (IUDs) are recommended.

The management protocol of MDR-TB during pregnancy is given in Figure 6.2

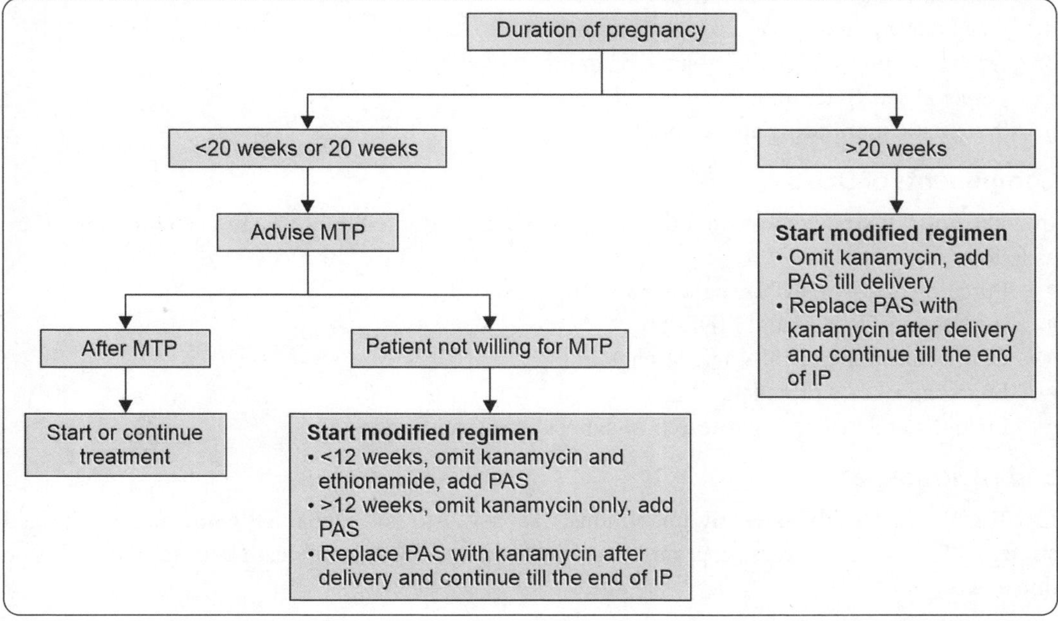

Figure 6.2: Management protocol of MDR-TB and pregnancy

Abbreviations: MTP, medical termination of pregnancy; PAS, para-aminosalicylic acid; IP, intensive phase

Strategic Implementation of RNTCP

The pilot study was conducted between 1993 and 1996 to test operational feasibility. The revised strategy was introduced in a phased manner.

Phase I	Phase II	Phase III
1997–2006	2006–2011	2012–2017

Phase I: 1997–2006

The Revised National TB Control Program launched in 1997 was based on WHO-DOTS strategy. The entire country was covered in March 2006.

Strategies of Phase I

- Augmentation of organization support at the central and state level for meaningful co-ordination.
- Increase in budgetary outlay.
- Use of sputum microscopy as a primary method of diagnosis among self-reporting patients.
- Standardized treatment regimens.
- Enhanced supervision at peripheral level through the creation of a subdistrict supervisory unit.
- Ensuring regular and uninterrupted supply of drugs up to most peripheral level.
- Emphasis on training IEC operational research and NGO involvement in the program.

DOTS Strategy

It was adopted by Revised National TB Control Program. The program initially had the following five main components:

1. Political will and administrative component
2. Diagnosis by quality ensured sputum smear microscopy
3. Adequate supply of quality assured chemotherapy drugs
4. Direct observed treatment
5. Systematic monitoring and accountability

Components of DOTS

In 2006 stop TB strategy was announced by WHO and adopted by RNTCP. The components are as follow:

- Pursuing quality DOTS expansion and enhancement
- Addressing TB/HIV and MDR-TB
- Contribution to health system strengthening
- Engaging all care providers
- Enabling and promoting research (diagnosis, treatment, vaccine)

End TB Strategies

In 2014, World Health Assembly unanimously approved to end global TB epidemic by "End TB strategy". This was a 20 years program with vision of a world with zero death diseases and suffering due to TB.

Phase II: 2006–2011

RNTCP phase II consolidated the achievement of Phase I to maintain its progressive trend and affect further improvement in its functions:

- Implementation of DOTS-plus for MDR-TB cases in a phased manner
- Distribution of pediatric drug boxes
- Institutional strengthening at national, state and district level
- Introduction of TB-HIV coordinator, urban coordinator and communication facilitator.

Components of the Strategy and Implementation Approaches

- Pursue high quality DOTS expansion and enhancement
- Address TB/HIV–MDR –TB and other challenges
- Contribute to health system strengthening
- Engage all care providers
- Empower people with TB and create awareness in the communities
  - Community participation in TB care
  - Advocacy, communication and social mobilization
  - Patient's right for tuberculosis care
- Enable and promote research.

Activities

- **Case finding:** Patients presenting themselves with symptoms of TB to be screened through sputum smear examination. Sputum examination is done in RNTCP microscopic centers at PHC, CHC or in TB dispensary.
- Implementation of DOTS-plus for multidrug-resistant TB cases in a phased manner. All patients are provided short course chemotherapy free of cost.

Phase III: 2012–2017

Objectives

- To ensure early and improved diagnosis of all TB patients, including drug resistant and HIV associated tuberculosis.
- To provide access to high quality treatment for all diagnosed cases of TB.
- To scale up access to effective treatment for drug resistance TB.
- To decrease the morbidity and mortality of HIV associated TB.
- To expand RNTCP services to patients diagnosed and treated in the private sector.

Strategies

- Strengthening and improving the quality of basic DOTS services.
- Further strengthening and aligning with health system under NRHM.
- Deploying improved rapid diagnostics to the field level.
- Expanding efforts to engage all care provider.
- Strengthening urban TB control.
- Expanding diagnosis and treatment of drug resistant TB.
- Improving communication, outreach and social mobilization.
- Promoting research for development and implementation of improved tools and strategies.

Achievements of RNTCP

RNTCP covers whole country since 2006.
- Phase II of RNTCP was launched in 1st October 2006.
- The treatment success rate has more than trebled from 25% in 1998 to 88% in 2015.
- Death rate has been brought down to seven fold from 29% to 4%.
  - 731 DTCs, 4888 TB units and 13,886 DMCs are functioning in the country.
- The program involves >1,813 NGOs, >13,926 private practitioners, over 319 medical colleges and >150 corporate health facilities.
  - >13,309 peripheral laboratories, designated microcopy centers, have been established.
- >6 lakhs public healthcare providers have been trained under the program.
- Master trainers on TB/HIV have been trained on TB/HIV related issues in 12 states.
- >6 million of patients have been initiated in treatment saving 2.8 million of lives.
- Four urban DOTS projects have also been launched to solve problem of inaccessibility of TB care faced by urban poor.

NATIONAL STRATEGIC PLAN FOR TB ELIMINATION (2017–2025)

Goal

To achieve a rapid decline in burden of TB, morbidity and mortality while working toward elimination of TB in India by 2025.

Objectives

- To achieve 90% notification rate for all cases.
- To achieve 90% success rate for all new and 85% for retreatment cases.
- To significantly improve the successful outcome of treatment for DRTB cases.
- To achieve decreased morbidity and mortality for HIV associated TB cases.
- To improve the outcome of TB care in the private sector.

Approaches of RNTCP, India (2019)

- Find TB cases with an emphasis on reading every TB patient in the private sector.
- Treat TB cases with high quality anti TB drugs.
- Prevent the emergence of TB in susceptible population and stop catastrophic expenditure due to TB.
- Build and strengthen supportive systems including enabling policies, empowered institutions and human resources with enhanced capacities.

Strategies of RNTCP, India (2019)

- Early diagnosis and prompt treatment with high quality anti TB drugs.
- Active case search for presumptive TB cases by house-to-house survey.
- Mandatory TB notification for diagnosing of TB and treatment for TB–NIKSHAY notification system.

- Starting of Nikshay Poshan Yojana for nutritional support for TB patients by Government of India.
- **Incentive-based system for treatment compliance:**
  - Private provider – ₹1000/-, ₹500 for notification and ₹500 to private practitioner/hospital for update patients treatment outcome.
  - Patients – ₹500/- per month for nutritional support during the period of anti TB treatment
  - Tribal patients – ₹750/- for tribal patients as transport allowance for patient from notified tribal area.
  - **Incentive for treatment supporter**
    - New cases ₹1000/- at completion of treatment.
    - Drug resistance cases ₹2000/- at completion of intensive phase and ₹3000/- at completion of treatment of TB cases.
- **Incentive for informant** ₹500 for notification of TB case to any health facility.

New Initiatives

- **Nikshay:** TB surveillance using care-based web-based IT system. The word Nikshay is the combination of two words Ni and kshay meaning eradication of TB.
  This software was launched in May 2012 and has the following components:
  - Master management
  - User details
  - TB patient's registration and details of diagnosis, DOTS provider, HIV status, follow-up contact tracing outcomes
  - Details of solid and liquid culture and DST, LPA, CBNAAT details
  - DR-TB patient registration with details
  - Referral and transfer of patients
  - Private health facility registration and TB notification
  - Mobile application for TB notification
  - SMS alerts to patients on registration
  - SMS alerts to program officer
  - Automated periodic reports:
    - Case finding
    - Sputum conversion
    - Treatment outcome: The program has started using IT enabled adherence tools like 99 DOTS of HIV-TB patients. This will be extended to all patients of TB with implementation of daily regimen.
- **TB notification:** Government of India notification dated 7th May 2012: "It is now mandatory for all healthcare providers to notify every TB case to local authorities, i.e., district health officer/chief medical officer of a district and municipal health officer every month in a given format. Notification is essential to ensure proper diagnosis and management of TB cases and to reduce the transmission and the spread of MDR-TB".
- **Ban on TB serology:** The serological test is based on antibody response which is highly variable. The currently available serological test is having poor specificity and should not be used for the diagnosis of pulmonary or extrapulmonary TB. Their import, manufacturing, sale, distribution and use are banned by the Government of India.

- **Direct benefit transfer scheme:** Direct beneficiary transfer system is being established by linking TB patients reported in NIKSHAY with AADHAR and PEMS to effectively deliver benefits to TB patients and their provider.

Organization of RNTCP at State Level

The structure of RNTCP at state level is as given follows:
- State tuberculosis officer heads the state tuberculosis office
- Director is the in charge of state tuberculosis training and demonstration center
- District tuberculosis officer is responsible for the management of district tuberculosis center
- Tuberculosis unit is managed by the following:
  - Medical officer TB control
  - Senior treatment supervisor
  - Senior TB laboratory supervisor
- Microscopy center
- Treatment center
- Dots provider

NATIONAL ANTIMALARIA PROGRAM

Introduction

National Antimalaria Program was started in 1999 by Indian government. The program originally was started as National Malaria Control Program in 1953 during the first Five-Year Plan. With the change in policies, the program was re-named as National Antimalaria Program in 1999.

Objectives

- To reduce the morbidity rate of malaria.
- To reduce malaria transmission at low level.

Strategies

- Residual insecticide spray with DDT was done twice a year.
- Malaria control team to survey and monitor incidence.
- No organized chemotherapy but was made available on demands.

Activities Undertaken for Malaria Control

The medical officer in charge PHC should be well-trained and he/she should take keen interest in malaria control activities and should carry out the following activities:
- Early diagnosis and complete, prompt and effective treatment
- Integrated vector control
- Supportive supervision
- Plan for IEC
- Recording and reporting
- Checking random sample of blood smears
- Cross-checking of activities from records

Achievements of the Program

There was decline of incidence from 75 million to only 2 million in 1958. The Government of India adopted Malaria Eradication Program in 1958 instead of malaria control program.

Activities of National Malaria Eradication Program

- Spraying operation
- Fortnightly active case detection
- Radical treatment
- Investigation of positive cases and remedial measures.

As a result of this program, only 0.009 million cases were registered till 1965. The success was really outstanding. In 1976, the malaria again bounced back and 6.47 million cases were registered. In 1977 a modified plan of operation (MPO) was initiated with the aim of establishing effective control on malaria and to bring the number of deaths due to malaria to zero. Implementation of this plan brought down the number of registered cases of malaria to 2.18 million in the year 1984.

Till 1993: This number remained stable and 2 million cases were reported. Since 1994 again there was increase in malaria cases and number of deaths due to malaria. The cases were between 2 and 3 million till 2001 and thereafter it started declining. About 88% of malaria cases were reported from high diseases burden states.

Malaria Action Plan (MAP)

Government of India formed an expert committee in 1994 and the committee identified malaria is a problem and recommended the adoption of special measures against it.

Objectives

- Management of critical and complicated cases of malaria.
- Checking of deaths due to malaria in high-risk groups.
- Reduce morbidity rate.
- Checking malaria endemic.
- Limiting the drug resistance malaria and falciparum infection.

Activities

- Treating the cases of malaria.
- Controlling the parasites.
- Taking anti-larva measures.
- Identifying primary areas facing problems.
- In urban area, the Malaria Eradication Program was also coupled with health education.

Surveillance System for Malaria Control

- The surveillance system is a component of modified plan of operation (MPO). Under this, malaria surveillance workers collect the blood slides for all fever cases and provide medical treatment which is found positive.

- **Active surveillance:** Malaria surveillance worker goes home to home in his/her area for collecting blood slides of all fever cases. After examination of slides at PHC, radical treatment to the positive cases and give chloroquine to all fever cases.
- **Passive surveillance:** The detection of malaria in hospitals/clinic, SC/PHC/CHC done by taking blood slides of all fever cases and sent for examination. A single dose of treatment for malaria is given. If malaria infection is found positive, message is sent to local surveillance workers for providing radical treatment.

Enhanced Malaria Control Project

Enhanced Malaria Control Project (EMCP) was started in 1997 with financial support of World Bank. EMCP is being run in 100 districts of 8 states which are more affected with malaria.

Components of EMCP

- Early diagnosis and prompt treatment.
- Selective vector control and individual protection.
- Information, education and communication.
- Developing capacity against infection.
- Epidemic planning and rapid response.

Under this project, state malaria society has been formed in all states. To create awareness among people to control malaria 1st-7th May is celebrated as malaria week. Fever treatment centers and medicine distribution centers have been set in rural areas.

In 1999, the name of the program was changed from National Malaria Eradication Program to National Anti-Malaria Program. Now this program is being conducted under the head of vector-borne diseases control program (VBDCP).

Intensified Malaria Control Project

This scheme was launched in July 2005 with assistance of global funds for AIDS, TB and malaria. It was introduced in high-risk malaria states, i.e., NE states, Odisha, Jharkhand and West Bengal.

Objectives

- To increase access to rapid diagnosis and treatment through community participation.
- To enhance awareness about malaria control program.
- To reduce transmission by the use of insecticides, treated bed nets and larvivorous fish.
- To promote the participation of community, NGOs and private sector.

Urban Malaria Scheme

Urban Malaria Scheme (UMS) was launched in 1971. The scheme is being implemented in 31 towns/cities in 19 states and UTs. About 7.2–7.4% of the total area of malaria were reported from urban area during 2007–2008 in the country. Death toll was also high in these cities and towns. Maximum number of cases were reported from Ahmedabad, Chennai, Kolkata, Mumbai, Vadodara, Vishakhapatnam and Vijayawada.

Objectives

Reduction of disease to a tolerable level in which the human population in urban areas can be protected from malaria transmission.

Aims

- Prevent death due to malaria.
- Reduction in transmission and morbidity.

Control Strategy

Must Know

Antimalaria month campaign

Antimalaria month campaign is observed every year in the month of June throughout the country.

To control parasite and vector, the following steps can be taken care of:
- In parasite control, treatment is done through passive agencies, e.g., hospitals, dispensaries, both in private and public sectors.
- Vector control consists of source reduction, use of larvicides, use of larvivorous fish, space spray, minor engineering and legislative measures.
- **Aerosol-space spray:** Space spraying of pyrethrum extract (2%) in and around houses to kill infective mosquitoes.

NATIONAL FILARIA CONTROL PROGRAM

Introduction

Filaria is a major health problem in many states of India. The disease is endemic in 255 districts, 16 states and 3 UTs. According to recent estimation about 630 million people are exposed to the risk of infection.

The National Filaria Control Program (NFCP) was launched in 1995 for the control of Bancroftian filariasis. Filariasis is caused by several rounds coiled and thread-like parasitic worms belonging to the family "Filarioidea". These parasites after getting deposited on the skin enter through the mosquito bite or penetrate on their own and reach the lymphatic system. Lymphatic filariasis is commonly known as elephantiasis is a disfiguring and disabling disease usually acquired in childhood. The long-term consequences are painful swollen limbs. Hydrocele in males also common in endemic area.

Objectives

- To control the disease in urban area through recurrent antilarval and antiparasitic measures.
- To reduce the problem in the area which has not been surveyed.
- To treat diagnosed cases and the carriers of microfilaria with diethylcarbamazine citrate. It has been proved that the extensive use of single dose of DEC medication is effective.

  In 1978 NFCP was emerged with urban malaria plan for maximum utilization of resources to be achieved. But now it is running under Vector-Borne Diseases Control Program (VBDCP).

Goal

Global elimination of this disease by the year 2020 has been envisaged by WHO and the Government of India is also the signatory to the World Health Assembly resolution in 1997 for its global elimination. National Health Policy in 2002 has envisaged elimination of lymphatic filaria in India by 2015.

Control Strategy

- Vector control through antilarva spray/application at weekly intervals with appropriate larvicides.
- Biological control through Larvivorous fishes.
- Environmental engineering through source reduction and water management.
- Antiparasitic measure through diagnosis and treatment of microfilaria carriers and cases.
- Information, education and communication to generate community awareness.

Revised Strategy

The revised strategy for elimination of lymphatic filariasis in India to eliminate lymphatic filaria by 2027, 3 years ahead of the global target through mission mode, multipartner, multisectoral targeted drive for which a roadmap to eliminate lymphatic filaria has been drawn.

Goal: To eliminate lymphatic filaria by 2027, 3 years ahead of the global target through five-pronged roadmap 2023–2027 (Fig. 6.3).

These prongs are described as follows:

1. **Mission mode MDA:** MDA campaign twice a year on 10th February and 10th August-celebration of deworming day. Health workers will go door to door to administer antifilaria medicine in 10 filaria affected states, i.e., Bihar, Chhattisgarh, Jharkhand, Maharashtra, Uttar Pradesh, West Bengal, Karnataka, Odisha, Madhya Pradesh and Andhra Pradesh.

   A single dose of Diethylcarbamazine citrate (DEC) 5 mg/kg body weight annually. Drug administration to 5-year-old and more to eligible population except pregnant mothers and children below 2 years of age, and seriously ill patients.

2. **Morbidity management and disability prevention (MMDP):** To reduce morbidity and mortality in infected cases by:
   - Early diagnosis
   - Engagement of medical colleges for strengthening MMDP services.

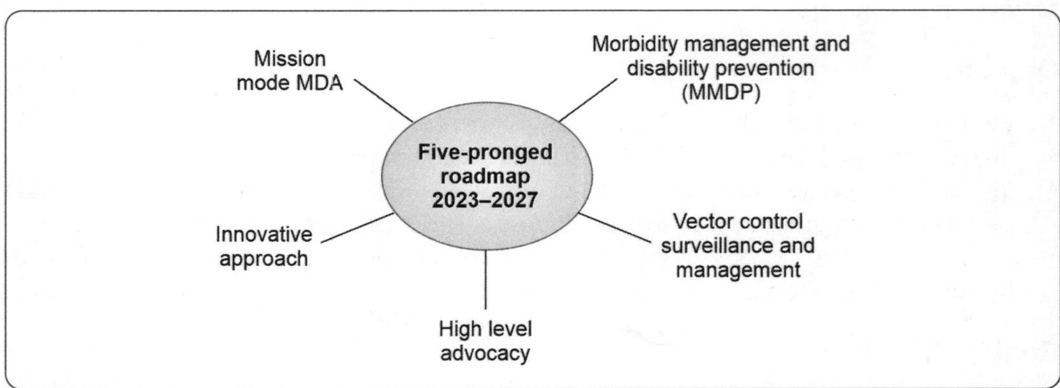

Figure 6.3: Roadmap of elimination of lymphatic filaria (2023–2027)

3. **Vector control surveillance and management:** Integrated vector control with multisectoral coordinated efforts.
4. **High level advocacy:** For better sectoral convergence and allied departments and ministries such as Ministry of Water and Sanitation, Ministry of Panchayati Raj, Ministry of HRD, Ministry of Rural Development.
5. **Innovative approach:** Leveraging existing digital platform for lymphatic filaria and explore additional diagnostics.

To sensitize people about the awareness and complication of lymphatic filaria, extensive IEC activities are to be carried on. The world filarial day is celebrated on 11th November every year to disseminate information about filaria, its prevention and treatment.

Basic Principles

The basic principles for the single dose of DEC administration are as follows:
- Interruption of diseases transmission.
- Home-based management of lymphedema cases and up-scaling of hydrocele operation in identified CHCs, district hospitals and medical colleges.

Salient Features

- Single dose mass therapy with DEC at a dose of 5 mg/kg body weight annually.
- Management of acute and chronic filariasis and self-care methods at door step.
- IEC to increase awareness on protective and preventive measures for filaria control.
- Anti-vector measures to continue in all the NFCP towns as complementary to antiparasitic measures. Microfilarial carriers detected in filaria clinics and elsewhere to receive the standard dose of DEC, i.e., 6 mg/kg body weight for 12 days.

Advantages of Single Dose Mass Therapy

- The single dose mass therapy is cost-effective in terms of manpower, material and time as it eliminates the blood smear examination.
- Ensures the treatment of all family members.

Functions of the Central Organization

- To plan and coordinate as per pattern to offer the financial and technical guidance to state/UTs for the implementation of the program.
- To train officer and staff for the program.
- To undertake research studies on epidemiology, newer methods of filaria control and related aspects.

Functions at State Level

NFCP is operated in 18 endemic states/UTs under a Joint Director (for malaria and filaria) by Director (for malaria and filaria) under the Director of Medical and Health Services of the concerned states. The states have been requested to identify a nodal officer for all vector borne disease control at state level for better coordination for VB-DCP.

NATIONAL GUINEA WORM ERADICATION PROGRAM

The guinea worm disease also known as the dracunculiasis is caused by nematode *Dracunculus medinensis*. The adult female guinea worm measures 60–100 cm in length emerges through the skin, usually the lower limbs causing swelling, ulceration and discomfort to the patients. Guinea worm disease is transmitted by drinking water containing copepods (water flea) that are infected with *Dracunculus medinensis*.

Global Scenario

The World Health Assembly adopted resolution in 1991 to eradicate dracunculiasis by 1995. A total of 180 countries and their territories were certified by WHO as eliminated dracunculiasis. Overall the annual incidence of the disease has declined from 892,055 cases reported in 1989 to 4619 in 2008. Two cases were reported to WHO in January–February 2014.

This was compared with three cases for the same period in 2013 with a decrease of 33%. Total number of cases in 2013 was 148 as compared to 542 in 2012, a decrease of 73% was noted.

Guinea Worm Eradication Program in India

Guinea Worm Eradication Program was started in 1984 with technical assistance from WHO, it was integrated into National Health System, India was able to reduce the disease in affected areas with intersectoral coordination and an efficient system of information and evaluation. The country reported zero case since August 1996. In February 2000, the International Commission for the certification of dracunculiasis eradication recommended that India would be certified free from dracunculiasis transmission.

Eradication Strategies

- Provision of safe drinking water
- Control of cyclops population
- Health education of the public with special emphasis on school children and women in rural area.
- Active surveillance for case detection
- Treatment of cases detected
- Trained manpower development
- Concurrent evaluation and operation research

WHO declared India as a guinea worm free country in February 2000 and advised the Indian government to maintain surveillance of guinea worm diseases till its global eradication.

NATIONAL LEPROSY ERADICATION PROGRAM

Introduction

Leprosy is caused by *Mycobacterium leprae* by close contact with infected patients or through droplet infection. It affects the peripheral nerves and causes total loss of cutaneous sensation in the affected area and thickening of the nerves and finally deformities in the affected area. It is one of the major health problems along with social stigma to the patient.

Prevalence

The average prevalence of disease in 1981 was 5.77 per 1000. The National Leprosy Control Program was launched in 1955 by the Government of India. Multidrug therapy came into use from 1982 and the program was redesignated as National Leprosy Eradication Program (NLEP) in 1983. Since then remarkable change has been achieved in reducing the disease burden. The NLEP is 100% centrally sponsored scheme. Multidrug therapy (MDT) is supplied free of cost by WHO. It was only in 1970 that a definite case was identified in the form of MDT. MDT came into wide use from 1982, following the recommendation by the WHO study group Geneva in October 1981. Government of India appointed a high power committee under the chairmanship of Dr Ms Swaminathan in 1981 for dealing with problems of leprosy. This was done based on the recommendations of the committee and NLEP was launched in 1983.

Goal of NLEP

To eradicate the disease by the year 2000.

Aim

To reduce case load to 1 or <1 per 10,000 population.

History

1955: National Leprosy Control Program was launched

1983: National Leprosy Eradication Program launched

1983: Introduction of multidrug therapy (MDT) in phases

2005: Elimination of leprosy at national level

2012: Special action plan for 209 high endemic districts in 16 states/UTs

2016: Leprosy case detection campaign in high endemic area

2017: Sparsh Leprosy Awareness Campaign

Revised Strategy

Early detection of cases by population surveys, school surveys, contact examination and voluntary reference. The strategy for leprosy eradication till 2027 is shown in figure. This is made effective based on the following factors:
* Short-term multidrug therapy
* Health education
* Ulcer and deformity care
* Rehabilitation activities
* Free domiciliary treatment in endemic districts through specially trained staff
* Treating leprosy cases with MDT, taken in phased manner
* Reconstructive surgery to improve functional status of the individual.

WHO Regimen of Leprosy Control

In 1982, WHO regimen of chemotherapy:
- Multidrug therapy includes (MDT):
  - Rifampicin – 600 mg once a month
  - Dapsone – 100 mg once a day
  - Clofazimine – 300 mg once a month
  - Duration of treatment 2 years
- Antibacillary Therapy (ABT)
  The recommended drug regimen under ABT is:
  - Rifampicin – 600 mg once in a month × 6 months
  - Dapsone – 100 mg once a day × 6 months
  - Duration of the treatment 6 months
- **Other measures include:**
  - Selective isolation
  - Follow-up cases, protection of children by BCG vaccination
  - Rehabilitation
  - Health education

To strengthen the process of elimination of leprosy in the country, first World Bank supported project was introduced in 1993. On completion of this project, the second phase supported by World Bank was started in 2001–02 which ended in 2004. Since then the program is continuing with Government of India funds and technical support from WHO and International Federation of Antileprosy Association (ILEP) organization. The program has been integrated with general healthcare system in 2003–2004 since then leprosy treatment and diagnosis is available with PHCs and government hospitals.

Components of the program: The components of the program are as follows:
- Decentralized integrated leprosy services through general healthcare system
- Capacity building of all general health services functionaries
- Intensified information, education and communication
- Prevention of disability and medical rehabilitation
- Intensified monitoring and supervision.

Major initiatives taken are as follows:
- More focus has been given to new case detection then prevalence which gives only the number of cases on record at a point in time. New case detection is the main indicator of the program.
- Treatment completion rate has been taken as an important indicator to be calculated by states at yearly basis.
- More emphasis on providing disability prevention and medical rehabilitation services to the leprosy affected persons. The aid provided is:
  - Dressing materials, supportive medicines and ulcer kits are provided to patients having ulcers and wounds.
  - Micro-cellular rubber foot wear are provided for protection of insensitive skin.
  - Patients from below poverty line (BPL) family undergoing reconstructive surgery are provided ₹8000/- out of this ₹500 as incentive to compensate for the loss of wages on discharge and traveling.

- ■ Support is also provided to government institutions and PMR centers in the form of ₹5000 per reconstructive surgery conducted.
- ASHA has been involved in bringing out suspected cases from villages for diagnosis and treatment at PHC and follow-up for their treatment completion.

Incentives to ASHA:

- ■ ₹250/- on confirmed diagnosis of case brought by ASHA without disability
- ■ Upon completion of treatment
  - ◆ PB leprosy (Paucibacillary) case ₹400/-
  - ◆ MB (Multibacillary) leprosy case ₹600/-
- ■ An early case before onset of any visible deformity ₹250/-
- ■ A new case with visible deformity in hands, feet or eye ₹250/-

Activities of ASHA:

- ■ Search for suspected cases of leprosy
- ■ Follow-up of all cases of leprosy for completion of treatment
- ■ Advise and motivate self-care practices, i.e., proper care of hands and feet during follow-up period
- ■ Spreading awareness
- Intensive IEC activities with a theme toward "Leprosy Free India"

Disability Prevention and Medical Rehabilitation

- Early treatment, physiotherapy, reconstructive surgery and providing microcellular rubber (MCR) foot wear.
- **Integrating DPMR services:** Provision of services to persons with disabilities by various departments under different ministries convergence of National Leprosy Eradication Program (NLEP) services into National Rural Health Mission (NRHM) facilitates their integration.
- To develop a referral system to provide prevention of disability services to all leprosy disabled persons. The referral is three tier system.
  1. At primary level care the institutions are PHCs, CHCs, subdivisional hospitals and urban leprosy centers
  2. Secondary level care institutions are district head quarter hospitals and district nucleus units.
  3. Tertiary level institution are as follows:
     - ◆ Central government institutions Chengalpattu and RLTRI at Aska (Gauripur and Raipur)
     - ◆ ICMR institute Jalma Agra
     - ◆ ILEP supported leprosy hospital
     - ◆ All PMR institutions and departments of medical colleges.

Other supporting units:

- Orthopedic and plastic surgery department of medical colleges
- Identified NGOs institutions
- All National Institutions under Ministry of Social Justice and Empowerment
- Contractual surgeons skilled in reconstructive surgery (RCS) and rehabilitation.

Program Implementation Plan for 12ᵗʰ Plan Period (2012–2013 to 2016–2017)

- Elimination of leprosy. To reduce the case found to one or less than one per 10,000 population in all districts of the country.
- Strengthen disability prevention and medical rehabilitation of persons affected by leprosy.
- Reduction in the stigma associated with leprosy.

Program Strategy

- Integrated leprosy services through general healthcare system.
- Early detection and treatment of new leprosy cases.
- Strengthening of disability prevention and medical rehabilitation services.

Case Detection

Detection of new cases at the early stage is the only solution to reduce the transmission of infection in the community. The following plans are suggested for early case detection:
- To improve access to the services.
- To involve women including leprosy affected persons in case detection.
- To organize skin camps for detecting leprosy patients while providing services for other skin conditions.
- To undertake contact survey to identify the source in the neighborhood of each child or multibacillary case.
- To increase awareness through health workers, i.e., ANM, AWW, ASHA and other health workers while visiting the village and people affected by leprosy.

Management

Integrated leprosy services through all the primary healthcare facilities will continue to be provided in rural area. Early case detection, prompt treatment and referral services of patients with deformities and medical rehabilitation.

Three pronged strategy was introduced in the National Eradication Program from 2016–2017. The components of the strategy are as follows:
1. Leprosy case detection campaign
2. Focused leprosy campaign
3. Special plan for hard to reach areas

Sparsh Leprosy Awareness Campaign

Sparsh leprosy campaign was launched on January 2017 through Gram Sabhas and carried out with the help of Panchayat and Village Health and Sanitation Committee. The aim was to generate awareness, reduce stigma and improve self-reporting of cases.
- **Survey education and treatment (SET) scheme:** Under this scheme, NGOs are involved in disability prevention and ulcer care, IEC, referral of suspected cases and referral for reconstructive surgery, research and rehabilitation.
- **Incentive to patients:** The leprosy patients undergoing major reconstructive surgery will be paid ₹8000/- irrespective of their financial status, payment will be made by the district leprosy officer.

- **Information, education and communication (IEC/BCC):** The IEC strategy during 12th plan period was focus on communication for behavior changes in general public against the stigma and discrimination against leprosy affected persons. Through IEC, providing awareness to people for MDT treatment, correction of disabilities through reconstructive surgery and about the facilities available at government institutions for primary, secondary and tertiary level of care so that persons can live normal life.
- **The International Federation of Antileprosy Association (ILEP):** ILEP is actively involved as partner in NLEP in India.

The Global Leprosy Strategy 2016–2020

Accelerating Toward Leprosy Free World

The strategy was released on April 2016. It is based around 3 core pillars (Fig. 6.4):
- **Pillar–1:** To strengthen government ownership coordination and partnership
- **Pillar–2:** To stop leprosy and its complications
- **Pillar–3:** To stop discrimination and promote inclusion

In endorsing the global strategy, three key targets have been agreed by all national programs:
1. Zero grade 2 disability (G2D) among children diagnosed with leprosy.
2. The reduction of new leprosy cases with G2D to <1 (less than one) case per million population.
3. Zero countries with legislation allowing discrimination on the basis of leprosy.

Early detection and complete treatment with MDT remain fundamental principle of leprosy control.

Major Initiative Under NLEP 2017–2018

- **Focus on** new case detection is main indicator for program monitoring
- **Treatment** completion rate as operational indicator
- **Emphasis** on disability prevention and medical rehabilitation (DPMR)
  - Dressing material, ulcer kit, supportive medicine
  - Providing microcellular rubber footwear
  - Incentive to leprosy patients from BPL families
  - Incentive to health facility as INR 5000 for reconstructive surgery.

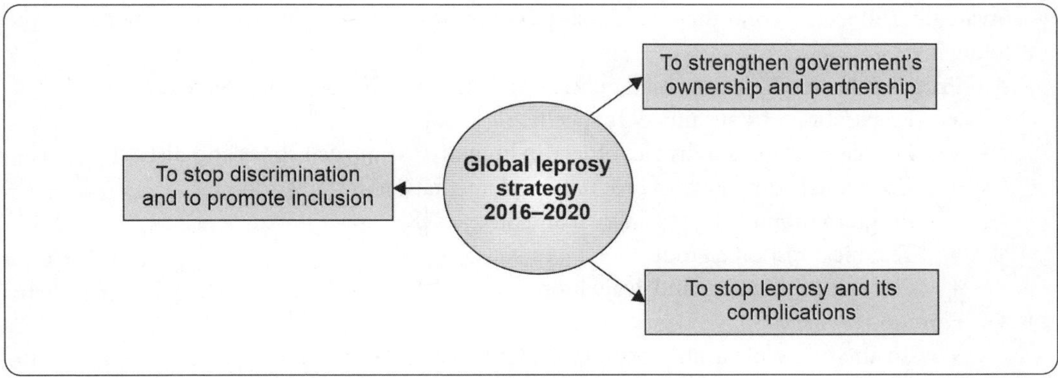

Figure 6.4: Global leprosy strategy 2016–2020

- ASHA incentives:
  - INR 250–confirmed diagnosis
  - INR 400 on completion of treatment of PB leprosy
  - INR–600 on completion of treatment of MB leprosy
- Intensive IEL—Awareness campaign

Must Know

Sparsh: Rolled on January 2017 for increasing awareness and address the issue of leprosy stigma in the society.
Sapna: It is a concept designed and developed keeping in mind a common girl living in community who will help to spread awareness in the community through key IEC message.
Who can become sapna: A local school girl who is willing to be sapna from same locality preferably.
World Leprosy Day (WLD) is celebrated on the last Sunday of January. The theme for World Leprosy Day 2024: "Beat Leprosy".

National Strategic Plan and Roadmap for Leprosy 2023–2027

The Government of India has launched National Strategic Plan and Roadmap for Leprosy 2023–2027 on 30th June 2023 to achieve zero transmission of leprosy by 2027, i.e., three years ahead of the Sustainable Development Goal (SDG) 3.3 (Figs 6.5 to 6.7).

Vision: Leprosy free India with zero infection and disease, zero disability, zero stigma and discrimination.

Goal: Acceleration toward achieving interruption of leprosy transmission in India.

Specific objectives:
- Strengthen leadership, commitment and partnership.
- Acceleration of case detection.
- Provision of quality services.
- Enhanced measures for prevention of disease, disabilities, stigma and discrimination and violation of human right.
- Digitalization of surveillance system.

Strategic Pillars and Roadmap for Leprosy

- **Strategic Pillar-1: Strengthen leadership community and partnership:** It includes the following:
  - **Program leadership:** Sustained politic commitment at National and State level
    - Preparation of state and WTs specific roadmaps.
    - Dedicated state and district officer in high disease burden states and district.
    - Creater accountability of program implementation in states and UTs
    - Program monitoring at National and State level
    - Technical resource group
    - Periodic monitoring and evaluation.
  - **Human resources:**
    - Ensure filling of vacant positions under NLEP
    - Human resource mapping and redistribution

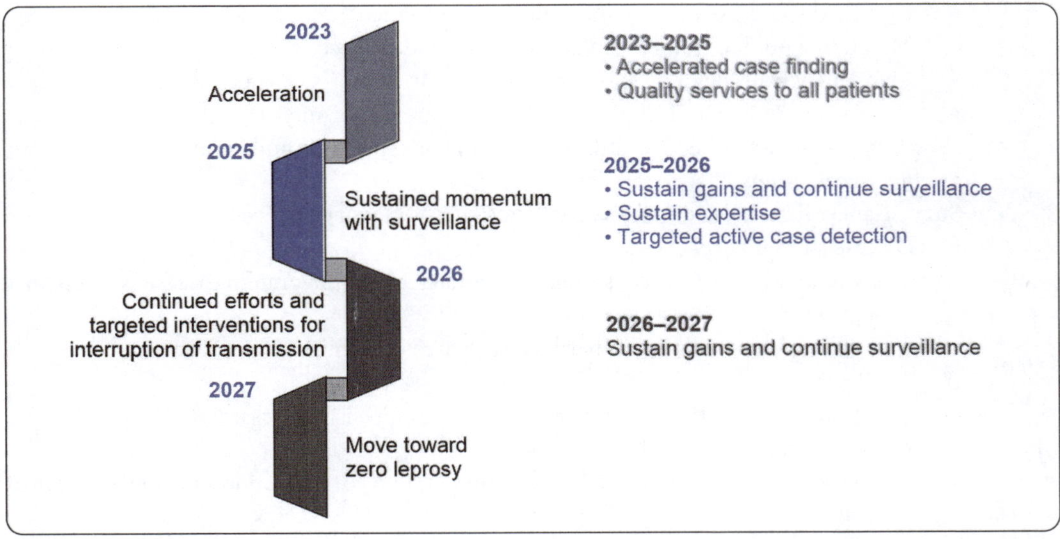

Figure 6.5: Strategy for leprosy eradication till 2027

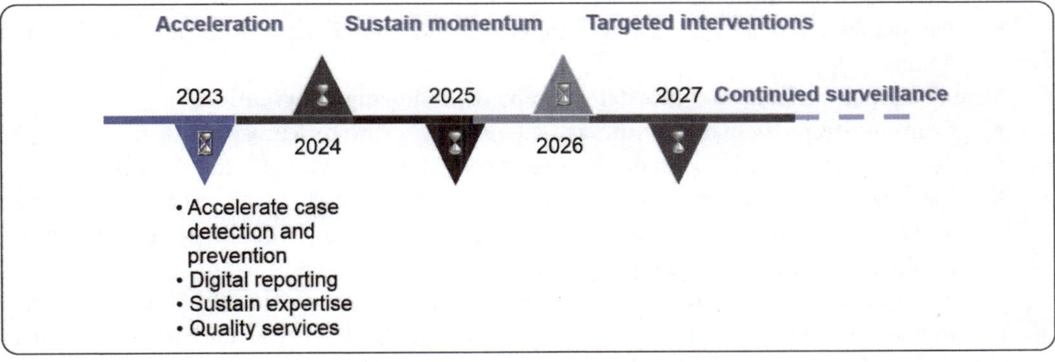

Figure 6.6: Timeline for leprosy eradication 2023–2027

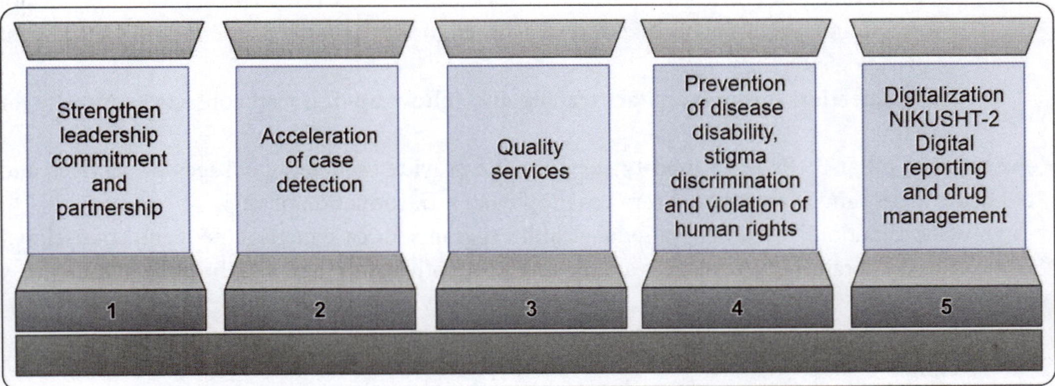

Figure 6.7: Strategic pillars and roadmap for leprosy 2023–2027

- ◆ Confined space assessment and training requirement
- ◆ Maintain a pool of trainers at national, state and district level
- ◆ Mandatory training of all skills every three years
- ◆ Review and update training material and ensure uniformity
- **Program financing:** Effective utilization an enhancement of budget at central and state level for acceleration.
- **Surveillance:** It includes disease surveillance and AMR surveillance.
  - I. Disease surveillance
    - ◊ Enhance surveillance system. Integrates with integrated disease surveillance program.
    - ◊ Strategic surveillance in hard to reach areas and migrant population.
  - II. AMR surveillance:
    - ◊ Enhance detection and management of drug resistance cases.
    - ◊ Build capacity of staff.
    - ◊ Develop collection and transportation system for collection of samples to AMR labs.
    - ◊ Enhance contact screening of cases with resistance.
- **Global and National New Evidence and Research:** Introduction of molecular tests for early diagnosis and confirmation for leprosy.
- **Partnership:** Strengthen existing partnership and collaboration with new partners and donors.
- **Strategic pillar-2: Accelerate case detection by the following interventions:**
  - **Community participation:** To make community aware to leprosy about its early signs detection, about the progress of disease and complications through extensive IEC activities. Importance of self-examination voluntary reporting and early treatment and interruption of transmission of disease incentive for any person reporting a confirmed case of leprosy facility for tele-helpline to support self-reporting.
  - **New case detection under NLEP program:** It includes active case detection, incentives to staff and any other persons reporting leprosy case and special plans for hard to reach areas and ASHA based surveillance for leprosy suspects (ABSULS).
  - **Other health programs and nonhealth institution and individuals:** Integrate case detection activities with house to house case detection and service delivery with other health program. Intersectoral coordination with other government departments and engagement of private sector.
  - **Case detection through contact tracing and follow-up** of traced contacts biannually for 5 years.
- **Strategic pillar-3: Provide quality services:** To provide complete packages of services and ensure access and availability of services prophylaxis. Introduction of any:
  - Coordination with other National Health Programs for case management and counseling.
  - Physiotherapists, psychiatrists and counselors of other programs may be utilized for leprosy services.
  - Coordination with medical colleges, private practitioners NGUs and private hospitals and clinics.

- Provide medical rehabilitation and mental well-being services to effected persons with leprosy.
- Establish criteria for diagnosis, clinical assessment classification, treatment and management of complication.
- Specialized services for persons affected by leprosy. Supportive treatment pharmacovigilance and post-treatment follow-up.
- **Strategic pillar-4: Prevention of disease, disabilities, stigma, discrimination and violation of human rights: It includes the following:**
  - **Disease prevention:** Expand coverage of contacts with postexposure prophylaxis. Introduction of any newer and more efficacious PEP regimens.
  - Research on more effective immune prophylaxis options. Introduction of newly available effective and approved vaccines.
  - Prevention of stigma, discrimination and violation of human rights through extensive IEC activities and by observing. Antileprosy day and Sparsh leprosy awareness campaign sensitization of leaders. Policy makers faith based leaders, Gram Panchayat, Gram Pradhan, ward members, members of Legislative assembly, member of Parliament, Resident welfare associations, council members of municipal corporations and members of social welfare organization.
- **Strategic pillar-5: Develop digital system for NLEP:**
  - Digitalization of reporting and recording system of programs and integrated with integrated health information platform (IHIP). Digitalize antileprosy drug management on IHIP.
  - Launch and rollout new version of NIKUSTH 2.0 for digitalization of individual patient records.

NATIONAL AIDS CONTROL PROGRAM

Introduction

Acquired immunodeficiency syndrome (AIDS) has emerged as one of the most serious public health problem in India. The first-case of AIDS was detected in 1986 in Chennai. AIDS is caused by a virus which belongs to retrovirus group.

Prevalence

The high prevalence states present in the country are Andhra Pradesh, Maharashtra, Manipur, Nagaland, Karnataka and Tamil Nadu. Disease is transmitted by the infected blood transfusion, use of infected needles which are common in drug addicts, sexual transmission, tattooing, piercing, acupuncture and maternal fetal transmission.

Burden of the Disease

According to National AIDS control organization of India, the prevalence of AIDS in India in 2013 was 0.27 which has come down from 0.41 in 2002. There are 2.39 million people living with HIV/AIDS in India as estimated in 2008–2009. According to more recent data, there is a reduction of 57% in estimated annual new HIV infections from 0.274 million in 2000 to 0.116 million in 2011. The four high prevalence states of India, Andhra Pradesh –500,000, Maharashtra –4,20,000, Karnataka –250,000, Tamil Nadu –150,000 account for 55% of all HIV infection in country. National

AIDS Control Program was launched in the year 1987. National AIDS control organization was set up by the Ministry of Health and Family Welfare as a separate cell to implement this program.

The aims of this project are as follows:

- Minimizing the HIV infections in the country
- Reducing the morbidity and mortality rate due to AIDS and to check the spreading of HIV/AIDS infection to achieve their objective.

National AIDS Control Organization

National AIDS Control Organization (NACO) is the "nodal organization" for formulation of policy and implementation of the program for the prevention and control of HIV/AIDS in India. It was established in 1992.

Objectives

- To control epidemic of AIDS in India.
- To facilitate and improve access to treatment for HIV positive people and also to promote and protect their human dignity.
- To create awareness about HIV/AIDS giving accurate and reliable information.
- To clear existing myths and misconceptions and providing practical skills that can be implemented at the individual level so as to lead to behavior changes that minimize the risk of HIV infection.

National AIDS Prevention and Control Policy

Union government approved the National AIDS Prevention and Control Policy (NAPCP) in April 2002.

Objectives of NAPCP

- To reduce the impact of epidemic.
- To bring about zero transmission rate of AIDS by 2007.

National Council of AIDS

National Council of AIDS (NCA) has been constituted to provide policy guidelines and political leadership to the NAPCP. NCA is chaired by the Prime Minister of India and consists of 31 ministries, seven chief ministers, representative of civil society, positive people network and private sector organization.

Objectives

- To mainstream HIV/AIDS issue in all ministries and departments by treating it as a development challenge and not merely a public health problem.
- To provide leadership to increase multisectoral response to combat HIV/AIDS in the country with special reference to youth, women and the workforce.
- Link Worker Scheme is one of the part of mainstreaming project, which is being implemented through different NGOs.

Phases of National AIDS Control Program

There are four phases of NACP (Fig. 6.8). Fifth phase NACP-V, will extend till 31 March 2026.

Phase I (1992–1999)

Phase I was implemented across the country with objective to slow the spread of HIV. To reduce future morbidity, mortality, and the impact of AIDS by initiating a major effort in the prevention of HIV transmission.

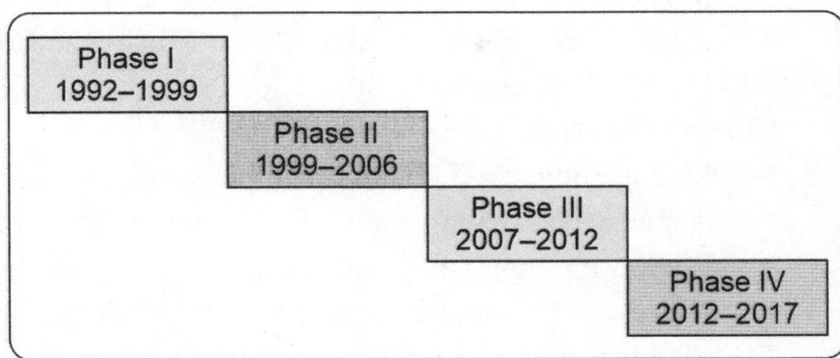

Figure 6.8: Phases of National AIDS Control Program

Phase II (1999–2006)

NACP phase II was aimed at:
- Reducing spread of HIV infection in India
- Strengthening India's capacity to HIV epidemic on long-term basis.

Phase III (2007–2012)

NACP phase III is based on experience and lessons drawn from NACP I and II and it is built upon their strengths. Its priorities and thrust area are drawn up accordingly. The strategic objectives of NACP phase III are as follows:
- Prevent infection through saturation of coverage of high-risk group (HRG) with targeted intervention and scaled up intervention in general population.
- Provide greater care, support and treatment to more people living with HIV/AIDS.
- Strengthen the infrastructure system and human resources in prevention, care, support and treatment programs at district, state and national level.

Phase IV (2012–2017)

The strategic plan for NACP-IV (2012–2017) has been developed through an elaborate and extensive process.

Goal

Accelerate reversal and integrated response.

Objectives

- To reduce new infections by 50% (2007) baseline of NACP-III
- To provide comprehensive care and support to all persons living with HIV/AIDS and treatment services for all those who require it.

Activities Under NACP

- **Blood safety:**
  - Provision of adequate safe and quality blood to every patient.

- Mandatory testing of every unit of blood of donors' blood against transfusion transmissible infection (TTIs), i.e., HIV hepatitis B, C, syphilis and malaria.
- Establishment of national blood transfusion authority.
- Blood storage units at FRUs.

- **STD/STI control:**
  - Management of STD/STI in an integrated manner.
  - A manual on management of STIs by NACO and RCH division jointly.
  - Facilitating the management of STIs in the peripheral health facilities.
  - A package for involvement of private physician.

- **Targeted intervention for population of high-risk:**
  - Interruption of the HIV transmission among highly vulnerable population.
  - Targeted high-risk group includes female sex workers, men who have sex with men (MSM), injection drug user (IDUs) and bridge population (truckers and migrants).
  - Components of targeted intervention are BCC, access to STI services, ensure safe sex practices, engaging community organization, needle syringe exchange program and linkage to care, etc.

- **Surveillance:**
  - Detection of spread of disease.
  - Pattern of behavior and making the appropriate strategy.
  - Various types of surveillance, e.g., HIV Sentinel Serosurveillance, AIDS surveillance, STD surveillance, behavioral surveillance, HIV-TB and other diseases integration surveillance, etc.

- **School AIDS education program:**
  - Developing a safe and responsible lifestyle.
  - University talk AIDS project.
  - Distribution of training modules "learning for life".

- **Family health awareness campaign:**
  - Creating awareness about HIV/AIDS and about available services for treatment of STDs/STIs.
  - Addressing the main issue of reproductive health in families especially in rural and vulnerable section.
  - Capacity building of medical, nursing and paramedical professional.

- **Condom promotion:**
  - Use of condom as a protection against STIs HIV/AIDS in addition to family planning.
  - Free distribution of condom through social market.
  - Availability of condom vending machines.

- **National pediatric AIDS initiative:**
  - Providing comprehensive care and support including ART to children infected by HIV.
  - Guidelines for antiretroviral therapy (ART).
  - Establishment of regional pediatric centers.
  - Free CD4 monitoring, treatment of opportunistic infections and micronutrient supplementation.
  - Care and support for children living with HIV/AIDS (CLHA), orphans and vulnerable children.

- **Care and support-ART center:**
  - Providing free antiretroviral therapy (ART).

- Establishment of ART center.
- Community care center across the community for providing care and support services to persons living with HIV/AIDS (PLHAs).
- **Integrated counseling and testing center (ICTC):**
  - Merging prevention of parent to child transmission (PPTCT) and voluntary counseling and testing centers (VCTC) into ICTCs.
  - Establishment of ICTCs at medical colleges, district hospitals, subdistrict hospitals and a few community centers.
  - ICTC in the obstetrics and gynecology department of such hospitals having large number of ANCs and institutional deliveries.
- **Information education and communication (IEC):**
  - Emphasis on behavior changes through awareness generation.
  - NACOs focus on reduction of stigma and discrimination, promotion of services, routine use of condom and blood safety.
  - A new cadre of Village Level Link Workers for BCC.
  - Intensive IEC among general population.
  - Life skill programs in schools.
  - Launching of red ribbon express (1.12.2007).
  - Set up of toll-free national AIDS telephone, helpline having computerized 4-digit number 1097.

> **Recent Update**
>
> The NACP-IV, started with a target of speeding up the process of reversal of the epidemic and making India's response against the virus stronger over its five years through a careful and well-defined integration process, has now been extended in its fifth phase, NACP-V, till 31st March 2026.

- **Community nursing centers:** NACO has started community nursing centers in the country to take care of HIV infected patients. The major activities of these nursing centers are as follows:
  - Providing shelter to patients suffering from HIV/AIDS.
  - Providing them balanced and therapeutic nutrition.
  - Providing appropriate nursing care.
  - Providing recreational facilities to patients and persons taking care of them.
  - Providing spiritual nursing.
  - Arranging referral services for the patients.
  - Providing appropriate and essential training to the families of the patients and community-based organization.

NATIONAL STRATEGIC PLAN FOR HIV/AIDS AND STI 2017–2024

Vision

AIDS-free India.

Mission

To attain universal coverage of HIV prevention, testing, treatment to care continuum that is effective, inclusive, equitable and adopted to population and local needs.

Goal

To achieve:
- Zero new infections
- Zero AIDS related deaths
- Zero discrimination

Objectives

The national strategic plan purposes—six objectives toward fulfilling its vision of an AIDS free India. These are as follows:

Objective 1: Reduce 80% new infections by 2024 (Baseline 2010).

Objective 2: Ensure 95% of estimated people living with HIV (PLHIV) know their status by 2024.

Objective 3: Ensure 95% PLHIV have ART initiation and retention by 2024 for sustained viral suppression.

Objective 4: Eliminate mother to child transmission of HIV and syphilis by 2020.

Objective 5: Eliminate HIV/AIDS related stigma and discrimination by 2020.

Objective 6: Facilitate sustainable NACP service delivery by 2024.

Broad Strategies

Test and treat policy relates as prevent, test and treat (PTT).

Prevent

- Increased coverage for improved prevention, testing and care linkage.
- Systematic evidence generation to reach 'at risk' population.
- Retain knowledge and practice (KP) with adequate and appropriate survey.

Test

- Geo-prioritized differential approach.
- Use graded approach to increase HIV testing.
- Pilot and scale-up newer modalities of testing (e.g., community-based testing (CBT) self-testing, etc.)
- Active use of IEC to increase demand for HIV testing.

Treat

- Accelerate update of ART.
- Improve ART retention by engaging community/NGO or private sector.
- Ensure supportive environment for achieving universal access to ART.
- Address comorbidities of HIV infection to lower mortality and morbidity.

NATIONAL STD CONTROL PROGRAM

Introduction

Sexually transmitted diseases are major health problems all over the world including India. The annual incidence of STD in India as reported to the central bureau of health intelligence during 1989 was approximately 14 million.

National STD Control Program was started in 1946 in India. With the arrival and spread of HIV infections in the country, it was brought under the purview of national AIDS organization in the year 1992.

Aims

The main aim of STDs Control Program is to prevent ill health caused by STDs infections through the following interventions:

- **Primary prevention:** It includes prevention of infection.
- **Secondary infection:** By early diagnosis and prompt treatment to prevent complications of the disease.

Objectives

- To prevent the transmission of the disease and minimize the incidence.
- Screening of cases and contacts.
- Early diagnosis and treatment of infected cases.
- To create awareness by IEC activities.
- To treat every newborn baby born to infected mother.

Strategies to Control STDs

- Strengthening the infrastructures for providing appropriate laboratory services for the diagnosis of STDs and establish STDs clinics in the hospitals and health centers for the consultation and treatment.
- Training of the healthcare workers for efficient case management.
- Screening of cases and contacts and ensuring their complete treatment. Priority to be given to pregnant mothers, blood donors, industrial workers, army, police refugees and prostitutes.
- **Primary healthcare:** Health education to the community through health workers on prevention of disease by personal prophylaxis. The use of condom and other chemical barriers to prevent the transmission of infection from sexual partner.
- **Information system:** Strengthening the IEC activities to create greater awareness among the general public to prevent and control the STDs.
- **Social welfare measures**
  - It includes counseling services by the expert professionals.
  - **Social therapy:** Provision of recreational facilities in the community, provision of descent living conditions, marriage counseling, prohibiting the sale of sexually stimulating literature, books and photographs, etc. Rehabilitation of the prostitutes.
- Surveillance, monitoring and evaluation of the program for its effectiveness.

NATIONAL PROGRAM FOR CONTROL OF BLINDNESS

Introduction

National Program for Control of Blindness (NPCB) was launched in the year 1976 as a 100% centrally sponsored scheme now 60:40 in all states and 90 in NE states with the goal to reduce

TABLE 6.4: Causes of blindness

Cataract counts for	62.6%
Refractive error	19.70%
Corneal blindness	0.90%
Surgical complication	1.2%
Posterior capsular opacification	0.90%
Glaucoma	5.80%
Posterior segment disorder	4.70%
Others	4.10%

the prevalence of blindness from 1.4% to 0.3% by 2020. As per survey in 2001–2002, prevalence of blindness is estimated to be 1.1%. Rapid survey on avoidable blindness conducted under NPCB during 2006–07 showed reduction in the prevalence of blindness from 1.1 (2001–02) to 1% (2006–07). Various activities/initiatives undertaken during the Five-Year Plans under NPCB are targeted toward achieving the goal of reducing the prevalence of blindness to 0.3% by the year 2020. Various causes which led to blindness are tabulated in Table 6.4.

Goals and Objectives of NPCB in the 12th Five-Year Plan

- To reduce the backlog of blindness through identification and treatment of blindness at primary, secondary and tertiary level based on assessment of the overall burden of visual impairment in the country.
- To develop and strengthen the strategy of NPCB for eye-health and prevention of visual impairment through provision of comprehensive eye care services and quality service delivery.
- To strengthen and upgradation of Regional Institute of Ophthalmology (RIO) to become center of excellence in various subspecialties of ophthalmology.
- To strengthen the existing and developing additional human resources and infrastructure facilities for providing high quality comprehensive eye care to all districts of the country.
- To enhance community awareness on eye care and lay stress on preventive measures.
- To increase and expand research by prevention of blindness and visual impairment.
- To secure participation of voluntary organizations, private partners in eye care.

Strategies of the Program

- **Surveillance:** To assess the magnitude, geographical distribution and causes of blindness in the country and take appropriate measures in those areas to prevent disease.
- Prevention of eye disorders resulting from nutritional deficiencies by proper diet and nutritional supplements.
- **Primary eye care:** Health workers at subcenters and PHC to provide treatment of conjunctivitis, ophthalmia neonatorum, removing of superficial foreign bodies and treatment of xerophthalmia to prevent these disease at the grass-root level.
- Screening of cases
    - **School eye health services:** Early detection and treatment of eye disorder among the school children during their routine health checkups.

- Case findings by arranging eye camps run by public, private, NGOs and volunteer health organization and their appropriate treatment.
- **Strengthening of infrastructure and training of manpower:** To provide secondary eye care by treating the blinding conditions such as cataract, trachoma, glaucoma, entropion, ocular trauma, corneal transplantation by the ophthalmologist at the district hospital and PHC.
- **Vitamin A prophylaxis:** Vitamin A 20,000 IU are administered orally to children of 1–6 years age at 6 months intervals under the vitamin A distribution scheme in India.
- **Occupational eye health services:** To prevent occupational eye hazards, the workers are educated to use protective devices, factories to improve working condition with proper lighting of the working area.
- Health education on eye care by strengthening IEC activities and raising living standard of people.
- Rehabilitation of incurable blindness.

Strategic Plan for Vision 2020—the Right to Sight in India

Strategic Plan for Vision 2020 is a global initiative to reduce avoidable blindness by year 2020. India is also committed to this initiative.

A meeting held in Goa on October 2001 and constituted a working group. The draft plan of action submitted by the 'working group' includes the following strategies:

- **Strengthen advocacy:** The activities include public awareness and information about eye care and prevention of blindness. Introduction of topics on eye care and health of eyes in school curriculum. Involvement of professional organizations such as All India Ophthalmological Society (AIOS), Eye Bank Association of India (EBAI) and Indian Medical Associated (IMA) in the NPCB, to strengthen the functioning of District Blindness Control Society (DBCS), to enhance involvement of NGOs, local community societies and community leaders, to strengthen hospital retrieval programs for eye donation through effective grief counseling by involving volunteers, forensic department and police, etc.
- **Reduction of disease burden:** The target diseases identified under "Vision 2020" are cataract, childhood blindness, refractive errors and low vision, corneal blindness, diabetic retinopathy, glaucoma and trachoma.
- **Human resources development:** Mid-level ophthalmic personnel are as follows:
  - **Hospital-based MLOP:** Ophthalmic nurses, technicians, optometrists, orthoptists.
  - **Community-based MLOP:** Primary eye care workers, ophthalmic assistants.
- Eye care infrastructure development includes primary, secondary and tertiary level of care.
  - Primary level includes:
    - Vision centers – 20,000.
      - Refraction and prescription of glasses
      - Primary eye care
      - School eye screening program
      - Screening at referral services
  - Secondary level includes:
    - Service centers – 2000
      - Cataract survey
      - Other common eye surgeries

- ◊ Facilities for refraction
- ◊ Referral services
- ■ Tertiary level includes:
  - ◆ Training centers – 200
    - ◊ Tertiary eye care including retinal surgery, corneal transplantation
    - ◊ Glaucoma surgery
    - ◊ Training and continue medical education
  - ◆ Center excellence – 20
    - ◊ Professional leadership
    - ◊ Continue medical education
    - ◊ Research
    - ◊ Laying of standards and QA
    - ◊ Strategy development

> **Recent Update**
>
> The United Nation's resolution in 2021 sets a target for eye care for all by 2030 – with countries set to ensure full access to eye care services for their populations, and, to support global efforts, to make eye care part of their nation's journey to achieving the sustainable development goals.

IODINE DEFICIENCY DISORDER CONTROL PROGRAM

Introduction

Iodine deficiency disorder is worldwide major health problem. These affect a large segment of the population in all continents and >1.5 billion people all over the world are at risk.

India commenced a Goiter Control Program in 1962 based on iodized salt. At the end of three decades, the prevalence of the diseases still remained high. As a result, a major national program "the IDD Control Program" was initiated. This program was designed to focus on provision of iodized salt in identified endemic areas. The nomenclature of the program was changed in August 1992 to National Iodine Deficiency Disorders Control Program (NIDDCP). This was done to emphasize wider implication of iodine deficiency. According to this program, nation-wide rather than area-specific use of iodized salt is being promoted. It was decided as a national policy to fortify all edible salt in a phased manner by the end of 8th Five-Year Plan. The essential components of the program are to use iodized salt in place of common salt, monitoring and surveillance, manpower training and mass communication.

Objectives

- Surveys to assess the magnitude of the iodine deficiency disorders in districts.
- Supply of iodized salt in place of common salt.
- Resurveys to assess iodine deficiency disorders and the impact of iodized salt after every 5 years in districts.
- Laboratory monitoring of iodized salt and urinary iodine excretion.
- Health education and publicity.

Significant Achievements

On liberalization of iodized salt production, salt commissioner has issued licenses to 824 salt manufacturer out of which 777 units have commenced production with annual production capacity of 222 lakhs metric tons of iodized salt. Notification banning the sale of noniodized salt for different human consumption in the entire country is already issued under "Food Safety and Standard Act 2006 and regulation 2011."

For effective implementation of National Iodized Deficiency Disorders Control Program, 34 states/UTs have established iodine deficiency disorders control cells in their state health directorate.

EXPANDED PROGRAM ON IMMUNIZATION

Introduction

Most of the communicable diseases of childhood are preventable by immunizing against certain diseases. Immunization program in India was introduced by WHO in 1978 as Expanded Program of Immunization. The program gained momentum in 1985 and was expanded as Universal Immunization Program (UIP) to be implemented in phased manner to cover all districts in the country by 1989–90. UIP has become a part of child survival and safe motherhood (CSSM) in 1992. Since 1997, UIP is an important component of reproductive and child health program and currently under National Health Mission. Under UIP, government is providing vaccination to prevent 7 vaccine preventable diseases, i.e., Diphtheria, pertussis, tetanus, polio, measles, tuberculosis and hepatitis.

Objectives

- To reduce the morbidity and mortality among children of major six childhood diseases.
- To achieve 100% coverage of eligible children by an ongoing integrated program.
- To achieve an integrated immunization services through healthcare centers, as primary healthcare services package.
- To develop a surveillance system and collect adequate information on the disease preventable by immunization.
- To minimize the efforts and cost of treatment.
- To promote a new healthy generation.

Strategies

- Integrate vaccination session with PHC centers.
- Appropriate measures to expand the vaccination coverage to the eligible population.
- Ensuring regular supply of potent vaccines.
- Strengthening the cold chain.
- Training of health personnel.
- Promotion of community participation.
- Incorporating health education activities related to EPI.
- Ensuring logistic support (supplies and equipment).

- Introducing a system for continuous monitoring and periodic evaluation.
- Undertaking operational research to find out deficiencies and difficulties in the program and suggest methods of improvement.

Pulse Polio Immunization Program

Pulse denotes sudden, simultaneous mass administration of oral polio vaccine on a single day to all children below five years of age.

Pulse polio immunization was launched in the country in 1995. Under this program children five years of age are given additional oral polio drops in December and January every year on fixed days. From 1999 to 2000, house to house vaccination of missed children was also introduced.

Milestone of the Immunization Program in India

1978 : Expanded program of immunization was introduced after smallpox eradication. Vaccination against BCG, DPT, OPV, typhoid was limited to only urban population.

1985 : Universal Immunization Program, introduced. Measles immunization was added.

1990 : Vitamin A supplementation as started.

1992 : Child survival and safe motherhood program was launched.

1995 : Polio National Immunization days were started.

1997 : Reproductive and Child Health Program (RCH-1) was launched.

2005 : RCH-II and National Rural Health Mission was launched.

2010–2011 : Hepatitis B vaccination was introduced.

2016 : Rotavirus vaccine was introduced.

Recent Update

Electronic Vaccine Intelligence Network (eVIN)

The Government of India has rolled out an Electronic Vaccine Intelligence Network (eVIN) system that digitizes the entire vaccine stock management, their logistics and temperature tracking at all levels of vaccine storage – from national to the subdistrict. This enables program managers to have real time view of the vaccine stock position and their storage temperature across all the cold chain points providing a detailed overview of the vaccine cold chain logistics system across the entire country. eVIN is to be scaled up to entire country.

Cold Chain

The "cold chain" implies to a system of storage and transport of vaccines at low temperature from the place of manufacturer to the actual vaccination site. Cold chain is necessary to prevent vaccines from getting denatured and preventing vaccine failure. The term C-4, complete care cold chain is also in vogue in maintenance of cold chain of vaccine. All vaccines must be stored under the recommended conditions of the manufacturer in the literature accompanying the vaccines otherwise they become denatured and ineffective. Vaccines which should be kept in freezer compartment are polio and measles, as polio is most sensitive to heat and must be stored at –20°C. Vaccines of typhoid, DPT, TT, DT, and BCG and diluents are stored in the cold part but never allowed to freeze.

According to WHO National Immunization Schedule (NIS) for infants, children and pregnant women (India) is given in Table 6.5.

TABLE 6.5: **National immunization schedule for infants, children and pregnant women**

Vaccine	Due age	Max age	Dose	Diluent	Route	Site
For pregnant women						
TT-1	Early in pregnancy		0.5 mL	No	Intramuscular	Upper arm
TT-2*	4 weeks after TT-1		0.5 mL	No	Intramuscular	Upper arm
TT-Booster*	If received TT doses in a pregnancy within the last 3 years		0.5 mL	No	Intramuscular	Upper arm
For infants						
BCG	At birth	Till one year of age	(0.05 mL until 1 month) 0.1 mL beyond age 1 month	Yes Manufacturer supplied diluent (Sodium chloride)	Intradermal	Upper arm — left
Hepatitis B birth dose	At birth	Within 24 hours	0.5 mL	No	Intramuscular	Anterolateral side of mid-thigh—left
bOPV-0	At birth	Within the first 15 days	2 drops	–	Oral	Oral
bOPV 1, 2 and 3	At 6, 10 and 14 weeks	Till 5 years of age	2 drops	–	Oral	Oral
Pentavalent 1, 2 and 3** (Diphtheria + pertussis + tetanus + hepatitis B + Hib)	At 6, 10 and 14 weeks**	1 year of age	0.5 mL	No	Intramuscular	Anterolateral side of mid-thigh—left
Fractional inactivated polio vaccine (IPV)	At 6 and 14 weeks	1 year of age	0.1 mL	No	Intradermal	Upper arm—right
Rotavirus + (Where applicable)	At 6, 10 and 14 weeks	1 year of age	5 drops	No	Oral	Oral

Contd...

Vaccine	Due age	Max age	Dose	Diluent	Route	Site
Pneumococcal conjugate vaccine (PCV) (Where applicable)	At 6 and 14 weeks at 9 completed months booster	1 year of age	0.5 mL	No	Intramuscular	Anterolateral side of mid-thigh—right
Measles/Rubella 1st Dose**	At 9 completed months–12 months	5 years of age	0.5 mL	Yes Manufacturer supplied diluent (Sterile water)	Subcutaneous	Upper arm—right
Japanese Encephalitis-1@ (Where applicable)	At 9 months–12 months@	15 years of age	0.5 mL	Yes Manufacturer supplied diluent (Phosphate Buffer solution)	Subcutaneous	Upper arm—left
Vitamin A (1st dose)	At 9 months	5 years of age (1 lakh IU)	1 mL	–	Oral	Oral
For children						
DPT booster -1	16–24 months	7 years of age	0.5 mL	No	Intramuscular	Anterolateral side of mid-thigh—left
Measles/Rubella 2nd dose#	16–24 months	5 years of age	0.5 mL	Yes Manufacturer supplied diluent (Sterile water)	Subcutaneous	Upper arm—right
bOPV Booster	16–24 months	5 years	2 drops	No	Oral	Oral
Japanese Encephalitis -2@ (Where applicable)	16–24 months@	Till 15 years of age	0.5 mL	Yes Manufacturer supplied diluent (Phosphate Buffer solution)	Subcutaneous	Upper arm—left
Vitamin A$(2nd to 9th dose)	At 16 months. Then, one dose every 6 months	Up to the age of 5 years	2 mL (2 lakh IU)	–	Oral	Oral

Contd...

Vaccine	Due age	Max age	Dose	Diluent	Route	Site
DPT Booster-2	5–6 years	7 years of age	0.5 mL	No	Intramuscular	Upper arm
TT	10 years and 16 years	16 years	0.5 mL	No	Intramuscular	Upper arm

*Give TT-2 or Booster doses before 36 weeks of pregnancy. However, give these even if >36 weeks have passed. Give TT to a woman in labor, if she has not previously received TT.

**Pentavalent vaccine is introduced in place of DPT and Hep B 1, 2 and 3

+Rotavirus vaccine is being introduced in phases

#MR vaccine introduced in phases replacing measles vaccine in the UIP schedule. If first dose delayed beyond 12 months ensure minimum one month gap between 2 MR doses

@JE vaccine has been introduced in selected endemic districts. If first dose is delayed beyond 12 months ensure minimum 3 months gap between 2 JE doses.

$The 2nd to 9th doses of Vitamin A can be administered to children 1–5-year-old during biannual rounds, in collaboration with ICDS.

→Human Papilloma Virus (HPV) Vaccine– presently not in schedule

→Td– Tetanus, diphtheria to replace TT – to be added in schedule

WHO recommendations for routine immunizations for children are given in Table 6.6.

TABLE 6.6: WHO recommendations for routine immunizations for children (updated April 2018)

Vaccine	Antigen	Age at 1st dose	Doses in primary series	Interval between doses 1st to 2nd	2nd to 3rd	3rd to 4th	Booster dose
Recommendations for all children							
BCG		As soon as possible after birth	1				
Hepatitis B	Option 1	As soon as possible after birth (<24 hr)	3	4 weeks (min.) with DTPcv1	4 weeks (min.) with DTPcv2	4 weeks (min.) with DTPcv3	
	Option 2	As soon as possible after birth (<24 hr)	4	4 weeks (min.) with DTPcv1	4 weeks (min.) with DTPcv2		
	bOPV + IPV	6 weeks	4 (IPV dose to be given with bOPV dose from 14 weeks)	4 weeks (min.) with DTPcv2	4 weeks (min.) with DTPcv3		

Contd...

Vaccine	Antigen	Age at 1st dose	Doses in primary series	Interval between doses			Booster dose
				1st to 2nd	2nd to 3rd	3rd to 4th	
Polio	IPV/bOPV Sequential	8 weeks (IPV 1st)	1–2 IPV 2 bOPV	4–8 weeks	4–8 weeks	4–8 weeks	
	IPV	8 weeks	3	4–8 weeks	4–8 weeks		
DTP-containing vaccine		6 weeks (min.)	3	4 weeks (min.) –8 weeks	4 weeks (min.) –8 weeks		3 Boosters 12–23 months (DTP-containing vaccine) 4–7 years (Td); and 9–15 years (Id)
Haemophilus influenza type b	Option 1	6 weeks (min.) 59 months (max.)	3	4 weeks (min.) with DTPcv2	4 weeks (min.) with DTPcv3		
	Option 2		2–3	8 weeks (min.) if only 2 doses, 4 weeks (min.) if 3 doses	4 weeks (min.) if 3 doses		At least 6 months (min.) after last dose
Pneumococcal (Conjugate)	Option 1	6 weeks (min.)	3	4 weeks (min.)	4 weeks		
	Option 2	6 weeks (min.)	2	8 weeks (min.)			9–5 months
Rotavirus	Rotarix	6 weeks (min.) with DTP 1	2	4 weeks (min.) with DTPcv2			
	RotaTeq	6 weeks (min.) with DTP1	3	4 weeks (min.)–10 weeks with DTPcv2	4 weeks (min.) with DTPcv3		
Measles		9 or 12 months (6 months min.)	2	4 weeks (min.)			
Rubella		9 or 12 months with measles containing vaccine	1				
HPV		As soon as possible from 9 years of age (females only)	2	6 months (min. 5 months)			

Contd...

Vaccine	Antigen	Age at 1st dose	Doses in primary series	Interval between doses			Booster dose
				1st to 2nd	2nd to 3rd	3rd to 4th	
Recommendations for children residing in certain regions							
Japanese encephalitis	Inactivated Vero cell-derived	6 months	2 generally	4 weeks (generally)			
	Live attenuated	8 months	1				
	Live recombinant	9 months	1				
Yellow fever		9–12 months with measles containing vaccine	1				
Tick-borne encephalitis		≥1 year FSME-IMMUN and Encepur	3	1–3 months FSME-IMMUN and Encepur	5–12 months FSME-IMMUN and Encepur 12 months		At least 1 Every 3 years
		≥3 years TBE–Moscow and Ence Vir		1–7 months TBE-Moscow and Ence Vir	TBE-Moscow and Ence Vir		
Recommendations for children in some high-risk populations							
	TCV (Typbar)	>6 months	1				Every 3 years
Typhoid	Vi PS	2 years (min.)	1				
	Ty21a	Capsules 5 years (min.)	3 or 4	1 day	1 day	1 day	Every 3–7 years
	Dukoral (WC-rBS)	2 years (min.)	3 (2–5 years) 2 (≥6 years)	≥7 days (min.) <6 weeks (max.)	≥7 days (min.) <6 weeks (max.)		Every 6 months Every 2 years

Contd...

Vaccine	Antigen	Age at 1st dose	Doses in primary series	Interval between doses			Booster dose
				1st to 2nd	2nd to 3rd	3rd to 4th	
Cholera	Shanchol, Euvichol and mORCVAX	1 year (min.)	2	14 days			After 2 years
	MenA conjugate	9–18 months (5 µg)	1				
Meningococcal	MenC conjugate	2–11 months ≥12 months	2 1	8 weeks			After 1 year
	Quadrivalent conjugate	9–23 months	2	12 weeks			
		≥2 years	1				
Hepatitis A		1 year	At least 1				
Rabies		As required	2	7 days			
Dengue (CYD-TDV)		9 years (min.)	3	6 months	6 months		
Recommendations for children receiving vaccinations from immunization programs with certain characteristics							
Mumps		12–18 months with measles containing vaccine	2	1 month (min.) to school entry			
Seasonal influenza (inactivated tri- and quadrivalent)		6 months (min.)	2 (<9 years) 1 (≥9 years)	4 weeks			Revaccinate annually 1 dose only
Varicella		12–18 months	1–2	4 weeks to 3 months per manufacturer recommendations			

Nursing Considerations

Remember

- Only disposable syringes should be used.
- Hepatitis B dose is given only within 24 hours after birth as it helps to prevent prenatal transmission of hepatitis B.
- OPV-0 dose is given within 15 days after birth. OPV can be given up to till 5 years of age.
- Pentavalent vaccines contain a combination of DPT, hepatitis B and Hib. Hepatitis B birth dose and booster dose of DPT will continue as before.
- Interval between 2 doses of pentavalent, OPV and hepatitis-B should not be less than one month.
- There is no restriction of vaccination in case of minor cough, cold and minor fevers.

Know about Hazards of Immunization

- **Local reaction:** At the site of vaccination there may be swelling, redness and pain which disappears after 48 hours.
- **General reaction:** It includes nausea, vomiting, fever, headache, uneasiness. If these signs appear, should be reported to the doctor.
- **Allergic reaction:** These are due to hypersensitivity of person toward immunizing agents. In case of anaphylactic shock, it can be life-threatening reaction. It can be immediate or delayed. Symptoms of anaphylactic reactions are tachycardia, dyspnea, cold and clammy skin, itching, rashes on the skin, fainting and low blood pressure. The symptom should be noted and immediate intervention is to be taken. Symptoms of serum sickness are fever, rashes on the skin, swelling, pain in joints develop after 7–12 days after vaccination.
- Abscess formation at the site of vaccination due to technical errors, due to defective sterilization or technique not following the cold chain.

Responsibilities of Community Health Nurse in Immunization

- Should have thorough knowledge and practice of immunization schedule.
- Should supervise the work of health team engaged in immunization.
- The hazards of vaccination should be prevented by accurate technique and precautions.
- Children or people with normal health should be vaccinated only.
- Children suffering from high fever, acute respiratory tract infection, seizure or during any severe illness, vaccination should be postponed.
- Malnourished children should be vaccinated but their parents should be advised regarding proper nutrition of the child.
- Before the administration of antitoxin or antiserum, allergy test should be done.
- Emergency medicine, equipment, oxygen and all antianaphylactic drugs should be ready at hand to handle emergency. All health workers dealing with immunization should have thorough practice for the management of anaphylaxis.
- Only disposable syringes and needles should be used.
- Cold chain should be maintained.
- Restraints can be used for vaccinating children.
- During pregnancy, precautions should be taken while administering vaccines other than tetanus toxoid
- Follow the six rights of medications, right patient, right drug, right dose, right route, right time and right person.
- Reassure children and mothers. Inform about next immunization sessions.

NATIONAL FAMILY WELFARE PROGRAM

Topic is discussed in Unit 7.

NATIONAL WATER SUPPLY AND SANITATION PROGRAM

National Water Supply and Sanitation Program was introduced in 1954, in the first year of Five-Year Plan. The objectives of the program were to provide safe water supply and adequate drainage facilities for the entire urban and rural population of the country. The states gradually built up the public health engineering departments (PHED) to tackle the problem of rural water supply and sanitation. In spite of this, it was found in mid 1960s that majority of the scheme was implemented in easily accessible villages whereas the remote villages are devoid of this facility where they have severe water scarcity. In 1972, a special program was started which was known as accelerated rural water supply program as a supplement to the National Water Supply and Sanitation Program. In spite of increased financial outlay, only a small dent was made on the overall problem. During the fifth Five-Year Plan, rural water supply was included in minimum needs program of the state plans. The Government of India requested the states to identify the problem villages through assistance under accelerated rural water supply program.

DRINKING WATER SUPPLY PROGRAMS AND POLICIES

1949 : The Environment Hygiene Committee recommends the provision of safe water supply to cover 90% of Indians.

1950 : The constitution of India confers ownership of all water resources to the government specifying it as a state subject, giving citizens the right to potable water.

1969 : National Rural Drinking Water Supply Program was launched with technical supply from UNICEF.

1972 : Introduction of the Accelerated Rural Water Supply Program (ARWSP) by the Government of India.

1981 : India as a party to the international drinking water supply and sanitation.

1986 : The national drinking water mission (NDWM) was formed.

1987 : Drafting of the first national water policy by the Ministry of Water Resources.

1991 : National drinking water mission (NDWM) is renamed as the Rajiv Gandhi National Drinking Water Mission (RGNDWM).

1994 : The 73rd constitutional amendment assigns Panchayati Raj institutions (PRIs) the responsibility of providing drinking water.

1999 : Paradigm shift from the "government-oriented supply-driven approaches" to the people-oriented demand-responsive approach.

2002 : Nationwide scaling up of sector reform in the form of Swajaldhara.

2004 : All drinking water programs are brought under the umbrella of the RGNDWM.

2005 : The Government of India launches the Bharat Nirman Program for overall development of rural areas.

2007 : Pattern of funding under the Swajaldhara scheme changes from the previous 90:10 central community share to 50:50 center state shares.

2007–2012: Eleventh Five-Year Plan foresees the provision of safe drinking water to all rural habitations.

> **Recent Update**
>
> The Government of India's centrally sponsored scheme, the National Rural Drinking Water Program (NRDWP), was restructured and subsumed into Jal Jeevan Mission (JJM) to provide Functional Household Tap Connection (FHTC) to every rural household, i.e., Har Ghar Jal, by 2024.

SWAJALDHARA

This program was launched by the Government of India on 25th December 2002. It is an initiative in the rural drinking water supply sector. It was opened up throughout the country as a community-based rural water supply program.

Principles of Swajaldhara

- Adoption of a demand-driven responsive and adaptable approach.
- Community participation based on empowerment of villages to ensure full participation in the project.
- Full ownership of drinking water assets at the Panchayat level.
- Panchayat/Communities to have the power to plan, implement, operate, maintain and manage all water supply and sanitation schemes.
- Partial capital cost sharing either in cash or kind including labor or both, 100% responsibility of operation and maintenance by the users.
- An integrated service delivery mechanism.
- Taking up conservation measures through rainwater harvesting and groundwater recharge system for sustained drinking water supply.

NATIONAL SANITATION PROGRAM

Rural Sanitation Program

The activities under this program are as follows:
- Demand-driven low-cost sanitation approach.
- Involvement of private bodies, NGOs, to provide sanitation facilities.
- Entrusting the responsibility of operation and maintenance of water supply and sanitation upon the Panchayati Raj institutions and local administrative.
- Improving the sanitation in rural areas through IEC programs.
- Converting all existing dry latrines to low-cost sanitary latrines.

Urban Sanitation Program

The activities considered under this program are as follows:
- To provide reasonable level of sanitation facility to a large population.
- Total elimination of dry latrines and manual scavenging.
- Onsite low-cost sanitation in unsewered parts of cities, small and medium towns.
- Technological innovation to improve the reusability of the recycled waste.

- Polluter paying principles should be applied to finance waste disposal program.
- Involvement of NGOs, private sector and community.
- Converting all existing dry latrines to low-cost sanitary latrine.
- Recycling the treated effluents for horticulture, irrigation and water harvesting and transport system for solid waste disposal.

NIRMAL BHARAT ABHIYAN

Nirmal Bharat Abhiyan (NBA) was launched in 2012 in the 12th Five-Year Plan.

Objectives

To achieve sustainable behavioral change with provision of sanitary facilities in entire communities. This must be done in a phased manner. Saturation mode with "Nirmal Grams" as outcomes.

SWACHH BHARAT MISSION

Swachh Bharat Mission (SBM) is a National campaign by the Government of India to clean roads, streets and infrastructure of the country. It was launched by the Prime Minister of India on 2nd October 2014.

Aims

- To eradicate open defecation by the year 2019 by construction 12 million toilets in rural India.
- Mission has two submissions, i.e., Swachh Bharat Mission–Urban and Swachh Bharat Mission–Gramin (SBM–G).

Swachh Bharat Mission–Gramin

The mission in rural India means improving the level of cleanliness in rural areas through solid and liquid waste management.

Objectives

- To bring improvement in general quality of life in rural area, promoting cleanliness, hygiene and eliminating open defecation.
- Accelerate sanitation coverage in rural area to achieve the Vision of Swachh Bharat by 2nd October 2019.
- Motivate communities and Panchayati Raj Institutions to adopt sustainable sanitation practice and facilities through IEC.
- Encourage cost-effective and appropriate technologies for ecologically safe and sustainable sanitation.
- Develop community managed sanitation system wherever required focusing on solid and liquid waste management system for overall cleanliness in the rural areas.

Swachh Bharat Mission–Urban

Swachh Bharat Mission–Urban (SBM–U) is being implemented by Ministry of Urban Development.

Objectives

- To eliminate open defecation.
- To eradicate manual scavenging.
- To manage modern and scientific municipal solid waste.
- To effect behavioral change regarding healthy sanitation practices.
- To generate awareness about sanitation and its linkage with public health capacity augmentation for urban local bodies (ULBs).
- To create an enabling environment for private sector participation in capital expenditure and operation and maintenance.

MINIMUM NEEDS PROGRAM

Introduction

The Minimum Needs Program (MNP) was introduced in the first year of fifth Five-Year Plan (1974–1978).

Objectives

- To provide certain basic minimum needs and thereby improving the living standard of the people.
- It is the expression of the commitment of the government for the "social and economic development of the community particularly the underprivileged and underserved population".

Components

The components of minimum needs program are (Fig. 6.9) as follows:

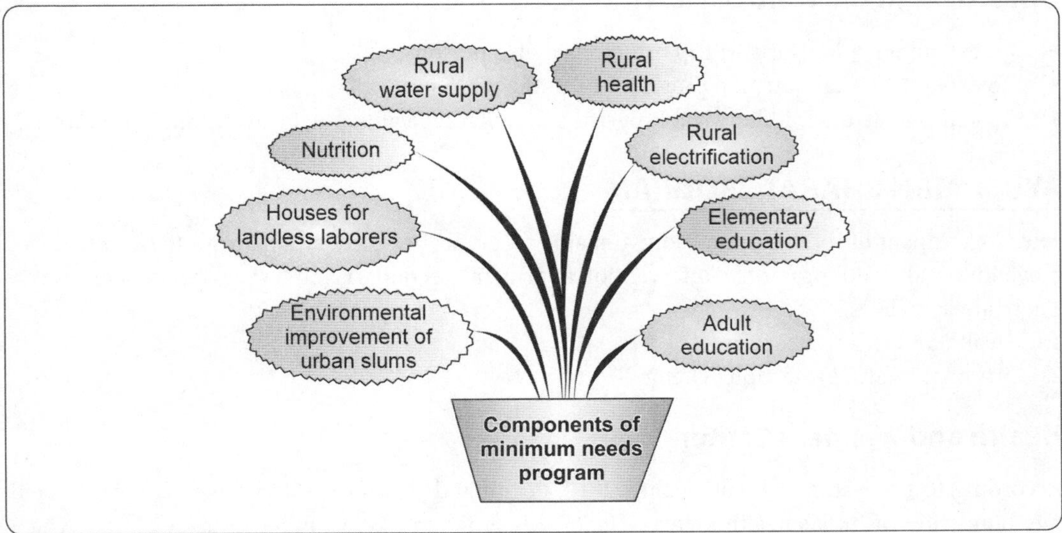

Figure 6.9: Components of minimum needs program

- Rural health
- Rural water supply
- Rural electrification
- Elementary education
- Adult education
- Nutrition
- Environmental improvement of urban slums
- Houses for landless laborers.

Principles

There are two basic principles which are to be observed in implementation of MNP:
1. The facilities under MNP are to be first provided to those areas which are at present underserved so as to remove disparities between different areas.
2. The facilities under MNP should be provided as a package to an area through intersectoral area projects to have a greater impact.

Goals to be Achieved

In the field of rural health, the objectives to be achieved by the end of the eighth Five-Year Plan under the minimum needs program were:
- One PHC for 30,000 population in plains and 20,000 population in tribal and hilly areas.
- One subcenter for 5000 population in the plains and 3000 in tribal and hilly areas.
- One community health center (rural hospital) for a population of one lakh or one community development block by the year 2000.

    The establishment of PHCs, subcenter upgradation of PHCs and construction of buildings thereof are all included in the state sector of the minimum need program.

Objectives in the Field of Nutrition Care

- To extend nutrition support to 11 million eligible persons.
- To expand "special nutrition program" to all the ICDS projects.
- To consolidate the Midday Meal Program and link it to health, potable water and sanitation.

AYUSHMAN BHARAT PROGRAM

The Government of India announced two major programs in February 2018 with the aim to cover preventive and health promotive intervention at primary, secondary and tertiary healthcare system. These are as follows:
1. Health and wellness center
2. National Health Protection Scheme

Health and Wellness Center

According to the National Health Policy 2017, health and wellness centers have been considered the foundation of India's health system. Under this program, there will be 1.5 lakh centers which will bring healthcare system close to the homes of people. These healthcare centers will deliver comprehensive healthcare including for communicable diseases and maternal and child health services. The centers will also provide free essential drugs and diagnostic services.

National Health Protection Scheme or Pradhan Mantri Jan Arogya Yojana

The second program under Ayushman Bharat is National Health Protection Scheme or Pradhan Mantri Jan Arogya Yojana (PMJAY). This scheme includes the following programs:

- The National Sample Survey Organization during its 71st round concluded that >17% of Indian population spends minimum 10% of their household budget on health services which leads the families into debt. About 82% of the urban and 85.9% of rural population have no access to healthcare insurance.
- PMJAY scheme will help to reduce out of pocket hospitalization expenses, fulfill unmet needs and improve access of identified families to quality inpatient care and day care surgeries.
- PMJAY will provide a coverage of ₹5 lakh per family per year for secondary and tertiary care hospitalization through a network of empaneled healthcare providers (EHCP).
- EHCP network will cover 1350 procedures including pre- and post hospitalization, diagnostics and medicine, etc. The access to EHCP services will be cashless and paperless to the beneficiaries.
- PMJAY beneficiaries will have access to services across the country anywhere through the provider network. No formal enrolment is required as the scheme is entitled based.
- PMJAY will target deprived rural families and identified occupational category of urban workers' families as per the latest Socio-Economic Caste Census (SECC) data covering both rural and urban.

  SECC will benefit:
  - Ragpickers, beggars, domestic workers, street vendors/cobblers/hawkers/other service providers working on streets, construction workers, plumbers, masonry workers/painters, welders/security guards.
  - Coolies and other head load workers.
  - Sweepers/sanitation workers/mali.
  - Home-based workers/artisan/handicrafts/helper to drivers and conductors, cart pullers, rickshaw pullers.
  - Shop workers/assistants/peon in small establishments/helpers/delivery assistants.
  - Electricians/mechanics/assemblers/repair workers.
  - Washer men/chowkidars.

  As per SECC 2011, automatically excluded are as follows:
  - Household having motorized 2/3/4 wheelers
  - Mechanized 2/3/4 wheelers agricultural equipment
  - Household with kisan credit card with limit ₹50,000/-
  - Any member earning >10000/ month
  - Household paying income tax, professional tax
  - Household with three or more pacca rooms owning telephone, refrigerator, and owning >2.5 acres land with irrigation equipment, all such enrolled families under Rashtriya Swasthya Bima Yojana (RSBY) that do not come under targeted groups as per SECC data, will also be included.

Categories Covered Under PMJAY

In rural population, the totally deprived household targeted for PMRSSM who come under six deprivation criteria are categorized as D_1, D_2, D_3, D_4, D_5, D_7.

D_1 : Only one room with kuccha walls and kuccha roof.

D_2 : No adult member between age 16 and 59.

D_3 : Female headed household with no adult male member between age 16–59

D_4 : Disabled member and no able-bodied adult member

D_5 : SC/ST household

D_7 : Landless households deriving major part of their income from manual casual labor.

Automatically included:

- Household without shelter
- Destitute/living on alms
- Manual scavenger families
- Primitive tribal group
- Legally released bonded labor.

NATIONAL DIABETES CONTROL PROGRAM

Introduction

Diabetes is a metabolic disease caused due to defective production or action of insulin hormone that controls glucose, fat and an amino acid metabolism. It is of two types:

1. **Type-I:** Insulin dependent diabetes mellitus.
2. **Type-II:** Noninsulin dependent diabetes mellitus.

Due to deficiency of insulin, there is an increased concentration of glucose in the blood. In type-I diabetes; pancreas fails to produce insulin that is essential for survival. However, in type-II noninsulin dependent diabetes, insulin produced is either not enough or the insulin produced is not effective enough. This type of diabetes occurs in adults.

Burden of the Disease

As per the estimation (2011 census) 61.3 million people aged 20–79 years live with diabetes in India. This number is expected to increase to 101.2 million by 2030 and 77.2 million people in India are expected to have prediabetes. The 2019 data showed that 77 million people above the age of 18 years are having type-2 diabetes which is 57% of individuals who remain undiagnosed. As per ICMR report 2023, prevalence of diabetes is 10.1 crore.

Program

Government of India started National Diabetes Control Program during the 7th Five-Year Plan in 1987 on pilot basis in some districts of Tamil Nadu, J&K and Karnataka, but due to deficiency of funds, in subsequent years, the program could not be expanded further in remaining years. A sum of 12 lakhs was allocated during 1995–96 for the program and in 1997–98, another one crore was allotted for the program.

Objectives of the Program

- To prevent and control diabetes through identification of high-risk cases and early intervention in the form of health education.
- To diagnose early and appropriate treatment of the cases.
- To prevent acute and chronic metabolic, cardiovascular, renal and ocular complications of the disease.
- To provide equal opportunity for physical attainment and scholastic achievement for the diabetic patients.
- To establish and develop capability for palliative care and rehabilitation to the partially or totally handicapped due to diabetes.

POLIO ERADICATION—PULSE POLIO PROGRAM

Introduction

Pulse Polio Program is being conducted all over the country with the objective of eradicating polio. Pulse denotes sudden, simultaneous, mass administration of oral polio vaccine (OPV) on a single day to all children below 5 years of age. This program is related directly to the pulse of polio, i.e., prevention of polio. So it is called pulse polio immunization.

Following world health assembly resolution in 1988, Pulse Polio Immunization Program was launched in India in 1995 with the aim to eradicate polio. Children in the age group of 0–5 years administered polio drops during national and subnational immunization rounds (in high-risk areas) every year. About 172 million children are immunized during each national immunization day (NID).

Objectives

The Pulse Polio Initiative (PPI) was started with an objective of achieving 100% coverage under oral vaccine. It aimed to immunize children through improved social mobilization, plan mop up operations in areas where polio virus has almost disappeared and maintain high level of morale among the public.

Aims

- The pulse polio-immunization aims at covering every child in the country. It aspires to reach children even in remote communities through an improved social mobilization plan.
- Not a single child should miss the immunization, leaving no chance of polio occurrence.
- Cases of acute flaccid paralysis (AFP) to be reported in time and their stool specimens to be collected within 14 days. Outbreak response immunization to be conducted as early as possible.
- Maintaining a high level of surveillance.
- Performance of good mop-up operations where polio has disappeared.

Activities

- Setting up of booths in all parts of the country.

- Initializing walk-in cold rooms, freezer rooms, deep freezers, ice lined refrigerators and cold boxes for a steady supply of vaccines to booths.
- Arranging employees, volunteers and vaccines.
- Ensuring vaccines by monitoring on each vaccine vial.
- Immunizing children with OPV on national immunization day.
- Identifying missing children from immunization process.
- Surveillance of efficacy.

Number of Polio Cases in India

Number of polio cases in India is given in Table 6.7.

Progress

- South-East Asia region of WHO including India has been certified polio free by "the regional certification commission (RCC) on 27th March 2014".
- India reported its last polio case from district of Howrah, West Bengal on 13th January 2011.
- WHO on 24th February 2012 removed India from the list of "Endemic countries with active polio virus transmission".
- There are 24 lakh vaccinators and 1.5 lakh supervisors involved in the successful implementation of the Pulse Polio Program.

Injectable Inactivated Poliovirus Vaccine

India joined 125 other countries to introduce inactivated poliovirus vaccine (IPV) into routine immunization as a part of polio eradication and endgame strategic plan. IPV is given along with third dose of oral polio vaccine (OPV) at 14 weeks of age for children under 1 year of age. The main aim of giving IPV along with OPV is to strengthen the children's immune system and to provide double protection against polio. It will be introduced along with routine immunization as per the world health assembly meeting on May 2012.

TABLE 6.7: Year-wise number of polio cases in India

Year	Number of polio cases	Year	Number of polio cases
1998	1934	2006	676
1999	1126	2007	874
2000	255	2008	554
2001	258	2009	741
2002	1600	2010	42
2003	225	2011	01
2004	134	2012	00
2005	66	2013	00
Contd...		2014 Till March	00

Steps Taken by the Government of India to Maintain Polio free Status in India

- Maintaining community immunity through high quality national and subnational polio rounds each year.
- An extremely high level of vigilance through surveillance across the country for any importation or circulation of poliovirus.
- By immunizing children under 5 year of age in spite of having received regular immunization
- Arranging pulse-polio immunization days at national level.
- Monitoring every case of polio through effective surveillance at national level.
- Involving ASHA as a team member for mobilization and vaccination of children.
- Conducting special rounds of vaccination in areas where polio has been detected.

NATIONAL CANCER CONTROL PROGRAM

Introduction

Cancer is an important health problem in the country. Every year about 10 lakh new cases are reported. It is estimated that there are about 2.8 million of cancer cases at any given point of time in the country. The Cancer Control Program was introduced in India in 1975–76. It was revised in 1984. In order to cater the changing needs of the disease, the program has undergone three revisions with 3rd revision in 2004. This program has now been integrated with program for prevention and control of cancer, cardiovascular disease, diabetes and stroke since 2010.

Objectives

- To promote primary prevention of cancer by health education especially regarding tobacco consumption and necessity for genital hygiene for prevention of cervical cancer.
- To promote secondary prevention, i.e., early detection and diagnosis of common cancer such as cervix, mouth, breast and tobacco related cancer by screening/self-examination method.
- Tertiary prevention, i.e., strengthening of the existing institutions of comprehensive therapy including palliative care.

Revised National Cancer Control Program

Under the revised program, the following schemes are there:

Regional Cancer Center Scheme

The existing regional cancer centers are being further strengthened to act as referral centers for complicated and difficult cases at the tertiary level. One-time assistance of ₹3 crore during the plan period is provided to regional cancer centers (except Tata Memorial Hospital, Mumbai and IRCH [AIIMS]) for strengthening and to the Chittaranjan National Cancer Institute (CNCI) Kolkata on the approved pattern of funding.

Oncology Wing Development Scheme

The scheme has been initiated to fill up geographical gaps in the availability of cancer treatment facilities in the country. The central assistance of ₹3 crore is provided for the purchase of equipment which include cobalt unit besides other equipment. A part of the grant can be used for the civil work but manpower to be provided by the concerned state.

Decentralized NGO Scheme

This scheme is meant for IEC activities. It is operated by nodal agencies. NGOs are given financial assistance, i.e., ₹8000 per camp in undertaking health education and early detection activities of cancer.

IEC Activities at Central Level

At the central level, IEC activities are initiated to provide wider publicity about anti-tobacco legislation for discouraging the consumption of tobacco in any form and its ill effects on health. Wider publicity would be given about rules being formulated for implementation of various provisions of the anti-tobacco legislation. November 7th is observed as National Cancer Awareness Day in the country.

Research and Training

Training program and research activities will be organized at the central level under this scheme. The training manuals developed are as follows:
- Manual for health professional
- Manual for palliative care
- Manual for cytology
- Manual for tobacco cessation

Cancer Services Under the NCCP

- Common diagnostic services, basic surgery, chemotherapy and palliative care are made available in 100 district hospitals.
- Each district is being supported with ₹1.66 crore per annum for the following:
  - Chemotherapy facilities for 100 patients in each district hospital.
  - Day care chemotherapy at 100 district hospitals.
  - Facilities for laboratory investigations including mammography in 100 district hospitals.
- Home-based palliative care.
- Support is being provided for contractual manpower through one medical officer (MO) oncologist, 1 cytopathologist, 1 cytopathology technician, two nurses for day care.
- State cancer institute (SCI) will provide comprehensive cancer diagnosis, treatment and care services. SCI will be apex institution in the state for cancer treatment activities.
- 45 centers were to be strengthened as tertiary cancer centers (TCCs) to provide comprehensive cancer care services at a cost of ₹6.00 crore each during 2011–12. At present, there are 62 cancer centers providing treatment to all states and UTs.

YAWS ERADICATION PROGRAM

Introduction

Yaws is a chronic bacterial infection caused by *Treponema pertenue*. It is a nonvenereal disease and spreads through direct contact with the skin of an infected person. The disease affects the skin, bones and cartilage causing disability. Skin exhibits early lesions followed by scarring on healing. Yaws most commonly affects the children in tropical regions. In India, it is reported from the tribal communities living in hilly, forest and difficult to reach areas in 49 districts of 10 states namely Andhra Pradesh, Assam, Chhattisgarh, Gujarat, Jharkhand, Madhya Pradesh, Maharashtra, Odisha, Uttar Pradesh and Tamil Nadu.

Objectives

- To achieve no case of transmission of yaws infection in the country.
- To eradicate yaws from the country.

The government of Andhra Pradesh, Gujarat, Madhya Pradesh and Odisha has taken several initiatives for interruption of infection by mass administration of single dose of penicillin in the affected areas. "Yaws cells" have been established in divisions of epidemiology to coordinate all activities.

Strategies of the Program

- Developing manpower
- Detection of cases
- Carry out treatment of cases and contacts
- IEC activities through multisectoral approach.

Activities of the Program

The case detection is carried out by active surveillance, i.e., house to house visit by trained paramedical workers and treatment of cases and contacts simultaneously and immediately after detection. In such cases a colored recognition cards are given to patients.

Treatment

Yaws can be cured by single injection of long acting penicillin (Benzathine benzyl).

WHO recommended three modes of treatment:

1. **Total mass treatment:** In areas where yaws is hyperendemic (>10% prevalence of clinically active yaws), treatment is given to all irrespective of disease status of person.
2. **Juvenile mass treatment:** In mesoendemic communities (6–10% prevalence), treatment is given to all cases and to all children under 15 years of age and other obvious contacts of infectious cases.
3. **Selective mass treatment:** In hypoendemic (<5% prevalence), treatment is confined to cases, their household and other obvious contacts of infectious cases.

Program Management

The National Institute of Communicable Diseases (NICD) has been identified as the nodal agency for planning, guidance, coordination, monitoring and evaluation of the program. The program is implemented by the state health directorate of yaws endemic states utilizing existing healthcare delivery system with the coordination and collaboration of tribal welfare and other related institutions. Director General of health services and Ministry of health form the task force to coordinate and review program.

NATIONAL NUTRITIONAL ANEMIA PROPHYLAXIS PROGRAM

Introduction

The National Nutritional Anemia Prophylaxis Program (NNAPP) was launched in 1970 to prevent nutritional anemia in pregnant and lactating mothers, infants and children. Under this program, the expectant and nursing mothers, and acceptors of family planning are given iron and folic acid tablets. The program is being taken up by maternal and child health (MCH) division of Ministry of Health and Family Welfare. At present, the National Nutritional Anemia Prophylaxis is operated as a part of RCH program. Under the revised policy, the target group has been expanded to include infants aged 6–12 months, school children and adolescent 11–18 years of age clinically found to be anemic.

Specific Objectives

- To assess the baseline of nutritional anemia in mother and young children through estimation of hemoglobin level.
- To put the mothers and children with low Hb levels <10 g and <8 g respectively on antianemia treatment.
- To put the mothers with Hb level >10 g and children with Hb level >8 g on the prophylaxis program.
- To monitor continuously the quality of the tablets, distribution and consumption of supplements.
- To assess periodically the Hb level of beneficiaries.
- To motivate mothers to consume the tablets through relevant nutrition education.

Activities

The program focuses on the following activities:
- Promotion of regular consumption of food rich in iron.
- Supply of iron and folic acid supplements in the form of tablets to the target group.
- Identification and treatment of severe anemia cases.
- The program also includes health and nutrition education to improve overall dietary intakes and promote consumption of iron and folate rich foods as well as food items that promote iron absorption.

Dosage Schedule

- **Children 6–60 months:** 20 mg elemental iron +100 µg folic acid (one table of pediatrics IFA or 5 mL of IFA syrup or 1 mL of IFA drops) for a total of 100 days if the child clinically found to be anemic.
- **School children 6–10 years:** 30 mg elemental iron + 250 mg folic acid for 100 days.
- **Adolescents (11–18 years):** 100 mg elemental iron + 500 µg (microgram) folic acid for 100 days.
- **Pregnant mothers:** One tablet of 100 mg elemental iron + 500 µg folic acid for 100 days.
- **Nursing mothers and acceptors of family planning:** One tablet containing 100 mg elemental iron + 500 µg folic acid for 100 days.

Organization

The program is implemented through the primary health centers and its subcenters. The multipurpose health workers female and other paramedical staff in PHCs are responsible for the distribution of IFA tablets (Adult and pediatric doses) to beneficiaries. The functionaries of ICDS scheme assist in implementation of the program.

TWENTY POINT PROGRAM

Twenty point program was started in 1975 by the Government of India to promote social justice and economic development of the country in addition to the running of Five-Year Plans and programs. The program was restructured in 1982 and again in 1986 with the introduction of new policies and program, it was finally restructured in 2006 and it has been in operation w.e.f. April 1, 2007.

The 20 points program consists of the following points:

- Point 1   :   Attack on rural poverty
- Point 2   :   Strategy for rained agriculture
- Point 3   :   Better use of irrigation water
- Point 4   :   Bigger harvest
- Point 5   :   Enforcement of land reforms
- Point 6   :   Special program for rural labor
- Point 7   :   Clean drinking water
- Point 8   :   Health for all
- Point 9   :   Two children norm
- Point 10 :   Expansion of education
- Point 11 :   Justice for SC/ST
- Point 12 :   Equality for women
- Point 13 :   New opportunities for women
- Point 14 :   Housing for the people
- Point 15 :   Improvement for slums
- Point 16 :   New strategy for forestry
- Point 17 :   Protection of environment
- Point 18 :   Concern for the consumer
- Point 19 :   Energy for the villages
- Point 20 :   A responsive administration

At least eight points out of the aforementioned 20 points are directly or indirectly related to health.

These 8 points are as follows:

- Point 1   :   Attack on rural poverty
- Point 7   :   Clean drinking water
- Point 8   :   Health for all
- Point 9   :   Two children norm
- Point 10 :   Expansion of education
- Point 14 :   Housing for the people
- Point 15 :   Improvement of slums
- Point 17 :   Protection of the environment

Twenty Points of the Restructured Program, 2006

The 20 points of the restructured program of 2006 are as follows:
1. Poverty eradication
2. Power to people
3. Support to farmers
4. Labor welfare
5. Food security
6. Clean drinking water
7. Housing for all
8. Health for all
9. Education for all
10. Welfare of Sc/ST/OBC and minorities
11. Women welfare
12. Child welfare
13. Youth development
14. Improvement of slums
15. Environment protection and afforestation
16. Social security
17. Rural roads
18. Energizing of rural areas
19. Development of backward areas
20. IT enabled and e-governance

INTEGRATED CHILD DEVELOPMENT SCHEME PROGRAM

Introduction

Integrated Child Development Scheme (ICDS) is the most important scheme in the field of child welfare. ICDS was launched on October 2, 1975 first on experimental basis of 33 projects in 4 urban areas, 19 rural and 10 tribal areas spread over 22 states and union territory of Delhi. The positive results of the scheme led to the expansion of the scheme to all the states of the country.

The ICDS scheme seeks to lay a solid foundation for the development of the nation's human resource by providing an integrated package of early childhood services. These services consist of:
- Supplementary nutrition
- Immunization
- Health checkup
- Medical referral services
- Nutrition and health education for women.
- Nonformal education for children up to the age of 6 years pregnant and nursing mothers of rural, urban, slums and tribal areas.
- ICDS scheme is designed to provide preventive and development effort.

Objectives

- To improve the nutritional and health status of children in the age group 0–6 years.
- To lay the foundation for proper psychological, physical and social development of the child.
- To reduce mortality and morbidity, malnutrition and school dropout.
- To achieve an effective coordination of policy and implementation among the various departments working for the promotion of child development.
- To enhance the capability of the mothers and nutritional needs of the child through proper nutrition and health education.

Funding of the Scheme

Central government provides 50% of the expenditure to the states and UTs.

Services are provided at Anganwadi centers, subcenter, PHC and CHC.

The population norms of setting up of Anganwadi center (AWC) and Mini-AWC have been revised to cover all habitation by SC/ST minorities. The revised norms are as follows:

For AWC in rural/urban projects:

- One Anganwadi center for 400–800 population.
- Two Anganwadi centers for 800–1600 population.
- Three Anganwadi centers for 1600–2400 population.

Thereafter one AWC for multiples of 800 population. Mini AWC – one mini AWC for150–400 population.

For tribal/desert/hilly and other difficult areas:

- One AWC for 300–800 population.
- One Mini AWC for 150–300 population.

Administrative Units

The ICDS is centered on Anganwadi workers who are from the local area. There is one supervisor for 20–25 Anganwadi workers, 4 supervisors for 100 Anganwadi workers are under one child development officer (CDPO).

Delivery of Services

- **Supplementary nutrition:** This includes supplementary feeding, growth monitoring and prophylaxis against vitamin A deficiency and control of nutritional anemia:
  - Each child 6–72 months of age gets 500 calories and 12–15 g of protein.
  - Severely malnourished child 6–72 months gets 800 calories and 20–25 g of protein.
  - Each pregnant and nursing mother to get 600 calories and 18–20 g of protein. Supplementary nutrition is given 300 days in a year.
- **Nutritional health education:** Education on nutrition and health should be given to all women in the age group 15–45 years, giving priority to nursing and expectant mothers. It is imparted by specially organized courses in village during home visits by Anganwadi workers.
- **Immunization:** Immunization against 6 vaccine-preventable diseases is being done. Expectant mothers are immunized against tetanus.

- **Health checkup:**
  - This includes antenatal care of expectant mothers and postnatal care including care of newborn babies.
  - Care of children under 6 years of age.
  - Besides antenatal and postnatal care, women are given iron and folic acid tablets along with protein supplements. High-risk mothers are referred to appropriate institutions for management. The healthcare of children under 6 years includes:
    - Height and weight record at periodical intervals.
    - Watch over milestone.
    - Immunization
    - General checkup in every 3–6 months to detect disease or malnutrition.
    - Treatment of diseases like diarrhea, dysentery and respiratory tract infections, etc.
    - Prophylaxis against deficiency of vitamin A and anemia.
    - Deworming.
    - Referral of serious cases to hospitals. Records are maintained and one card containing records of health is given to parents.
- **Preschool nonformal education:** The nonformal preschool education component of the ICDS may be well-considered backbone of the ICDS program since all its services are covered at the Anganwadi center.
- **Referral services:** During health checkups and growth monitoring, sick or malnourished children in need of prompt medical attention are referred to the primary health center or its subcenters.

MIDDAY MEAL PROGRAM

Midday Meal Program was started in 1961. It is also known as school lunch program. The program has been in operation throughout the country.

Major Objectives

- To attract more children for admission to the schools.
- To improve the school attendance and reduce dropout.
- To improve the literacy of children.
- To promote social integration.
- To improve the nutrition of children and inculcate good food habits.
- To prevent malnutrition of children.

Principles

- The meal should be supplement and not a substitute of the home diet.
- The meal should provided at least one-third of the total calorie requirement and half the protein needed.
- The cost of the meal should be reasonably low.
- The locally available food items should be included to reduce the meal cost.
- The menu should be such that it can be prepared easily.
- Variety of menu should be provided to avoid monotony.

Goals to be Achieved

- Incorporating nutritional education to the school curriculum.
- Improve school attendance and retention of children.

A model menu prepared by National Institute of Nutrition, Hyderabad

Food stuffs	g/day/child
Cereal and millets	75
Pulses	30
Oils and fats	8
Leafy vegetables	30
Nonleafy vegetables	30

As per the view of National Institute of Nutrition, Hyderabad, the minimum feeding days in a year should be 250 to have a desired impact on children.

Midday Meal Program became a part of Minimum Needs Program in 5th Five-Year Plan.

MIDDAY MEAL SCHEME

Introduction

Midday Meal Scheme is also known as National Program of Nutritional Support to Primary Education. It was launched as a centrally sponsored scheme on 15th August 1995 and revised in 2004. It was implemented in 2,408 blocks in the first year and covered the whole country in a phased manner by 1997–98. The program originally covered the children of primary stage (class I–V) in government local body and government aided schools and was expanded in October 2002 to cover children studying in Education Guarantee Scheme and alternative and innovative education centers also.

Objectives

- To increase enrolment, improve school attendance as well as retention.
- To promote school integration.
- To improve nutritional status of the primary school children.
- To inculcate good food habits in children.
- To protect children from classroom hunger.
- To improve socialization among children.
- To improve the issues of malnutrition among the children.
- To encourage children from poor background to attend school regularly and help them to concentrate in school activities.
- To provide nutritional support to students in drought ridden areas throughout summer vacation.

The central assistance provided to states under the program is byway of free supply of food grains from nearest Food Corporation of India godown at the rate of 100 g per student per school per day and subsidy for transport of food grains. To achieve the objectives a cooked midday meal with minimum 300 calories and 8–12 g of protein content will be provided to all children in class I–V.

Revised Midday Meal Scheme

In October 2007, the scheme was extended to cover children of upper primary section of classes VI to VIII studying in 3479 educationally backward blocks since 2008–2009 the scheme covers all children of VI to VIII classes of the country studying in government schools, education guarantee schemes and alternative and innovative centers. The minimum nutrition provided to upper primary section per child per day is given as follows:

Calories   – 700
Protein   – 20 g
Food grains   – 150 g

NATIONAL MENTAL HEALTH PROGRAM

Introduction

The National Mental Health Program (NMHP) was launched in 1982 in order to ensure availability and accessibility of minimum mental healthcare services for all to encourage mental health knowledge and skill and to promote community participation in mental health services development and to motivate self-help in the community.

Aims

- Prevention and treatment of mental and neurological disorders and their associated disabilities.
- Use of mental health technology to improve general health services.
- Application of mental health principles in total national development to improve quality of life.

Objectives

- To ensure availability and accessibility of minimum mental healthcare for all in the foreseeable future, particularly to the most vulnerable and underprivileged section of population.
- To encourage application of mental health knowledge in general healthcare and social development.
- To promote community participation in the mental health services department and to stimulate efforts toward self-help in the community.

MENTAL HEALTH POLICY

Mental Health Policy was launched on October 10, 2014 with the vision of promoting general mental health, preventing mental illness, enabling recovery and socioeconomic inclusion of persons affected by mental illness by providing accessible, affordable and quality health and social care to all persons through their life span. The goal is to reduce stress, disability, exclusion, morbidity and premature mortality associated with mental health problems.

Strategies

- The integration of mental health with primary healthcare through NMHP.
- Provision of tertiary care institutions for treatment of mental disorders.

- Eradicating stigmatization of mentally ill patients and protecting their rights through regulatory institutions like the Central Mental Health Authority and State Mental Health Authority.

Components of NMHP

The components of NMHP are shown in Fig. 6.10.

Treatment

The treatment program is planned in keeping with primary healthcare as the sheet of anchor. It consists of an appropriate referral system.

Rehabilitation

Rehabilitation of patients with mental disorders will be facilitated at the community level.

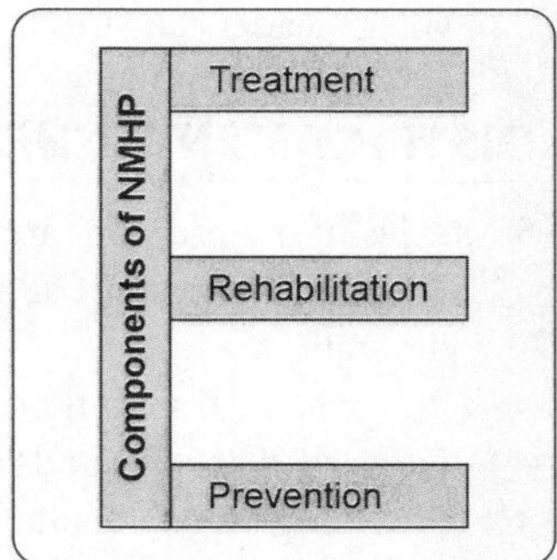

Figure 6.10: Components of NMHP

Prevention

This component of the service program will be community-based with a united involvement of the health service personnel.

Activities of NMHP

- Integration of mental health services to all existing general health services.
- Early detection and treatment and follow-up of cases.
- Increase the awareness of mental health problems.
- Eradicating stigmatization of mentally ill.
- Providing rehabilitative services for chronically ill patients.
- Providing counseling services for the alcoholic, drug addicts and delinquents.
- Establishing of tertiary care institutions for treatment of mental disorders.
- Training mental health team at nodal institutions in the state.
- Training to the trainers from states at NIMHANS Bengaluru.
- Protection of mentally ill patients and their rights.
- Providing rehabilitative services for chronically disabled mental patients.

INTEGRATION OF MENTAL HEALTH WITH PRIMARY HEALTHCARE

- This was initiated by training healthcare personnel in PHC services to detect and manage mental illness.
- Active liaison with the government health and medical services departments established (well-sustained effort at ensuring a supply of basic psychotropic medicines at PHC).
- Awareness program held periodically using local folklore, dance and music.
- The emphasis is on early recognition of mental illness and prompt treatment.
- Community volunteers are to be identified and trained.
- Involvement and training to lay community workers facilitate easier acceptance by the patients and their families.

- The intervention offered as a part of this program has facilitated community integration of the mentally ill.
- Establishment of rapport with the family and the community through the involvement of local village leaders ensures the acceptance of such a program by the population.

DISTRICT MENTAL HEALTH PROGRAM

Strategies of the program are as follows:
- Training program of all workers in the mental health team at the identified nodal institute in the state.
- Public education in the mental health to increase awareness and to reduce stigma.
- For early detection and treatment, the OPD and indoor services are provided.
- Providing valuable data and experience at the level of community to the state and center for future planning, improvement in services and research.

Services Provided

District Mental Health Program has now incorporated promotive and preventive activities for positive mental health which includes the following:
- Daily out patients (OPD) services.
- Ten-bedded in services facility (IPD).
- Referral services.
- Liaison with primary health center.
- Provide follow-up services.
- Community survey if feasible.
- Remove stigma of mental illness by creating awareness in community.

School Mental Health Services

- Life skills education in school.
- Counseling services.
- Focus on educational performance and difficulties.
- Focus on special children.

College Counseling Services

- Issues related peer groups.
- Issues related to family.
- Issues interfering with education.
- Drug abuse.
- Sex experimentation.
- Issues related with job and future plans.

Workplace Stress Management

- Stress in formal and informal sectors including farmers and women, etc.
- Stress of various groups of employees.

Suicide Prevention Services

Counseling center at district level, sensitization workshops, IEC, help lines, etc.

Thrust Areas

- District Mental Health Program in an enlarged and more effective form covering the entire country.
- Streamlining/modernization of mental hospitals in order to modify their present custodial role.
- Upgrading departments of psychiatry in medical colleges and enhancing the psychiatric content of the medical curriculum at the undergraduate as well as postgraduate level.
- Strengthening the central and state mental health authorities with a permanent secretariat. Appointment of medical officer at state headquarters in order to make the monitoring role more effective.
- Research and training in the field of community mental health, substance abuse and child adolescent psychiatric hospitals.

ADOLESCENT HEALTH PROGRAM

Introduction

Taking into consideration of the diverse nature of adolescent health needs, a comprehensive adolescent health strategy has been developed.

The components of the health needs of adolescent:

- Nutrition
- Sexual and reproductive health
- Mental health
- Gender-based violence
- Noncommunicable diseases
- Substance use.

Strategies of Intervention

- Health promotion
- Prevention
- Diagnosis
- Treatment
- Referral

These strategies of intervention can help toward building protective factors that can help adolescents and young people develop resilience to resist negative behaviors and operate at four major:

1. Individual
2. Family
3. School
4. Community by providing a comprehensive package of information, commodities and services.

Priority Interventions

- Adolescent nutrition, iron and folic acid supplementation.
- Facility-based adolescent reproductive and sexual health services (ARSH) adolescent health clinic.
- Information and counseling on adolescent sexual reproductive health and other health issues.

- Menstrual hygiene.
- Preventive health checkup.

Adolescent Reproductive and Sexual Health Program

The package of services included under adolescent reproductive and sexual health is promotive, preventive, curative and counseling services for married and unmarried girls and boys. These services are made available at:

- Facility-based health services—adolescent friendly health clinics.
- Facility-based counseling services—dedicated ARSH and Integrated counseling and testing center (ICTC).
- Community-based intervention outreach activities.

Adolescent Friendly Health Clinics (AFHC)

These clinics provide routine checkup at primary, secondary and tertiary level of care on fixed days. At present 6,302 AFH functioning and provide information and commodities to > 2.5 million adolescents for health-related needs such as contraceptive provision, management of menstrual problems, management of antenatal care and anemia.

Facility-Based Counseling Services

Counseling services on nutrition, puberty, prevention and contraception, delaying marriage and Childbearing and concerns related to contraception, abortion services, premarital concerns, substance misuse, sexual abuse and mental health problems are being provided through recruitment and training of dedicated counseling.

Outreach Activities

These are conducted at schools, colleges, teen clubs, vocational training centers, during village health nutrition day, health melas and collaboration with self-help groups to provide adequate and appropriate information to adolescent in spaces where they normally congregate.

Weekly Iron and Folic Acid Supplementation

Ministry of Health and Family Welfare launched the weekly supplementation of iron and folic acid tablets to prevent the incidence of anemia among the adolescent girls and boys. The key interventions of the program are as follows:

- Administration of supervised weekly iron-folic acid supplements 100 mg elemental iron + 500 µg folic acid on fixed day of the week.
- Screening for moderate and severe anemia and their referral to appropriate health facility.
- Biannual deworming, i.e., Albendazole 400 mg tablets to control helminths infestation.
- Information and counseling for improving diet and taking action for prevention of intestinal worm infestations.

Menstrual Hygiene

To provide adequate knowledge on menstrual hygiene and have access to high quality sanitary napkins and safe disposal mechanism. The Ministry of Health and Family Welfare launched the

scheme for promotion of menstrual hygiene for adolescent girls of 10–19 years in rural areas. The activities of scheme include:
- Community-based health education and outreach in the target population to promote menstrual hygiene.
- Sourcing and procurement of sanitary napkins.
- Storage and distribution of sanitary napkin to the adolescent girls.
- Training of ASHA and nodal teachers in menstrual health.
- Safe disposal of sanitary napkins.

TRIBAL HEALTH

There are about 104 million tribal people spread over 706 tribes in India. It accounts for 8.6% of Indian population. These people remained under privileged socioeconomically and politically. About 90% of the tribal population live in rural areas and mostly in hilly and forested areas. The tribal health and their healthcare needs remained unsolved.

Demographic Profile of Tribal Population

Habitation

The tribal population is found in ten states and in eight North-East states. About 90% of population live in rural areas. Madhya Pradesh alone accounts for 15 million of rural population followed by Maharashtra—10 million, odisha—9 million and Rajasthan also 9 million. The concentration of population is highest in North-East states. They live in hilly areas surrounded by forests.
- The male population of tribal is 52.5 million.
- Female population of tribal is 52 million.

Sex Ratio

According to the Census 2011, the sex ratio for the tribal population is 990 females per 1,000 males, compared to the national average of 943.

Life Expectancy

The life expectancy at birth of tribal people is 63.9 years as against 67 years for the general population.

Maternal and Child Health

Maternal Mortality

There is no recent estimate of maternal mortality available among tribal women. However, early marriage, early child birth, anemia, low body mass index (BMI) accounts for high maternal mortality. The institutional deliveries among tribal women are 68% which is lower than the national average of 78.9%, 71.5% deliveries are conducted by skilled health personnel. The postnatal care within 48 hours after delivery is only 37%.

Infant Mortality

According to NFHS-4, the estimated infant mortality rate was 44.4 per 1000 live births.

Child Mortality Rate

Child mortality rate of 1–4 years was 13.4.

Under-Five Mortality Rate

Under-five mortality rate was 57.2. The time trend shows major improvement in the mortality rate.

Immunization

Immunization coverage of tribal children was lower than general population.

Nutrition Status of Tribal Children

Malnutrition in the tribal children was found higher than the general population children. The percentage of stunting, wasting and underweight is reduced.

Burden of Disease in Tribal Population

The tribal population faces malnutrition, communicable and noncommunicable diseases. In addition, the rapid urbanization, environmental distress and changing life style have resulted in increased prevalence of noncommunicable diseases such as hypertension, diabetes, cancer, mental illness and addiction.

The main communicable diseases in tribal communities are tuberculosis, malaria, leprosy, sexually transmitted diseases, AIDS/HIV, skin infections, diarrheal diseases and hepatitis, etc.

Tuberculosis

The prevalence of pulmonary tuberculosis among tribal population is significantly higher than the general population. It is found to be 703 per 100,000 population as compared to national average 316 per 100,000 population in rest of the country. RNTCP provides free diagnosis and treatment to all the patients. The RNTCP has started active case finding to improve case detection rate in difficult to reach areas. To improve access to tribal and other marginalized areas, there is a provision for:

- Additional TB unit and designated microscopy center in tribal/difficult areas.
- Compensation for transportation for patients and attendants in tribal areas.
- Higher rate of salary to contractual staff posted in tribal area.
- **Provision of TB health visitors for urban area:** A mobile TB diagnostic van equipped with X-ray facilities and sputum microscopic facilities have been deployed. This offers diagnostic services for tuberculosis at the door steps of the patient's home in difficult to reach areas of the tribal population. This intervention is expected to improve the standard of care among extremely deprived population. This helps to improve early case detection, treatment and to reduce out of pocket expenditure of individual patient.

Leprosy

Leprosy services are uniformly provided to all scheduled castes and scheduled tribes irrespective of caste and religion under National Leprosy Eradication Program. These services are allotted to NGOs and they are encouraged to work in tribal areas for providing IEC services, prevention of deformities and follow-up of cases. IEC services are also taken up through various media so that inaccessible and remote tribal areas are covered.

Malaria and Other Vector-Borne Diseases

The tribal population accounts for about 30% of all malaria cases in the country under the National Vector-Borne Disease Control Program, services for prevention and control for malaria, kala-azar, filaria, Japanese encephalitis, dengue/dengue hemorrhagic fever and chikungunya are provided to all sections of the community without any discrimination. Since the prevalence of vector-borne diseases is more in low socioeconomic groups, focused attention is given to areas dominated by tribal population in north-eastern states and parts of Andhra Pradesh, Chhattisgarh, Gujarat, Jharkhand, Karnataka, Madhya Pradesh, Maharashtra and Odisha. Additional inputs under externally assisted projects from global funds to North-eastern states and from World Bank to other states especially for control of malaria are provided. North-eastern states are being provided 100% central assistance for implementation of the program.

Noncommunicable Diseases

The increase in incidence of noncommunicable diseases has been observed due to rapid urbanization, environmental distress and changing life style.

- **Hypertension:** It is very common among the tribals. One out of four adults suffers from hypertension. The prevalence of the disease increases with age, consumption of alcohol, tobacco and sedentary life style. Most of the adult men and women even did not know the signs and symptoms of the disease.
- **Blindness and visual impairment:** The goal of National Program for Control of Blindness and Visual Impairment is to reduce the prevalence of blindness to 0.3% by the year 2020. It is a centrally sponsored scheme and meant for all including SC/ST population. But keeping in view the needs of North-Eastern states including Sikkim, which are tribal prominent, the following initiatives have been implemented and National Program for Control of Blindness and Visual Impairment (NPCBVI):
    - Assistance has been provided for construction of dedicated eye units in N-E states including Sikkim and other hilly states.
    - Appointment of contractual ophthalmic manpower to meet the shortage of ophthalmic manpower in the states.
    - Assistance of setting up of multipurpose district mobile ophthalmic units for diagnosis and medical management of eye diseases for coverage is difficult to reach areas.
    - Besides cataract, assistance for treatment and management of other eye diseases like diabetic retinopathy, glaucoma, refractive errors, corneal transplantation, Vitreoretinal surgery and childhood blindness is provided.
- **Genetic disorders:** The genetic disorders vary 1–40% in different communities. The prevalence of sickle cell anemia and thalassemia is 1 in 86 births among the tribal communities in central India. Another genetic disease prevalent in tribal groups is G6PD.
- **Mental health and addiction:** Consumption of tobacco and alcohol is more as compared to nontribal population. Both these addictions are risk factors for noncommunicable diseases and cause serious diseases and increase mortality.
- **Animal attacks and violence in conflict areas:** Animal bites, snake bites, dog bites and scorpion bites are common in tribals as the tribal areas are often surrounded by forests.

Healthcare Infrastructure of the Tribals and their Development

The traditional life style, remoteness of habitation, dispersed population and displacement make it difficult for health planners and policy makers to plan and implement accessible and equitable health services. During the fifth Five-Year Plan, a tribal sub plan (TSP) strategy was adopted, now it is known as schedule tribal component (STC). This STC was adopted for the accelerated development of tribal people Ministry of Tribal Affairs and Ministry of Health and Family Welfare are working to improve tribal development through tailored educational, infrastructural and livelihood schemes in terms of various indicators relating to literacy, health and socioeconomic status.

Healthcare Infrastructure of Tribals Under National Health Mission

According to the present policies and programs of National Health Mission to increase universal access to the decentralized health system, the infrastructure in tribal and hilly areas is given as follows:

- One health subcenter per 3000 population
- One primary health center per 20,000 population
- One community health center per 80,000 population

Human Health Resource

The human health resources in the health centers of tribal areas are very poor. This is because of limited scope of professional growth of staff, poor working conditions, limited social infrastructure feeling of social and professional isolation and weak human resources policies. To overcome the shortage of doctors and other medical staff, the various measures have been tried but remained impractical. In October 2013, an expert committee was constituted on tribal health under the chairmanship of Dr Abhay Bang. The committee had its members, prominent academicians, civil society members and policy makers who have been working with the tribal people. The expert committee suggested the following measures to improve human resources for the tribal health:

- The healthcare providers to the tribal should be from the local tribal communities.
- To improve the human health resources in the tribal area, the local tribal people to be trained and deployed in the health force.
- The specialists and doctors should be deployed closer to the community.
- The role of ASHA in the tribal area should be expanded. He/she should work for four hours daily to perform eight type of functions.
- Mid-level care providers should be trained and placed at subcenters.
- The salary of the doctors working is tribal area should be increased.
- The committee recommended creation of dedicated medical colleges in the tribal districts exclusively to train tribal students in the scheduled areas.

ROLE OF A NURSE IN NATIONAL HEALTH PROGRAMS

Nurses have key role in the implementation of National Health Programs and are closely related with all National Health Programs. They are needed to take active participation. Nurses should know the aims of participation, needed equipment and resources, her activities and general instructions related to each National Health Programs.

Aims of Participation

- To understand and identify the feeling, attitude and adaptability of community toward specific health programs.
- To implement the policies and programs related to the health of the people and to get the cooperation of the community.
- To assist the community in changing undesirable habits and adopt healthy habits.
- To convert a local person into an effective health worker through good training and assisting the people in identifying and solving their problems.
- To motivate local people.
- To keep the relevant and latest information about National Health Programs.

Resources Required for Participating in the Program

- To identify the problems:
  - It is essential to maintain morbidity register, clinical register, survey register, personal card and family card.
  - Making arrangement for laboratory test.
- Equipment and articles for taking weight, height, BP instrument. TPR tray, immunization tray, vaccines, instruments and other devices as needed.
- Medicines as per the requirements.
- Health education material (cards, films, charts, etc.).
- For the examination of the patient availability of doctor/specialist/assistant workers/health worker/vaccinator, etc.

Activities

A nurse is expected to do the following activities:
- Quick identification of patients.
- Assisting in the diagnosis and laboratory examinations.
- Giving treatment to patients.
- Providing care to patients at home.
- Health education.
- Assisting in achieving the targets.
- Providing supervision and training.
- Preparation and maintenance of reports.
- Evaluation of health programs.

General Instructions

Community health nurse should pay attention to the following facts while implementing the health program. These are as follows:
- Ensuring participations of community and its leaders for the success of the program.
- Try to change unhealthy religious faiths and superstitions, which are resisting the program.
- Exchange knowledge and information so that receptivity for the program can increase.
- Health programs should be beneficial to the majority of people, not for some people only.

- Time of implementation of the program should be convenient for the community.
- Health education should be provided to public regarding the health programs.
- It is essential to get political support and help in implementation of national programs.

The role of community health nurse in National Health Programs is vast and varied. She is an investigator, educator, communicator, trainer, coordinator and provider of care.

Summary

- India is a developing country and it is facing many health problems.
- Soon after independence several measures have been taken by the Government of India to improve the health status of the people.
- The noncommunicable disease control program and control and eradication programs of communicable diseases have been started. Many diseases are controlled.
- These National Control Programs and development programs have been undertaken by the central government and implemented by the concerted effort of central as well as state government to combat various communicable and noncommunicable diseases and nutritional problems.
- Government of India has also launched several development programs and National Health Development Programs, i.e., Rural Development Program and Family Welfare Program; Mental Health Program; and Adolescent Health Program, etc.
- It is very important for the community health nurse to know and understand the various problems and national program which are planned, organized and implemented.
- This need to be ensured so that the community health nurse could give effective and integrated services to people in need and can contribute in bringing down the mortality and morbidity and help people improve their life and longev ty.

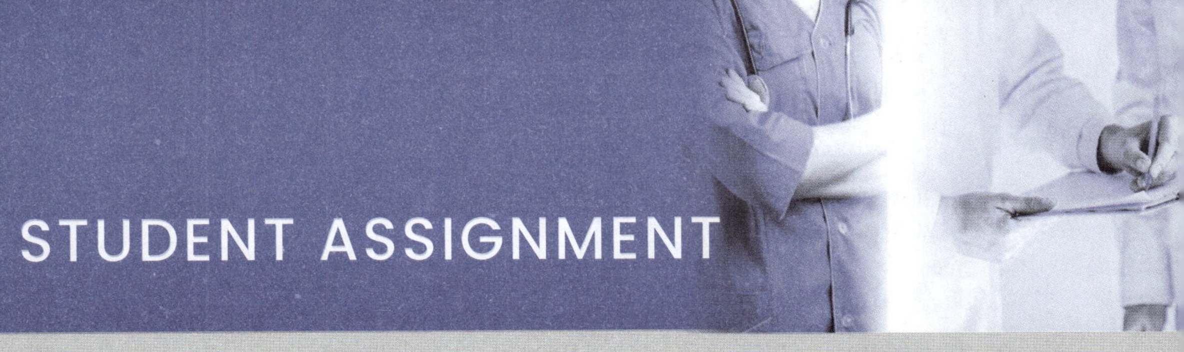

LONG ANSWER TYPE QUESTIONS

1. Enlist the National Health Program in India. Describe any two programs in detail.
2. Describe Revised National Tuberculosis Control Program in detail.
3. Discuss the Acute Respiratory Infection Control Program.
4. Explain the expanded program of immunization.
5. List the National Disease Control Program. Write any two programs in detail.
6. Explain the role of community health nurse in National Health Programs.

SHORT ANSWER TYPE QUESTIONS

1. Write short notes on the following:
   a. 20-point program
   b. ICDS program
   c. Midday meal program
2. Enlist various disease control program.
3. Write an account of any one of the following:
   a. National Program for Control of Blindness.
   b. Yaws Eradication Program.
4. Write short notes on any two of following:
   a. National Cancer Control Program.
   b. National STD Control Program.
   c. National AIDS Control Program.
   d. National Filaria Control Program.
5. a. Enlist various diseases control program.
   b. Enlist nutritional problems in India.

MULTIPLE CHOICE QUESTIONS

1. **Acute Respiratory Disease Control Program was launched in India in the year of:**
   a. 1981
   b. 1985
   c. 1990
   d. 1994

2. **A revised strategy for national TB control program (RNTCP) was evolved by a committee of expert after reviewing NTCP in the year:**
   a. 1992
   b. 1996
   c. 2002
   d. 2006

3. **Cancer Control Program was started in 1975 in limited form but it was revised, strengthened and converted to National Cancer Control Program in the year:**
   a. 1979
   b. 1984
   c. 2002
   d. 2005

4. National Malaria Control Program was converted into National Malaria Eradication Program in the year:
   a. 1958
   b. 1963
   c. 1968
   d. 1973

5. National Leprosy Control Program was renamed as National Leprosy Eradication Program in the year:
   a. 1963
   b. 1973
   c. 1983
   d. 1993

6. National Guinea Worm Eradication Program was launched in India with technical assistance from WHO in the year:
   a. 1974
   b. 1979
   c. 1984
   d. 1994

7. Yaws Eradication Program was started in 1996–97 for Koraput district Odisha but was extended to all endemic states in the year:
   a. 1999
   b. 2001
   c. 2004
   d. 2007

8. National Program for the Control of Blindness was established in:
   a. 1970
   b. 1976
   c. 1980
   d. 1986

9. Which of the following are avoidable blindness diseases?
   a. Cataract and refractive errors
   b. Childhood blindness and corneal blindness
   c. Glaucoma and diabetic retinopathy
   d. All of these

10. National Goiter Control Program was launched in:
    a. 1962
    b. 1957
    c. 2002
    d. 2006

11. National AIDS prevention and control policy was announced in:
    a. 2002
    b. 2005
    c. 2007
    d. 2012

12. National STD Control Program was started in:
    a. 1942
    b. 1946
    c. 1950
    d. 1952

13. Expanded immunization program was introduced in India in the year of:
    a. 1972
    b. 1978
    c. 1980
    d. 1981

14. Swajaldhara Program was launched in India in the year:
    a. 2001
    b. 2002
    c. 2005
    d. 2007

15. The Universal Immunization Program at present being conducted under:
    a. RCH-II
    b. CSSD
    c. RCH-I
    d. None of these

16. **The minimum need program was introduced in the year:**
    a. In the first year of fifth Five-Year Plan
    b. During the second Five-Year Plan
    c. During the eleventh Five-Year Plan
    d. None of the above

17. **The Pulse Polio Immunization Program in India was launched in the year:**
    a. 1970
    b. 1995
    c. 1980
    d. 1976

18. **The Midday Meal Program was started in the year:**
    a. 1984
    b. 1976
    c. 1982
    d. 1961

19. **National Nutritional Anemia Prophylaxis Program was launched in India in the year:**
    a. 1962
    b. 1968
    c. 1970
    d. 1971

20. **Integrated Child Development Scheme was launched in India in the year:**
    a. 1972
    b. 1975
    c. 1976
    d. 1978

21. **National Mental Health Program was launched in India in the year:**
    a. 1982
    b. 1983
    c. 1990
    d. 1994

Note

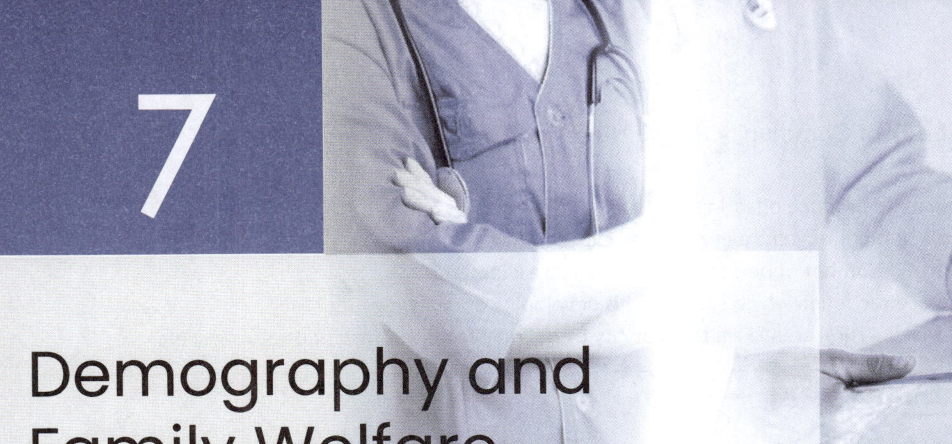

7

Demography and Family Welfare

LEARNING OBJECTIVES

After the completion of the unit, the readers will be able to:
- Explain the concepts of demography.
- Discuss the demographic trends in the world and India.
- Discuss the strategies of National Family Welfare Program.
- Describe the role of nurse in Family Welfare Program.

UNIT OUTLINE

Demography
- Introduction
- Concepts
- Definition
- History of Demographic Studies
- Demographic Cycle
- Demographic Processes
- Sources of Demography
- Demographic Trends in the World
- Demographic Trends in India
- Population Explosion
- National Population Policy, 2000 (NPP 2000)
- New National Population Policy, 2000 (NNPP 2000)
- Concepts of Fertility and Infertility
- Small Family Norms

Family Welfare
- Concepts of Family Welfare
- Services Included in the Family Welfare Program
- Importance of Family Welfare
- Aspects of Family Welfare
- Aims and Objectives of Family Welfare
- Family Planning
- Method of Family Planning
- Types of Contraceptives
- Elements of Success in Family Planning
- Family Planning Counseling
- National Family Welfare Policy
- National Family Welfare Program
- National Family Planning Insurance Scheme
- Role of Nurse in Family Welfare Program

KEY TERMS

Birth control: Limiting the pregnancies
Census: Official counting of country's population
Conception: Fertilization of female ovum by male sperm
Demography: Scientific study of human populations in terms of size composition and distribution
Family size: The number of children in the family
Fertility: Ability to produce viable offspring or actual bearing of children
Growth rate: It is obtained by subtracting crude death rate from crude birth rate.

Infertility: Inability to produce offspring
Life expectancy: Number of years a person may expect to live
Population density: Number of persons living per square kilometer
Trends: A general direction in which something is developing or changing.
Urbanization: Making rural area like a town or city by building factories, new houses, roads, etc.

Abbreviations

ASFR: Age-Specific Fertility Rate

GFR: Gross Fertility Rate

NIHFW: National Institute of Health and Family Welfare

NRR: Net Reproduction Rate

SIHFW: State Institute of Health and Family Welfare

TFR: Total Fertility Rate

DEMOGRAPHY

INTRODUCTION

The term "demography" refers to the study of human population as regard to their size, composition and distribution. There is a significant relationship between community medicine, community health nursing and population. An individual is the basic unit of community healthcare. Health problems of the community can be assessed and strategies can be planned to solve these problems only after studying the population. The population of the world is increasing very fast because of decline in death rate and increase in birth rate. This fast-increasing population is creating imbalance in ecosystem globally. This imbalance is affecting the socioeconomic aspects and quality of life. As a result, it is neutralizing the development achieved in agriculture, industries, housing, employment and healthcare facilities. This rapid increase in the population and its consequences on socioeconomic development and the resource management are global concerns now and almost all the countries across the globe expressing their anxiety on the issue and the measures taken to resolve it. It is a dire need to focus on the population growth through family welfare and family planning services.

CONCEPTS

- Demography is the scientific study of human population. In demography, the following three elements of population are given special attention:
  1. Changes in the size of population, i.e., increase or decrease in the size of population.
  2. Structure of population on the basis of sex or age group
  3. Geographical distribution of population on the basis of state or territory.
- Demography is derived from two Greek words, "*Demos*" meaning the people and "*Graphin*" meaning the record.
- Demography deals with the study of the size, its composition and the distribution of human population.
- The population size, its composition and distribution are determined by the number of births, deaths and migration which are occurring all the time in any place.

DEFINITION

Demography is the branch of science, which studies the human population and their elements. The elements are changes in the size, structure and geographical distribution of population.

HISTORY OF DEMOGRAPHIC STUDIES

The demography had been studying over centuries. The census records had been traced as far back as 4000 BC in Babylonia, 3000 BC in China and 2500 BC in Egypt. Canada was the first country to conduct census in 1666, United States in 1790 and England in 1801. In India, census operation was introduced in 1881. During the 17th century, the awareness was growing about vital registration and laws enforcing compulsory registration of vital events therefore the importance of vital registration was spread in the region of the world. India had introduced the act of registration of vital events in 1866. Further, the voluntary registration of birth, death and civil marriage act for compulsory vital registration was passed in 1969.

DEMOGRAPHIC CYCLE

The history of world population since 1659, suggests that there is a demographic cycle of five stages through which a nation passes (Fig. 7.1).

First Stage: A High Stationary Stage

In this stage, there is no change in the size and composition of population. This is because of high birth and death rate, which cancel each other and the population remains stationary. Until the middle of the 17th century, the world's population was in this stages and India was in this stage till 1920.

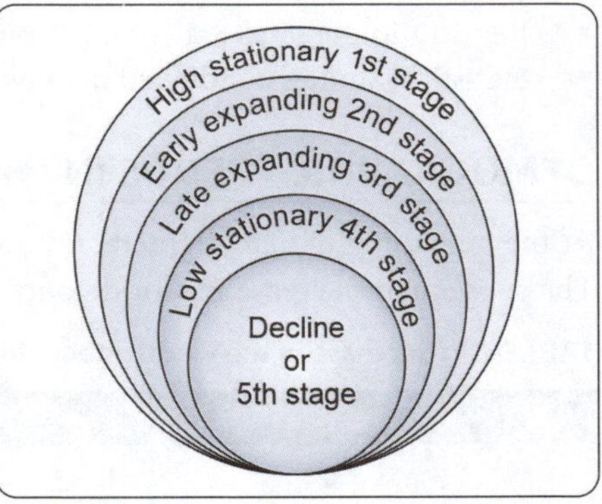

Figure 7.1: Stages of demographic transition

Second Stage: Early Expanding

In this stage, the death rate begins to decrease because of improvement in health condition and the birth rate remains unchanged. Therefore, there is some increase in population size. The world population was in this stage from middle of 17th to middle of 19th century. India was in this stage from 1921 to 1950.

Third Stage: Late Expanding

The death rate declines still further and the birth rate tends to fall. The population tends to grow because births exceed deaths. There is a tremendous natural increase in population. In number of developing countries birth rates have declined rapidly, India has entered in this phase.

Fourth Stage: Low Stationary

In this stage, there is low birth rate and low death rate with the result that population becomes stationary. Most of the developed and industrialized countries are in this stage. Zero population growth has been recorded in Australia during 1980–1985. In UK, Sweden and Belgium it has been recorded 0.1 during 1980–1985.

Fifth Stage: Declining Stage

In this stage, the birth rate is lower than death rate and population begins to decline. Germany and Hungary are experiencing this stage.

DEMOGRAPHIC PROCESSES

Demography is influenced by the following processes:
- Fertility
- Marriage
- Social mobility
- Mortality
- Migration

SOURCES OF DEMOGRAPHY

- Census
- National sample survey
- Registration of vital statistics, i.e., birth, death, etc.
- Statistical studies conducted in between the census

DEMOGRAPHIC TRENDS IN THE WORLD

At the beginning of Christian era, the world's population was estimated to be around 250 million. The subsequent increase in world's population is given in Table 7.1.

TABLE 7.1: Increase in the world population from 1750 to mid 2024

Year	Population (millions)	Average annual growth rate (%)
1750	791	–
1800	978	0.4
1850	1,262	0.5
1900	1650	0.6
1950	2526	1.1
1960	3,037	1.79
1970	3,696	1.92
1975	4,066	1.89
1980	4,432	1.72
1987	5,000	1.63
1991	5,385	1.7
1998	5,884	1.6
2000	6,054	1.4
2003	6,313	1.1

Contd...

Year	Population (millions)	Average annual growth rate (%)
2007	6,655	1.4
2008	6,734	1.2
2010	6,908	1.23
2014	7,238	1.2
2016	7,418	1.2
2018	7,621	1.2
2019	7,764	1.06
2020	7,850	0.98
2021	7,909	0.87
2022	7,975	0.83
2023	8,045	0.88
2024	8,122	0.91

Approximately 75% of the world's population lives in developing countries. The population of USA stands third in the world after China. It has been estimated by the United Nations that the world's population grew at an annual rate of 1.23% during 2000–2010. Growth rate of China was 0.6% during 2002–2012 as compared to India (1.4%). Three countries of South-East Asia Region (SEAR), i.e., India—population 1442.4 million, Indonesia—population 279.8 million and Bangladesh—population 174.8 million are among the most populous 10 countries of the world. Population of India stands first. As per UN estimation India's population will reach 1.53 billion by the year 2050 and will be the highest populated country in the world. The trends of population increase in SEAR countries are shown in Table 7.2.

Birth and Death Rate

Birth rate in the world fell below 30 in 1975 and had declined to 19 during 2015. In most countries of the world, this decline in birth rate is due to adopting small family norms. In Singapore the birth

TABLE 7.2: Trends in increase of population of SEAR countries (in millions)

Country	1991	2018	2024
India	843.9	1359.8	1442.4
Bangladesh	118	167.04	174.8
Bhutan	1.5	0.820	0.81
Indonesia	187.7	267.9	279.8
Maldives	0.221	0.447	0.517
Myanmar	42.5	54.04	54.964
Nepal	19.6	29.75	31.24
Sri Lanka	17.4	20.97	21.5
Thailand	56.4	66.2	71.9

Abbreviation: SEAR, South-East Asia Region

rate came down from 23 to 10 in 1970 and in Thailand from 37 to 10 in 1970. The crude birth and death rate in selected developed and developing countries are given in Table 7.3.

TABLE 7.3: Crude birth and death rates in selected developed and developing countries in 2018 mid 2024

Country	Crude birth rate		Crude death rate	
	2018	2024	2018	2024
India	20	16.75	6	7.4
Bangladesh	19	16.4	5	5.5
Pakistan	26	25.59	7	5.9
Sri Lanka	16	14.39	6	7.5
Thailand	11	9.39	8	8.4
Myanmar	16	16.37	8	8.9
Nepal	20	17.86	6	6.6
China	12	10.47	7	7.7
Japan	8	6.99	11	12.9
Singapore	9	8.22	5	5.4
UK	12	11.17	9	9.1 (2022)
USA	12	12	8	8.5

TABLE 7.4: Reduction in crude birth and death rates in selected countries in 1990–mid 2024

Country	Crude birth rate		Crude death rate	
	1990	2024	1990	2024
Bangladesh	35	16.4	10	5.5
Nepal	38	17.86	13	6.6
India	31	16.75	11	7.4
Sri Lanka	21	14.39	7	7.5
Thailand	19	9.39	8	8.4
Singapore	18	8.22	5	5.4
China	23	10.47	8	7.7
Pakistan	40	25.5	11	5.9

Table 7.4 shows the reduction in the crude birth and death rates in selected countries from 1990 to 2024.

In all these countries, the decline in birth rate is due to education, woman's employment, improved health services, availability of contraception and extension of services offered through family planning programs and changes in the marriage patterns. The decline in global death rate from 11 per 1,000 (1975–1980) to 7.9 per 1,000 populations during 2024, i.e., reduction of 23% and decline in crude death rate of SEAR is more marked from 14.1 to 7 per 1,000 population. The crude death rate is affected by infant and child mortality. The infant and child mortality rate has reduced due to improved maternal and child health services, implementation of expanded programs on immunization, infection control programs as well as with control of other infectious diseases. This decline in infant and child mortality rate has brought decline in death rate.

Growth Rate

The annual growth rate is obtained by subtracting the crude death rate from the crude birth rate. This annual growth rate is exclusive of migration. The world's population growth rate was at peak around 1970. It was around 1.92%. The most recent date shows a slight decline since then to 0.91% in mid 2024.

The growth rate is not uniform in the world. It is higher in developing countries. In European countries, it is 0.3% per year where as in developing countries, it is 2.6% per year. The difference in growth rate is due to fertility and mortality pattern. The salient features of population growth at a glance are as shown in Box 7.1.

Box 7.1

Salient Features of Population Growth

- About 95% of growth is occurring in the developing countries.
- Currently, one-third of the world's population is under the age of 15 and will soon enter the reproductive phase thereby increasing the population growth.
- The United Nations Fund for Population Activities (UNFPA) estimates that world population is most likely to reach 10 billion by 2050 and 20.7 billion a century later.
- The expected number of births per woman at current fertility rate (2016) is, for industrialized countries 1.6, in developing countries 2.8 and in least developed countries 4.2. The global fertility rate is 2.4.
- This increased population growth is an obstacle to the social and economic development in the under developed world.

DEMOGRAPHIC TRENDS IN INDIA

With a population of 1442.4 million in the mid 2024, is the number one populous country in the world, second is China and seventh in the land area, with only 2.4% of world's land area and is supporting about 17.5% of world's population. India has more arable land area than any country except United States and more water area than any country except Canada and United States. The Indian life revolves around agriculture and allied activities in small villages. Some important facts related to population as per the census 2011 are given in Table 7.5.

TABLE 7.5: Population of India 1901–2011 as per census

Year	Total population (in millions)	Average annual exponential growth rate (%)	Decadal growth rate (%)
1901	238.4	–	–
1911	252.1	0.56	0.75
1921	251.3	(–) 0.03	(–) 0.31
1931	279.0	1.04	11.00
1941	318.7	1.33	14.22

Contd...

Year	Total population (in millions)	Average annual exponential growth rate (%)	Decadal growth rate (%)
1951	361.1	1.25	13.31
1961	439.2	1.96	21.64
1971	548.2	2.20	24.80
1981	683.3	2.22	24.66
1991	846.4	2.16	23.87
2001	1028.6	1.7	21.52
2011	1210.1	1.64	17.64
2021	1407.5 (Historical data)	0.8	(Data not available)

- The population of India at 1210.2 million is almost equal to the combined population of USA, Indonesia, Brazil, Pakistan, Bangladesh and Japan (1214.3 million).
- The percentage decadal growth during 2001–2011 has registered the sharpest decline since independence, a decrease of 3.90% points from 21.54 to 17.64%.
- Uttar Pradesh is the most populous state in the country. Its population is more than the population of Brazil.
- The population density is highest in Delhi followed by Chandigarh. It is lowest in Dibang Valley in Arunachal Pradesh.
- Population of Uttar Pradesh and Maharashtra (312 million) is greater than population of USA.
- The total number of children in the age group 0–6 is 158.8 million which is 5 million less since 2001.
- The census indicated a continuing preference for male children over female children. The latest sex ratio is 914 females against 1,000 male children.
- The proportion of child population in the age group of 0–6 years to total population is 13.1% as compared to 15.9% in census 2001. There is a decline of 2.8 points.
- Overall sex ratio has increased 7 points since census 2001 to reach at 940 at census 2011. This is the highest sex ratio recorded since census 1971 and a shade lower than 1961.
- Literacy rate has increased from 64.83% in 2001 to 74.04% in 2011, showing an increase of 9.21% points.
- Literates constitute 74% of the total population aged seven and above and illiterate 26%. Kerala is the most literate state of the country.

Growth Rate

The population of India since 1971, average annual exponential growth rate (%) and the decadal growth of population (%) is already shown in the Table 7.5. Population in India has been steadily increasing since 1921. The year 1921 is called "big divide" because the absolute number of people added to the population. Since 1921, India's population is increasing at the rate of 16 million each year.

In 1901, the population of India was 238 million and doubled in 60 years, i.e., 439 million 1961 and again doubled in 30 years to reach 846 million by 1991. It crossed 1 billion mark on 11 May 2000 and is projected to reach 1.53 billion by the year 2050 making India the most populous country in the world surpassing China. With the division of some states the rank of most populous states has changed as shown in the Table 7.6. In this most populous states in the country are shown by rank.

TABLE 7.6: Ranking of most populous states of India by population size—2011 census

Rank	States	Population on 31.3.2011 (in million)	Percent to total (in million) population of India 1.3.2011
1	Uttar Pradesh	199.581	16.49
2	Maharashtra	112.372	9.29
3	Bihar	103.804	8.58
4	West Bengal	91.347	7.55
5	Andhra Pradesh	84.665	7
6	Madhya Pradesh	72.597	6
7	Tamil Nadu	72.138	5.96
8	Rajasthan	68.621	5.67
9	Karnataka	61.130	5.05
10	Gujarat	60.383	4.99

Uttar Pradesh comes first with about 199.581 million people, Maharashtra comes second with 112.372 million and Bihar comes third with 103.804 million. These 10 states account for about 71% of the total population of India.

It has been estimated that with current trend the population in India will increase from 1.210 billion to 1.4 billion during the period from 2011 to 2026, an increase of 13.57%. There is substantial difference in total fertility rate in between and within the states. Southern states like Kerala, Tamil Nadu, Karnataka and Andhra Pradesh are with total fertility rate at or below zero the replacement level. On the other hand, Uttar Pradesh, Chhattisgarh, Uttarakhand, Rajasthan, Jharkhand, Bihar, Madhya Pradesh and Odisha with an estimated combined fertility rate of 4.2 in 2000. The estimated year by which these states will reach the replacement level of fertility if current trend continues, is given in Table 7.7.

These States will delay the attainment of replacement level of fertility until 2021. These high fertility States are anticipated to contribute about 50 percent to the nationwide increase in population.

TABLE 7.7: States that will reach the replacement level of fertility

States	Expected years
Uttar Pradesh	2027
Madhya Pradesh	2025
Chhattisgarh	2022
Uttarakhand	2022
Bihar	2021
Rajasthan	2021
Jharkhand	2018
India	2021

Age and Sex Composition

The age and sex composition in Indian population is shown in Table 7.8 (0–14). The male population is 0.5% more than female in the age group of 0–14 years. In the age group of 60 and above female population is 0.7% more than male population. The proportion of 0–14-year age group is higher in rural areas (29.10%) than in the urban areas (24.30%) for both males and females. The proportion of population below 14 years of age showing decline whereas the elderly population is increasing. This trend will continue in the time to come. This increase in elderly population will impose a greater burden on health services in the country.

The table shows India's population of 2023, the percentage of males and females in the total population.

Sex Ratio

Sex ratio is defined as the number of females per 1,000 males. One of the basic demographic characteristic of the population is the sex composition as it plays a vital role in population. The sex composition of the population is affected by the differentials in mortality conditions of males and females, sex selective migration and sex ratio at birth. A low sex ratio indicates strong preference for

TABLE 7.8: Percent distribution of estimated population by age and sex, India 2023

Age group	Population percentage		
	Total	Males	Females
0–4	8.5	7.9	7.8
5–9	8.9	8.3	8.33
10–14	9.6	8.83	8.5
15–19	10.1	9.0	8.6
20–24	10.4	9.09	8.77
25–29	9.7	8.71	8.4
30–34	8.1	8.19	8.06
35–39	7.1	7.63	7.5 (mid 2024)
40–44	6.1	6.76	6.73
45–49	5.3	5.91	5.97
50–54	4.3	5.7	5.2
55–59	3.6	4.32	4.49
60–64	3.1	3.53	2.9
65–69	2.2	2.73	2.9
70–74	1.5	1.89	2.1
75–79	0.9	1.02	1.76
80–84	0.5	0.867	–
85+	0.3	–	–
Total	**100.0**	**100.0**	**100.0**

TABLE 7.9: **Sex ratio in India 1901 onward**

Year	1901	1911	1921	1931	1941	1951	1961	1971	1981	1991	2001	2011
Females per 1,000 males	972	964	955	950	945	946	941	930	934	927	933	940

male child and consequent gender inequalities, neglects of girl child resulting in higher mortality at younger age, female infanticide, female feticide, higher maternal mortality and bias in enumeration of population.

The sex ratio in India has been generally adverse to woman, i.e., number of women per 1,000 men generally been <1,000. Apart from being adverse to woman, sex ratio has also been declined over the decades. The trends in the sex ratio in India from 1901 onward are given in the Table 7.9.

Table 7.9 shows decline in sex ratio from 1901 to 2001. There is slight increase in 2011, i.e., the number of females per 1,000 males.

Sex Ratio at Birth

Sex ratio at birth can be affected by sex selectivity at birth. The sex ratio of India for the period 2014–2016 has been estimated at 898. It varies from 902 in rural areas to 888 in urban areas. Among the bigger states, the sex ratio at birth varies from 963 in Chhattisgarh to 852 in Haryana. In the rural areas, the highest and lowest sex ratio at birth is in the states of Chhattisgarh (995) and Haryana (835) respectively. The sex ratio in urban areas varies from 957 in Madhya Pradesh to 820 in Gujarat.

Table 7.10 shows the number of females per 1,000 males at birth in rural and urban areas of the states mentioned during 2014–2016.

TABLE 7.10: **Sex ratio at birth by residence in India 2014–2016**

Bigger State	Number of females per 1,000 males		
	Total	Rural	Urban
Andhra Pradesh*	913	923	888
Assam	896	898	880
Bihar	908	912	871
Chhattisgarh	963	995	833
Delhi	857	917	856
Gujarat	848	867	820
Haryana	832	835	824
Himachal Pradesh	917	921	852
Jammu and Kashmir	906	903	919
Jharkhand	918	927	882
Karnataka	935	965	883
Kerala	959	972	946

Contd...

Bigger State	Number of females per 1,000 males		
	Total	Rural	Urban
Madhya Pradesh	922	913	957
Maharashtra	876	872	882
Odisha	948	959	871
Punjab	893	876	921
Rajasthan	857	862	838
Tamil Nadu	915	926	903
Uttar Pradesh	882	871	923
Uttarakhand	850	857	832
West Bengal	937	938	932
India	898	902	888

*Andhra Pradesh including Telangana; Telangana is a separate State now.

Dependency Ratio

The proportion of person above 65 years of age and children below 15 years of age are considered to be dependent on the economically productive age group of 15–64 years.

Total Dependency Ratio

The ratio of the combined age group 0–14 years +65 years and above to the 15–65 years age group is referred to the total dependency ratio. It is also referred to as societal dependency ratio and reflects the need for a society to provide for their younger and older population group.

The dependency ratio can be subdivided into young age dependency ratio (0–14 years) and old age dependency ratio (65 years and above). It is given by the formula:

$$\text{Total dependence ratio} = \frac{\text{Children } 0-14 \text{ years of age} + \text{Population} > 65 \text{ more}}{\text{Population } 15-64 \text{ years}} \times 100$$

For India the dependency ratio for the year 2023 is 47%.

Density of Population

One of the important indices of population concentration is the density of population. It is the ratio of total population to the surface area (land). This ratio can be calculated for any territorial unit for any point of time depending on the surface of population data.

Census of India defines population density as the number of persons living per square kilometer. The population density varies in different cities of India as per census 2011; the population density of Mumbai, Kolkata and Delhi are 31700 km^2, 24252 km^2 and 1197 km^2, respectively. The trends of population density in the country from 1901 onward are shown in Table 7.11.

Table 7.11 shows that density of population has increased with increase in decadal growth.

TABLE 7.11: Density of population in India 1901–2021

Years	1901	1911	1921	1931	1941	1951	1961	1971	1981	1991	2001	2011	2021
Persons living per square kilometer	77	82	81	90	103	117	142	177	216	267	325	382	428

Urbanization

Urbanization is increasing in the developing countries. By definition, urban locality varies from country to country. In Indian context, urban areas are the towns (places with municipal corporation, municipal area committee, town, notified area committee or cantonment board) with 5,000 or more inhabitants, a density of not <625 person per square kilometer, pronounced urban characteristics and at least three-quarters of the adult male population employed in pursuits other than agriculture. As per the census of 2011, of the total population, the rural population is 833.1 million (68.84%) and urban population is 377.1 million (31–80%) an increase of 3.35% in urban population. In absolute numbers, rural population has increased by 90.47 million and urban population has increased by 91.00 million in the last decade.

Uttar Pradesh has largest rural population of 155.11 million, i.e., 18–62% of country's rural population whereas Maharashtra has the greatest urban population of 50.83 million, i.e., 13.48% of country's urban population.

This increase in urban population has resulted due to natural growth (through births) and migration from villages to seek employment, attraction of better living conditions and availability of social services, such as education, health, transport, entertainment, etc. The continuous migration of people from countryside to urban areas in India constitutes a social crisis. It may eventually impair the quality of life. Figure 7.2 indicates the level of urbanization is increasing with increase in population in the country.

Family Size

The family size refers to the total number of persons in a family. In demography, family size means the total number of children born to a woman at a point in time. The completed family size indicates the total number of children born by woman during her child-bearing age, i.e., between 15 and 45 years of age. The total fertility rate gives the approximate magnitude of the completed family size. The family size depends upon a number of factors:

- Age of woman at marriage
- Duration of marriage
- Education of the couple
- Number of live births and living children
- Preference of male child
- Desired family size.

The family size is important from demographic point of view to bring down the fertility rate. Family planning program campaign is currently based on the theme of a "two children" family norm with a view to reach the long-term demographic goal of NRR is a demographic indicator explained on subsequent pages. Family planning involves both the decision regarding the desired family size and the effective limitation of fertility, once that size has been reached.

The decline in fertility rate (completed family size) in India and selected countries is shown in Table 7.12. The decrease in family size is not due to reduction in fertility rate but it is due to result of deliberate family planning.

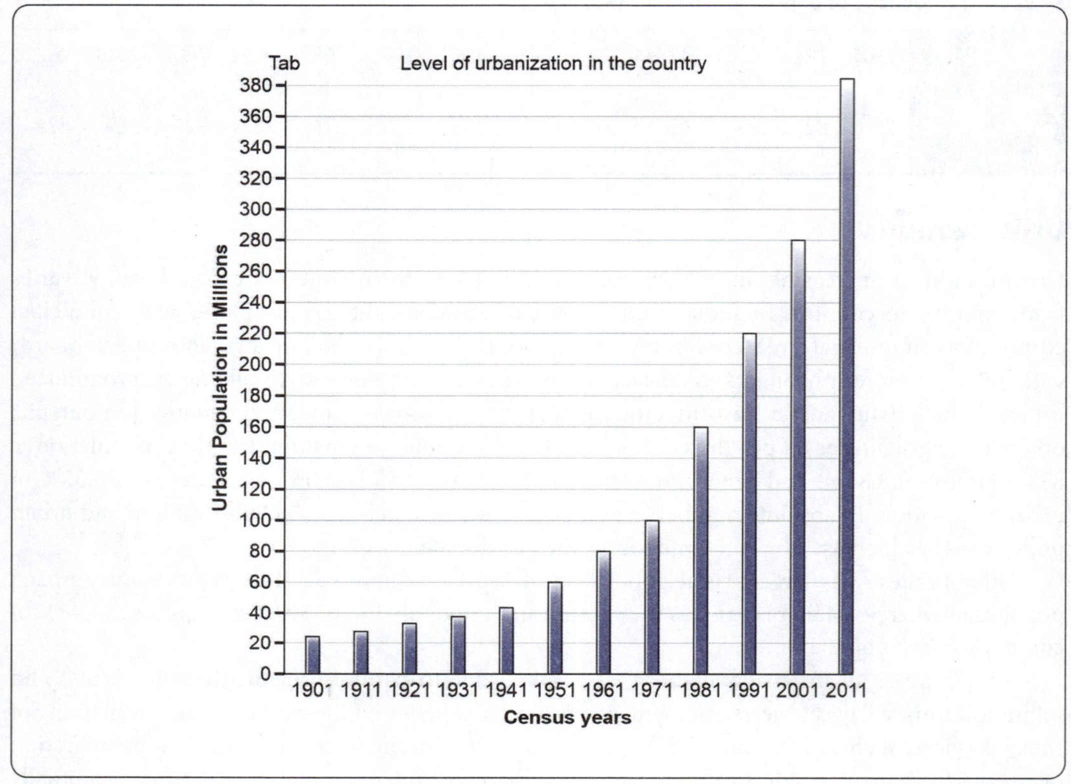

Figure 7.2: Level of urbanization in the country in census years

TABLE 7.12: Decline in fertility rate from 1994 to 2023

Countries	1994	2023
India	3.7	2.13
Bangladesh	3.9	1.93
Nepal	4.8	1.79
Sri Lanka	2.3	1.99
Myanmar	3.6	2.15
China	1.9	1.76
Pakistan	5.5	3.23
UK	1.8	1.75
USA	2.0	1.62
Japan	1.5	1.20
Switzerland	1.5	1.55

Literacy and Education

The Universal Declaration of Human Rights in 1948 stated that everyone has right to education. Yet, even today this right is being denied to millions of children. Education is a crucial element in economic and social development of any country. Without education, development neither can be broad based nor sustained. The benefits of literate population are multidimensional. Spread of education is associated with modernization, urbanization, industrialization, communication and commerce. It forms an overall development of individuals enabling them to comprehend their social, political and cultural environment better and respond it appropriately. Higher level of education and literacy lead to a greater awareness and also contribute to improvement of economic conditions and is prerequisite of acquiring various skills and better use of health facilities.

It was decided in 1991 census to use the term literacy rate for population relating to 7 years of age and above. A person is said to be literate, if he/she can read and write in any language. But a person who can only read and cannot write is not considered literate. The same concept has been confined in the census of 2001 and 2011 also.

The literacy rate taking in account the total population in the denominator has now been termed "crude literacy rate" the literacy rate taking into account the 7 year and above population in the denominator is called the affective literacy rate. The rate is given by the formula:

$$\text{Crude literacy rate} = \frac{\text{Number of literate persons}}{\text{Total population in a given year}} \times 100$$

$$\text{Effective literacy rate} = \frac{\text{Number of literate persons aged 7 and above}}{\text{Population aged 7 and above in a given year}} \times 100$$

The significant milestone reached in census 2011 is that the total number of illiterates has come down from 304.1 million in 2001 to 272.9 million in 2011 showing a decline of 31.1 million. The decadal increase in number of literates among males is 31.9% points and the corresponding increase among females is of 49.1% points. This shows that the gender gap in literacy is declining.

Literacy rate in India after independence has increased from 18.33 in 1951 to 74.04 in 2011 (Fig. 7.3).

The national average of literacy rate is misleading as wide variation exists between the states. The literacy rate in different states in India is shown in Table 7.13. The national percentage of literate's population above 7 years of age is about 74.04 with literate males 82.14% and female 65.46.

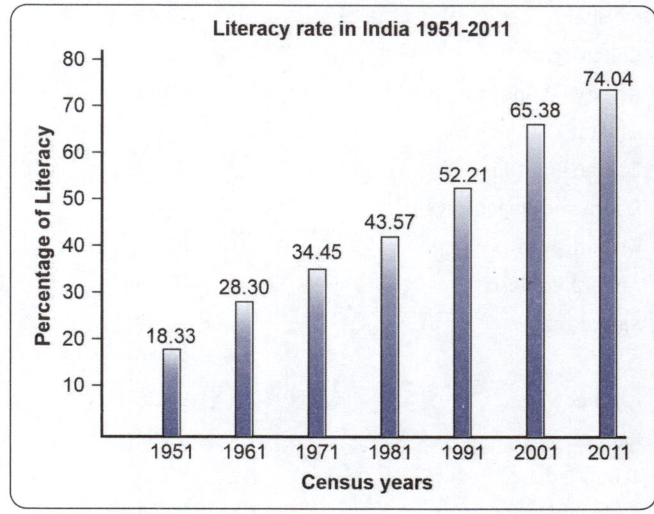

Figure 7.3: Literacy rate in India 1951–2011

TABLE 7.13: State-wise literacy rate in India—2011

State/union territory	Literacy rate		
	Total	Males	Females
Jammu and Kashmir	68.74	78.26	58.01
Himachal Pradesh	83.78	90.83	76.60
Punjab	76.68	81.48	71.34
Chandigarh	86.43	90.54	81.38
Uttarakhand	79.63	88.33	70.70
Haryana	76.64	85.38	66.77
NCT of Delhi	86.34	91.03	80.93
Rajasthan	67.06	80.51	52.66
Uttar Pradesh	69.72	79.24	59.26
Bihar	63.82	73.39	53.33
Sikkim	82.20	87.29	76.43
Arunachal Pradesh	66.95	73.69	59.57
Nagaland	80.11	83.29	76.69
Manipur	79.85	86.49	73.17
Mizoram	91.58	93.72	89.40
Tripura	87.75	92.18	83.15
Meghalaya	75.48	77.17	73.78
Assam	73.18	78.81	67.27
West Bengal	77.08	82.67	71.16
Jharkhand	67.63	78.45	56.21
Odisha	73.45	82.40	64.36
Chhattisgarh	71.04	81.45	60.59
Madhya Pradesh	70.63	80.53	60.02
Gujarat	79.31	87.23	70.73
Daman and Diu	87.07	91.48	79.59
Dadra and Nagar Haveli	77.65	86.46	65.93
Maharashtra	82.91	89.82	75.48
Andhra Pradesh	67.66	75.56	59.74
Karnataka	75.60	82.85	68.13
Goa	87.40	92.81	81.84
Lakshadweep	92.28	96.11	88.25
Kerala	93.91	96.02	91.98
Tamil Nadu	80.33	86.81	73.86
Puducherry	86.55	92.12	81.22
Andaman and Nicobar Island	86.27	90.11	81.84
India	74.04	82.14	65.46

Table 7.13 shows that Kerala has got highest literacy rate of 93.91% literate. The second highest is Lakshadweep 92.28% and third is the Mizoram with 91.58% literate population. The lowest literacy rate state is Bihar with 63.82%, and Arunachal Pradesh with 66.9% literacy rate.

Government of India has made education compulsory up to the age of 14 year but the major concern is high dropout rates in the first few years of schooling.

Life Expectancy

Life expectancy or expectation of life at a given age is the average number of years which a person of that age may expect to live, according to the mortality pattern prevalent in that country. Demographers consider it as one of the best indicators for a country's level of development and of the overall health status of its population.

Life expectancy at birth has continued to increase globally over the years. For 1950–1955, the combined life expectancy at birth for both sexes was 46.5 years. Five decades later by 2008, it was 69 years, an increase of 22.5 years.

The increase has been more marked in less developed regions of the world than in the developed regions. Most countries of the world show sex differential life expectancy, i.e., favoring woman, females live longer than males.

This increase in life expectancy in India is due to increasing awareness of better living conditions education and health. There is a need for health policy makers to recognize the changing demographic pattern and plan for prevention and control of diseases associated with old age. Tables 7.14 and 7.15 show the life expectancy at birth in selected countries.

Table 7.14 shows that the life expectancy has greatly increased from 1901 to 2011 in both sexes. Females show slightly higher life expectancy than males

Expectation of life at birth, years, in selected countries in 2017 is given in Table 7.15. This Table 7.15 also shows that life expectancy of female is longer than males.

TABLE 7.14: **Expectation of life at birth, years in India**

Year	1901	1911	1921	1931	1941	1951	1961	1971	1981	1991	2001	2011
Males	23.63	22.59	19.42	26.91	32.09	32.45	41.89	46.40	54.10	59.70	63.90	64.00
Females	23.96	23.31	20.91	26.56	31.37	31.66	40.55	44.70	54.70	60.90	66.90	67.00

TABLE 7.15: **Expectation of life at birth, years in selected countries 2017**

Developing countries	2017		Developed countries	2017	
	Males	Females		Males	Females
Nepal	70	71	UK	79	83
Bangladesh	70	73	USA	76	81
Myanmar	64	69	Sweden	81	84
India	67	70	Sweeter land	82	85
Sri Lanka	72	79	Russian Federation	66	78
Thailand	72	79	Japan	81	87
Pakistan	66	68	Singapore	81	85

POPULATION EXPLOSION

India is densely populated country. India has shown a rapid growth of population especially after independence. It is due to the inadequate implementation of family planning due to lack of resources in the country at right time. If the education is kept first priority of girls and boys with equal rights irrespective of cast religion and free education made compulsory up to 10th standard, most of the basic health problems and family planning problems can be solved from the beginning. Unemployment, poverty, low literacy, high prices, low status of health, pitiable conditions of woman, etc., all are clear indicators of over population and population explosion. In fact due to this rapid increase in population the building of India's economy has collapsed and the dream of economic progress is still a distant one. According to the census 2011, the growth rate has slightly decreased. The next proposed census was to happen in 2021 but it was postponed due to COVID-19 pandemic.

The replacement level means the total fertility rate that will result in stable population. This is possible due to the implementation of family welfare services and family planning programmers and other projects related to social development of the country. the population explosion can be controlled once the people are educated and realize the value of small family norm for better living.

Causes of Population Explosion

During the 20th to early 21st century, the Indian population has increased more than four times. The main reasons for this population explosion and fast increase rate are as follows:
- High birth rate
- Sharp fall in death rate.

The reason for population explosion in the country may be classified as under:
- **Reasons related to high birth rate are as follows:**
  - Child marriage
  - Illiteracy
  - Joint family system
  - Poverty
  - Lack of recreation
  - Polygamy
  - Lack of social security
  - High infant mortality rate
  - Neglect of family planning
  - Unavailability of family planning services
  - Religious superstitions
  - Preference for male child
  - Dependency of women
  - Marriage being essential
  - Housing problems
  - Poor status of woman in the family
  - Fatalistic attitude
  - Erotic literature.
- **Reasons for reduced death rate**
  - Improvement in medical and health services
  - Control of epidemics/untimely deaths
  - Improvement in economic conditions
  - Awareness about health
- **Political reasons for increase in population**
  - Illegal refugees
  - Return of migrants to India
  - Lack of political determination and will power regarding family planning
  - Failure to motivate people about small family norms

- Poor economy of the country
- Failure to provide basic amenities to the people.

Impact of Population Explosion

Population explosion impacts the growth of a country in the following ways (Fig. 7.4):

- **Inadequate resources:** With the increase in population the resources are decreasing:
  - **Lack of food production:** According to the Food and Agriculture Organization (FAO) of the United Nations that world food production requires an increase of 70% to meet the needs of the projected population of 9.1 billion by 2050. The food production in developing countries needs to be doubled to meet the requirement of increased population.
  - **Energy resources:** If the growth rate continued to occur in the same pace, 50% of more energy is required for increased population for industrialization and urbanization. The natural resources like wood, fossil fuel, oil, gas and coal will diminish.
- **Unemployment:** The jobs will not be sufficient for growing youth and there will be unemployment.
- **Poverty:** Unemployment leads to poverty and starvation. People will not be able to meet their minimum needs.
- **Lack of housing:** Due to increased density people will not have sufficient place for accommodation. They will be compelled to live in poor and overcrowded houses resulting in poor standard of living and become prey to many diseases.

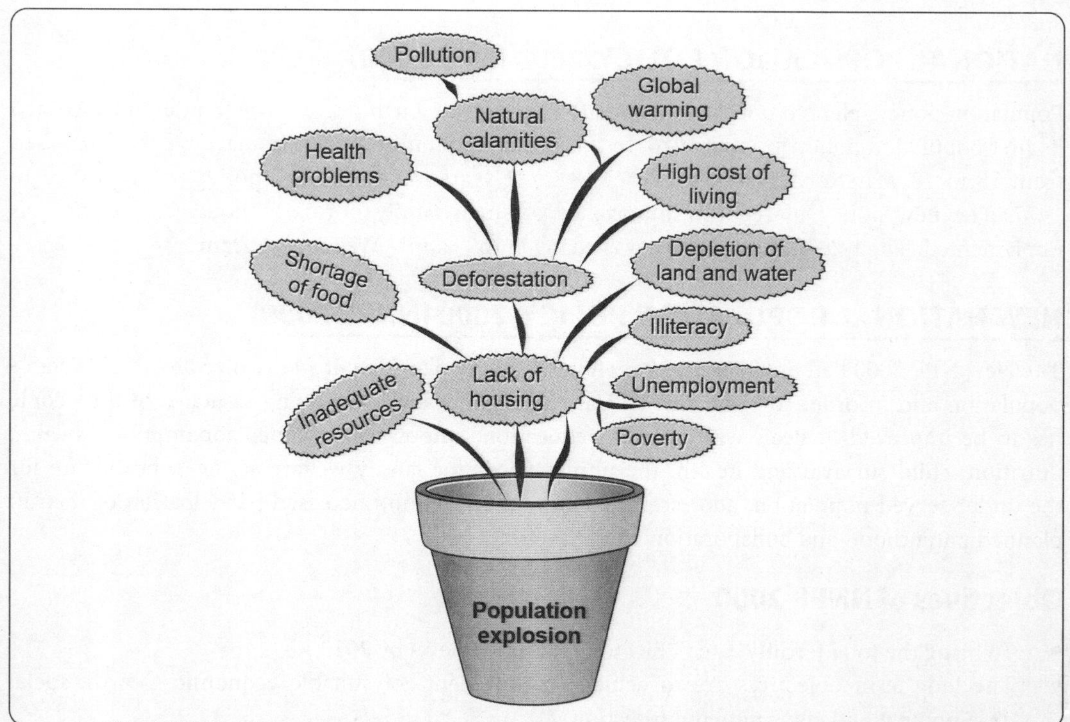

Figure 7.4: Impact of population explosion

- **Health problems:** Lack of food, unemployment, poor housing and overcrowding, and lack of health facilities for a large population result in many health problems.
- **Depletion of land and water:** The land area will diminish due to increased building, industrialization and urbanization. There will be increased demand of water and gradually there will be deficiency of water also.
- **Illiteracy:** The educational institutions will not be enough for increased population and also due to poverty people will not have access to education.
- **Pollution:** Overpopulation, deforestation, industrialization, urbanization, and lack of water resources will lead to air, water, noise, and land pollution.
- **Deforestation:** The forest has to be axed to need the housing demands of increasing population. It will again result in soil erosion, increase in temperature, melting of ice and lack of rain and water.
- **Global warming:** The burning of coal, gas, oil in increased motor vehicles will emit unburnt harmful gases, increased amount of carbon dioxide will increase the atmospheric temperature. This increased temperature with lack of trees can result into global warming.
- **Accidents:** Increased population, increased motor vehicles and lack of proper roads and traffic system can cause more accidents.
- **High cost of living:** Due to unemployment, poverty and lack of natural resources, the cost of living will increase and sustaining of normal life will be difficult.
- **Natural calamities:** Due to soil erosion, deforestation, there will be earthquakes, storms, draughts and famines and floods due to melting of glaciers.

NATIONAL POPULATION POLICY, 2000 (NPP 2000)

Population policy refers to policies intended to decrease the birth rate or growth rate. India formed its first population policy in April 1976. In this policy, the minimum age of marriage was increased from 15 to 18 years for females and from 18 to 21 years for males. The policy was modified in 1977. The new policy placed the importance of small family norms without compulsion was implemented. The title of the program was changed to "Family Welfare Program".

NEW NATIONAL POPULATION POLICY, 2000 (NNPP 2000)

The New NPP 2000 had broader aspect then just a family planning. It was realized to achieve stable population and in order to bring the TFR at replacement level, the living standard of the people has to be improved. It deals with women's education, empowering women for improved health, nutrition, child survival and health, the unmet needs for family welfare services, healthcare for the under-served population, adolescent health and education, increased participation of men in planned parenthood and collaboration with NGOs.

Objectives of NNPP 2000

- To bring the total fertility rate (TFR) to replacement level by 2010.
- The long-term objectives are to achieve requirements of suitable economic growth, social development and environment protection.

The national sociodemographic goals to be achieved by 2010 were:

- Reach the replacement level for TFR = 2.1
- Attain the net reproduction rate (NRR) of 1
- Address unmet needs of family planning
- Promote small family norms compulsory up to the age of 14 years
- Make school education free and compulsory up to the age of 14 years and reduce the dropout at primary and secondary school level below 20% for boys and girls
- Age of marriage for girls not <18, preferably >20 years
- 100% registration of births and death
- Reduce infant mortality rate to below 30/1000 live births
- Reduce maternal mortality ratio to below 100/100,000 live births
- Achieve 80% institutional deliveries and 100% deliveries by trained persons
- Achieve universal immunization of children against all vaccine preventable diseases
- Prevent and control communicable diseases
- Contain the spread of acquired immunodeficiency syndrome (AIDS) and promote greater integration between the management of reproductive tract infections (RTI) and sexually transmitted infections (STI) and the National AIDS Control Program
- Integrate Indian System of Medicine (ISM) in the provision of reproductive and child health services and in reaching out to the house hold
- Bring about the convergence in implementation of related social sector programs so that family welfare becomes a people centered approach.

The long-term goal of NPP 2000 is to stabilize population growth by 2045 at a level that satisfy demands of societal development, environmental preservation and sustainable growth.

CONCEPTS OF FERTILITY AND INFERTILITY

Fertility

Fertility refers to the ability to produce viable offspring. Fertility may be defined as the actual bearing of children. Some demographers use the word natality in place of fertility. A woman's reproductive period is roughly from 15 years to 45 years, i.e., a period of 30 years. A woman married at the age of 15 years and living with her husband till 45 years, she is exposed to the risk of pregnancy for 30 years and may give birth to 15 children, but this max is rarely achieved.

Fertility depends upon several factors. The higher fertility in India is attributed to universality of marriage:

- Low age at marriage
- Low level of literacy
- Poor level of living
- Limited use of contraceptives
- Traditional ways of life

The National Family Health Survey-3 conducted in India during 2005–2006 provides the following information about the fertility trends in India.

Determinants/Factors

Fertility is a multifaceted phenomenon. It may be affected by different factors which may be social, cultural, biological or physical in nature. India is a country of diversity in culture and social values. Therefore, the fertility rate is also different in different societies. Some important but common factors affecting fertility are universality of marriage, lower age of marriage, low literacy or illiteracy, less use of contraceptives, lifestyle of the people, widow marriage, industrialization, technology development, healthcare facilities, woman abuse, desire of a son, breastfeeding, customs, etc. The National Family Health Survey-2 (1998–1999) and NFHS-3 (2005–2006) provide various valuable information about fertility trends in India. These factors are described as:

- **Age at marriage:** The age at which a woman marries and enters the reproductive period of life has a great impact on her fertility. The data collected on a national scale on fertility by the Registrar General of India, found that females who marry before the age of 18 years gave birth to a larger number of children than who married after the age of 18 years. It has been also estimated by some demographers that if the marriage is delayed from 16 to 20–21 year, the number of births would decrease by 20–30%. The Child Marriage Restraint Act, 1978 raises the age of marriage for girls from 15 to 18 years and for boys from 18 to 21 years. This act has impact on fertility.
- **Duration of married life:** It has been shown in studies that 10–25% of all births occur within 1 to 5 years of married life and 50–55% of all birth within 5–15 years of married life. After 25 years of married life the birth declines to achieve that target of family planning. Therefore, the family planning should be emphasized in early years of married life.
- **Spacing of children:** Studies showed that when all the births are postponed by one year in each age group. There was a decline in total fertility. Therefore, spacing of children has a significant impact on general reduction in the fertility rate.
- **Education:** Lower fertility rate has been found in educated couples. There is an inverse association between fertility and educational status. Education provides knowledge, awareness and increased information and media exposure. Employment of woman increases participation in decision-making about family planning.
- **Economic status:** Survey indicates that high fertility rate is found in poor income group whereas rise in economic status decreases fertility. The world population conference held at Bucharest in 1974 stressed that economic development is the best contraception. It will take care of population growth and bring about reductions in fertility.
- **Religion:** Hindus have a lower fertility than Muslims. It is lowest among the Christians. NFHS-3 reported that a total fertility rate of 3.09 among Muslim as compared to 2.65 among Hindus and 2.35 among Christians.
- **Caste:** Lower castes of Hindus have higher fertility rate in comparison to the higher castes.
- **Nutrition:** There is a relationship between nutrition and fertility level. It has been found that all well-fed societies have low fertility and poor fed societies have high fertility. The effect of nutrition on fertility is largely indirect.
- **Family planning:** It is a key factor in declining fertility in the developing countries. It should be initiated rapidly and it requires only limited resources as compared to other factors.
- **Cultural beliefs and practices:** There are number of cultural and social factors such as lifestyle, place of women in society, value of children in society, breastfeeding, customs and beliefs, etc., influence the reproductive behaviors and fertility outcome.

Principles of Fertility Regulation

- **Avoid untimely pregnancies:** Untimely pregnancies are those pregnancies that occur at two extreme ends of reproductive phase of woman, i.e., before the age of 20 years and above the age of 35 years. There is an increased risk of morbidity and mortality of their untimely pregnancies.
- **Avoid too close pregnancies:** The short interval between the pregnancies undermines the health of mothers as the mothers have not recovered from the stress of previous pregnancies. An adequate inter-pregnancies interval is essential for the health of the mother and the baby.
- **Avoid unwanted pregnancies:** These are associated with high maternal and infant mortality. Unwanted pregnancies usually end in unsafe abortions with super added risk.
- **Avoid too many pregnancies:** Too many pregnancies impose a continued drain on the nutritional reserves of woman leading to maternal deprivation, depletion, reduced maternal competence and lowered resistance to infections, anemia, etc.
- **Avoid risk pregnancies:** Mothers having medical disease like hypertension, rheumatic heart disease, diabetes mellitus, chronic cerebral thrombosis and renal diseases with pregnancies are high-risk pregnancies and increase the risk of maternal and fetal morbidity and mortality.

Benefits of Fertility Regulation

- **Benefit to the mother:** The physical and mental stress of pregnancies are eliminated. Her body recovers from the physiological changes of previous parturition. Her nutritional status is improved and it leads to reduction in maternal morbidity and mortality.
- **Benefit to the child:** Baby born with adequate birthweight and reduced risk of congenital anomalies. Baby grows in an affectionate family environment and gets adequate breastfeeding and weaning diet. Risk of infection to the baby is much reduced, when care has been taken properly by the mother.
- **Benefit to the family:** There is economic security, improved nutritional status, educational status, proper housing and social status. All these raise the living standard of the family and reduce the incidence of sickness in the family thereby improving the health status of the family.
- **Benefit to the community:** Reduced demand for community facilities like housing, education, healthcare, water supply, communication, waste disposal services and marketing facilities.
- **Benefits to the country:** Stabilization of population, economic development and increased resources for providing better facilities of education, nutrition, healthcare, housing and communication decrease in the overall morbidity, mortality and fertility statistics of the country.

Approaches Toward Fertility Regulation

- **Educational approach:** Education provides awareness and makes the couple aware of the benefits of small family. Education helps couple to select methods of contraceptive to regulate fertility.
- **Services:** This approach demands continuity of care as provided in antenatal, intranatal. Postnatal and under-five clinics. Services approach implies maintaining contact with acceptors of contraception and also involves follow-up cases.
- **Motivational:** Incentives may be offered to the acceptors on individual basis or on community basis. Those who volunteer for sterilization operations are paid extra increment. They may be paid compensation for loss of wages beside a cash incentive.

- **Legal:** The most important legal measure is the Child Marriage Restraint Act, 1978. It has raised the legal age of marriage of boys and girls. Liberalization of Abortion Act (MTP Act) is another legal measure to promote fertility control.
- **Integrated:** It includes the elements of all other approaches and addresses all the problems connected with maternal and child health, inclusive of fertility control.
- **Methods to regulate fertility:**
  - **Contraception:** It is the process of interruption of conception at any stage preceding, accompanying or immediately following copulation. The methods used may be physiological, mechanical, chemical, hormonal or combination of all these. Contraception may be achieved by using rhythm method, barrier contraception, intra-uterine devices, hormonal contraception or postcoital contraception.
  - **Termination:** It is a process of dislodging the implantation of a fertilized ovum and disabling the continuation of an established pregnancy. Termination can be done within a few days of missing period or much later in pregnancy before the fetus is viable.
  - **Sterilization:** It is a surgical procedure that arrests the fertility of an individual on permanent basis. It creates mechanical barriers to the movement of ovum or sperms. It comprises vasectomy in males or no-scalpel vasectomy (NSV) and tubectomy in females.

Fertility Related Statistics or Indicators

Fertility is measured by a number of indicators. Some of the indicators are given as under:

- **Birth rate:** It is the simplest indicators of fertility and can be defined as the "the number of live births per 1,000 estimated mid-year population, in a given year." It is given by the formula:

$$\text{Birth rate} = \frac{\text{Number of the live births during the year}}{\text{Estimated mid-year population}} \times 1000$$

Birth rate is an unsatisfactory measure of fertility as the total population is not exposed to child bearing.

- **General fertility rate (GFR):** It is defined as "number of live births per 1,000 women in the reproductive age group of (15–44 years or 49 years) in a given year."

$$\text{GFR} = \frac{\text{Number of live births in an area during the year}}{\substack{\text{Mid-year married female population of} \\ \text{age (15–44 years or 49) in a given year}}}$$

General fertility rate is better measure of fertility than crude birth rate as the denominator is restricted to the number of women in child-bearing age.

- **General marital fertility rate (GMFR):** It is the "number of live births per 1,000 married women in the reproductive age group (15–44 or 49 years) in a given year".

$$\text{GMFR} = \frac{\text{Number of live births in a year}}{\substack{\text{Mid-year married female population} \\ \text{in the age group 15–49 years}}} \times 1000$$

- **Age-specific fertility rate (ASFR):** It is defined as the number of live births in a year to 1,000 women in any specified age group.

$$\text{ASFR} = \frac{\text{Number of live births in a particular age group}}{\text{Mid-year female population of the same age group}} \times 1000$$

- **Age-specific marital fertility rate (ASMFR):** It is the number of live births in a year to 1,000 married women in any specific age group.

$$\text{ASMFR} = \frac{\text{Number of live birth in a particular age group}}{\text{Mid-year married female population of the same age group}} \times 1000$$

- **Total fertility rate (TFR):** Total fertility rate represents the average number of children a woman would have if she were to pass through her reproductive years bearing children at the same rate as the woman now in each age group. It is computed by summing the age-specific fertility rate for all ages. If 5 years age groups are used the sum of the rates is multiplied by 5. This measure gives the approximate magnitude of "completed family size."

$$\text{TFR} = \frac{5 \times \sum_{15-19}^{45-49} \text{ASFR}}{1000}$$

- **Total marital fertility rate (TMFR):** It is defined as the average number of children that would be born to a married woman if she experiences the current fertility pattern throughout her reproductive span.

$$\text{TMFR} = \frac{5 \times \sum_{15-19}^{45-49} \text{ASMFR}}{1000}$$

- **Gross reproductive rate (GRR):** Average number of girls that would be born to woman if she experiences the current fertility pattern throughout her reproductive span (15–44 or 49) assuming no mortality.

$$\text{GRR} = \frac{5 \times \sum_{15-19}^{45-49} \text{ASFR for female live births}}{1000}$$

- **Net reproduction rate (NRR):** It is defined as the number of daughters a new born girl will bear during her life time assuming fixed age specific fertility and mortality rates of a given year. NRR is similar to GRR but takes into account that some females will die before completing their reproductive span of life. An NRR one means that each generation of methods is having exactly enough daughters to replace themselves in the population exactly. An NRR one can be achieved by adopting two child norms. If the NRR is <1 then the reproductive performance of the population is said to be below the replacement level. Replacement level refers to the fertility rate that with result in stable population. NRR is a demographic indication.
- **Child-woman ratio:** It is the number of children 0–4 years of age per 1,000 women of child bearing age, usually defined as 15–44 years or 49 years of age. This ratio is used where birth registration statistics either do not exist or inadequate. It is measured through data derived from censuses.
- **Pregnancy rate:** It is the ratio of pregnancies in a year to married woman in the age 15–44 years or 49 years. The number of pregnancies includes all pregnancies whether those had terminated as live births, stillbirths, abortions or had not yet terminated.

- **Abortion rate:** It is defined as the annual number of all type of abortions usually per 1,000 women of child-bearing age (usually defined as 15–44 years).
- **Abortion ratio:** This is calculated by dividing the number of abortions performed during the particular time period by the number of live births over the same period.
- **Marriage rate:** It is the number of marriages in the year per 1,000 population.

$$\text{Crude marriage rate} = \frac{\text{Number of marriages in the year}}{\text{Mid-year population}} \times 1000$$

- **General marriage rate:** It is defined as the number of marriages within 1 year per 1000 populations to the number of unmarried persons of age 15–19 years.

$$\text{General marriage rate} = \frac{\text{Number of marriages within one year}}{\text{Number of unmarried persons of age 15-49 years}} \times 1000$$

Trends of Fertility in India

India is a country of diversity in cultural, social, customs and religious beliefs which play a role in fertility. It has been indicated by National Family Health Surveys and census that level of fertility in India is beginning to decline. The crude birth rate which was about 49 per 1,000 populations during 1901–1911 has declined to about 25.0 per 1,000 populations in 2002 and was 20.0 per 1,000 populations in 2015. The rural urban differential has narrowed. However, crude birth rate has continued to be higher in the rural areas as compared to urban areas in last 3 decades.

The total fertility rate has declined from 3.6 in 1991 to 2.3 in 1994. TFR in rural areas has declined from 5.4 in 1971 to 1.2 in 2014, where the corresponding decline is in urban areas has been from 4.1 to 1.8 during the same period. However there is a considerable variation between the states in total fertility rate (Fig. 7.5).

Birth and death rates: The death rate has considerably declined from 27.4 in 1951 to an estimated 7.0 per 1,000 population in 2015, the birth rate has declined from 39.9 in 1951 to estimated 20 per 1,000 in 2015. The fifth Five-Year Plan's (1974–1979) objective was to reduce birth rate from 35 per 1,000 at the beginning to 30 per 1,000 by 1978–1979. During 1979–1984, the birth rate was stagnated at 33 per 1000 with no obvious decline. During 1990, however the birth rate showed slight decline of 30.2 per 1000 and further decline to 26.4 per 1000 by 1998. The table shows that birth and death rate in India are declining as shown in the Table 7.16.

Table 7.17 shows that birth rate was at peak from 1952 to 1970 and thereafter it has declined to 16.20 in 2023. Death rate was also maximum 27.4 per 1000 in 1941–1950 and thereafter it started declining and reached 6.4 per 1000 in 2016 and started increasing to 7.41 in 2023.

High birth rate: India also like other developing countries facing the problems of high birth rate and declining death rate. The causes of high birth rate are as follows:

- Universality of marriage
- Early marriage
- Early puberty in Indian girls between 12 and 14 years of age
- Low standard of living
- Low level of literacy
- Traditional customs and habits
- Absence of family planning habit.

TABLE 7.16: Birth and death rate in India

Year	Birth rate	Death rate
1941–1950	39.9	27.4
1951–1960	41.7	22.8
1961–1970	41.2	19.0
1971–1980	37.2	15.0
1981	33.9	12.5
1991	29.5	9.8
1995	28.3	9.0
1998	26.8	9.0
1999	26.1	8.7
2002	25.0	8.1
2004	24.1	7.5
2006	23.5	7.5
2008	22.8	7.4
2010	21.1	7.2
2012	21.6	7.0
2015	20.0	7.0
2016	20.4	6.4
2017	17.9	7.242
2018	17.65	7.237
2019	17.05	7.273
2020	16.57	7.309
2021	16.42	7.344
2022	16.27	7.380
2023	16.20	7.416

Declining death rate due to:
- Advancement in medical facilities
- Availability of health services
- Control of communicable diseases
- Universal Immunization Program
- Impact of National Health Program
- Absence of natural checks, e.g., famines, floods, cyclones and large scale epidemics
- Improvement in food supply and nutrition
- Improved maternal and child health services
- International aid in several directions.
- Improvement in social status.

Growth rate: The population of India prior to 1921 grew at slow rate due to operations of natural checks like epidemics, floods, famine, earthquakes, etc., which took a heavy toll of human life.

After 1921, the occurrence of famines and epidemics was effectively controlled through improved healthcare services; affective management of epidemics and natural calamities, better nutrition, immunization, etc., that resulted in decline in death rate steeply than the birth rate. Consequently, there was a net gain in birth over deaths leading to rapid growth in population which rose from 1.25% in 1951 to 1.96% in 1961, 2.20% in 1975, 2.22% in 1981, 2.14% in 1991, 1.93% in 2001 and 1.64% in 2011 and 0.8% in 2021.

Growth rate is shown in table of population of India 1901 to 2011 as per census in Table 7.5 under the heading demographic trends in India.

India is projected to be the most populated country in the world in 2024, with China coming in second adding 17.5 million every year to her 1210 million as per 2011 census. However, the most recent data indicates a decline in India's population growth rate. The estimate for the year 2023 was 1442.4 million.

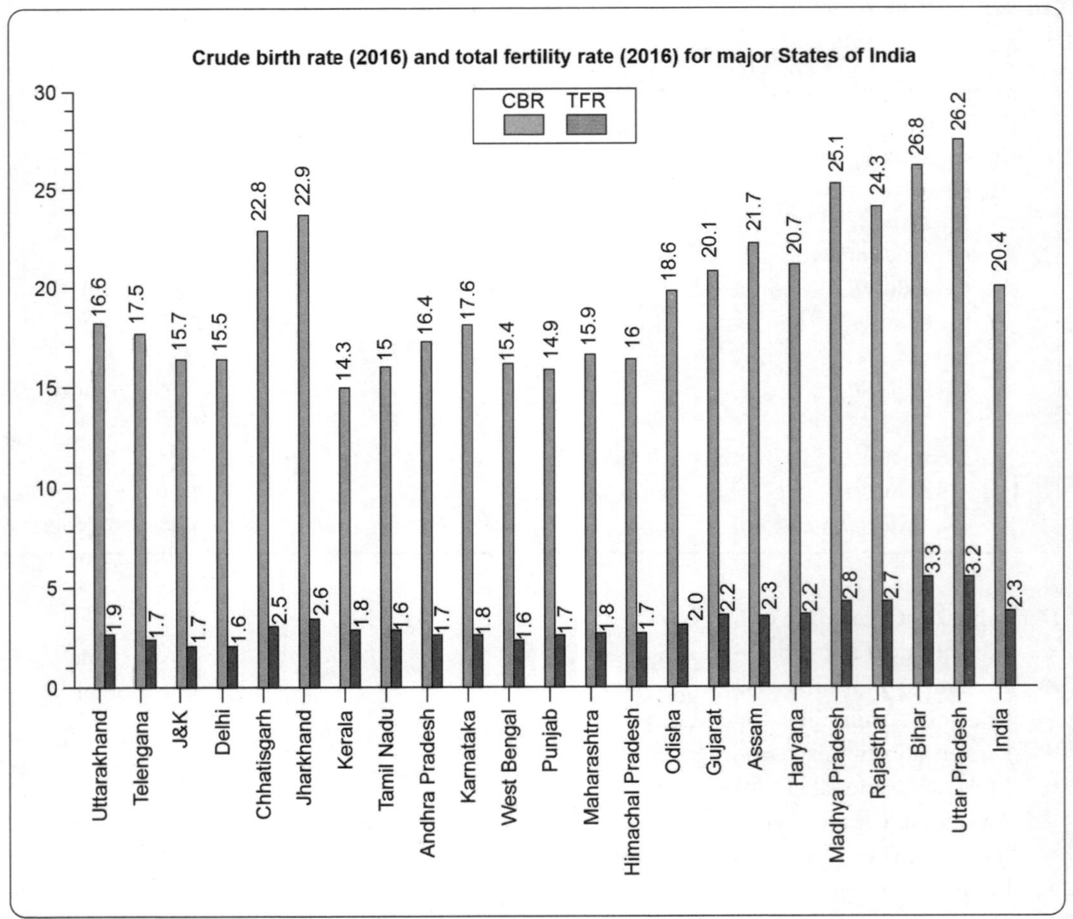

Figure 7.5: Crude birth rate (2016) and total fertility rate (2016) for major States of India

Infertility

Infertility is defined as a failure to conceive within one or more years of regular unprotected intercourse or it is the inability to produce offspring.

Incidence of infertility: It is estimated that worldwide one in seven couples have problems in conceiving.

Types of Infertility

Infertility may be primary or secondary:

- **Primary infertility:** Denotes couples who have never been able to conceive.
- **Secondary infertility:** It is defined as the failure to conceive after already having one or more pregnancy.

The term infertility also indicates the inability to produce children, generally because of a physical abnormality or often the absence of spermatogenesis in male or blockage of fallopian tubes in a woman.

Causes of Infertility

- Infertility may be due to problems of conception in male or female or both.
- Male factor contributes 30–40% female factor contributes 40–55%.
- **Combined:** In 10% of the people cause is unexplained.
- **Causes of male infertility**
  - Defective spermatogenesis
  - **Hypospadias:** It causes failure to deposit sperms high in the vagina
  - Obstruction of efferent ducts
  - **Gonadotrophic suppression:** This is found in chronic debilitating diseases. Malnutrition, heavy smoking and high intake of alcohols
  - Loss of sperm motility.
  - **Genetic:** Common chromosomal abnormality in azoospermic male is Klinefelter syndrome (47 XXY).
  - **Iatrogenic:** Radiation and cytotoxic drugs
    - **Congenital:** Undescended testes
    - **Infections:** Mumps orchitis after puberty may permanently damage spermatogenesis
    - **Endocrine factors:** Follicle-stimulating factors (FSH) level is raised in idiopathic testicular failure.
- **Causes of female infertility:**
  - Anovulation or oligo-ovulation, ovarian activity depends on gonadotrophins which are related to the release of gonadotropin-releasing hormone (GnRH) from hypothalamus. Disturbance of these may result in anovulation
  - Salpingitis
  - Too long fallopian tubes or kinks in the tubes
  - Tubal spasm
  - Uterine abnormalities like endometritis and fibroid, etc.
  - Cervical factors—chronic cervicitis
  - Scanty vaginal mucus
  - Vaginal abnormalities

- **Combined factors**
  - Age of wife above 35 years
  - Apareunia and dyspareunia
  - Anxiety
  - Immunological factors
  - Unexplained causes.

Management of Infertility

Management includes thorough investigations of the couple and identify the cause:
- If curable
  - Psychological support to couple
  - Proper therapeutic intervention
  - Follow-up care
- Counseling for genetic problems
- Adoption services for causes who cannot conceive.
- Artificial insemination if primary and secondary infertility cannot be treated, In vitro fertilization and embryo transfer. In vitro fertility can be used as both diagnostic and therapeutic tool in couples with unexplained infertility.

SMALL FAMILY NORMS

The family size plays an important role in the health and welfare of not only the individuals, family and community but also of the nation as a whole because it affects the population growth rate. A small difference in family size will make a big difference in the birth rate. The difference of only one child per family over a decade will have a large impact on population growth.

The voluntary acceptance of small family norm is the objective of family planning in India. In 1970, the slogan for small family was "Two or Three is enough" symbolized by the inverted red triangle; the program initially adopted the model of three child family. In view of the seriousness of the situation, the 1980 campaign has adopted the two-child norm. The current emphasis is on three themes:

1. Sons or daughters, two will do
2. Second child after 3 years, and
3. Universal immunization

A significant achievement of the Family Welfare Program in India has been the decline in the fertility rate from 6.4 in the 1950, to 2.3 in 2015. The national target was to achieve a net-reproduction rate of 1 by the year 2006 which is equivalent to attaining approximately 2 child norm.

The main objective of the Family Welfare Program in India is that people should adopt the "small family norm" to stabilize country's population at the level of some 1,533 million by the year 2050 AD.

Effects of Family Size

The size of the family affects the followings:
- **Basic human needs:** These include food, clothing, shelter, basic education and primary health. These are essential needs to be met by all the members. If the family size is large and resources are limited and shared by all. The per capita share will get smaller and will not fully meet the needs of the members. If the size of the family is small the per capita share will be more and helps in meeting all the basic needs of the family members.

- **Income, saving and resources:** If the family size is large, the per capita income will not be sufficient to meet all basic needs, low income, low saving and large family size will not help in further development.
- **Food and nutrition:** The larger the size of the family in proportion to the income and resources, the less will be quantity of food and inferior in quality will not meet the nutritive requirement of the member of the family. This will result in malnutrition, nutritional deficiency diseases and poor general resistance. This will predispose the family member to many more diseases and poor health.
- **Socioeconomic effect:** The larger family size will result in migration of rural people to urban areas in search for employment resulting urban slums and associated socioeconomic problems.
- **Fragmentation of family land:** Large family size end up into fragmentation of land holding in rural communities resulting in low per capita productivity. This again results in migration of rural people to urban areas for employment and creates burden on urban society.
- **Health:** Large family size has shown higher morbidity and mortality among mothers and children. This is because of early marriage, too early and frequent pregnancies, without proper gap and pregnancies continue till late reproductive age of the mother.
- **Education:** It is difficult for the large family to give proper education to all the children with limited resources and income which in turn will affect the size of their future families. The parent's education especially of woman affects the size of the family.

Hazards of Unplanned Large Family

The hazards are mainly due to early marriage, early pregnancy, frequents and too many pregnancies till late age. Some of the hazards are as follows:

- **Hazards due to early marriage and early pregnancy include:**
  - Health hazards of the mother in pregnancy and childbirth
  - Ill health of the mother
  - Low birthweight of the baby
  - Perinatal mortality
  - Abortion and miscarriage
  - Fetal and neonatal death
  - Incidence of cancer of cervix
  - Economic hardships
  - Difficulties in meeting the basic needs of the family members
  - Unhappiness and disharmony in the family.
- **Hazards due to frequent and too many pregnancies:**
  - Increased risk from pregnancy and childbirth
  - Ill health of the mother due to complications associated with pregnancies
  - Low birthweight baby
  - Divided attention between children
  - Increased risk of cancer of cervix
  - Economic hardships
  - Discontinuing education of children due to lack of finance
  - Unhappiness and domestic violence.

- **Hazards due to pregnancy at late age or till late age:**
  - Increased risk of pregnancy and childbirth
  - Congenital abnormalities of the child, i.e., mongoloid child
  - Loss of social status.
- **Overall hazards include:**
  - Increased maternal mortality and morbidity
  - Increased child mortality and morbidity
  - Increased congenital problems due to late pregnancies
    - Unemployment, illiteracy and poverty
    - Increased psychosocial problems
    - Increased diseases and disabilities.

Advantages of Planned Small Family

A small planned family has many advantages and benefit to couple, child, family as a whole, community and nation:

- **Advantage to couple:** Proper timing of birth, spacing of births and limiting the size of family will help husband and wife both.
- **Advantages to the wife include:**
  - Promotion of health, preparing for pregnancy regain her bodily strength, vigor and health after previous pregnancy
  - Be free of unwanted pregnancy
  - Less risk of maternal morbidity and mortality due to pregnancy and childbirth
  - Less risk of fetal death, abortion, miscarriage, birth defects, premature births, mortality in infancy and childhood
  - Have better opportunity for education, vocational training and employment
  - More time and strength to nurture the children and give proper attention to family.
- **Advantages to the husband:**
  - To have less family burden and be able to provide better nutrition, clothing, care, comfort, recreation, love and education to the children and other members of the family
  - To have family saving and develop resources for economic development in the long run
  - To be physically, mentally and socially healthy.
- **Advantages for the child:** Planned size of the family will help:
  - Child to have congenial atmosphere for wholesome growth and development of the child.
  - Child gets proper nutrition, education, parental care and love.
  - Child has less chance of infection especially gastrointestinal infections, respiratory infections and contagious infection.
  - Child will develop optimum level of intelligence.
  - Less risk of mortality.
- **Advantages to the family:** Small family norms will promote health, happiness, peace, harmony and prosperity in the family.
- **Advantages to the community and nation:**
  - Maintain natural resources
  - Maintain environmental health by controlling pollution, supplying adequate and safe water, proper sanitation and housing

- Maintain balance in ecosystem
- Reduce unemployment
- Promote adequacy of manmade resources, organization, institution and facilities, etc.
- Improve availability and accessibility of various facilities and services to the people
- In the long run, it will improve the living status of people and development of national economy
- Helps in reduction of population growth.

Barriers of Small Family Norms

- Children are considered God's gift and social security in old age especially the sons.
- Beliefs that "more hands more work" and considering that children are the wealth of poor people.
- Believing that children will support the parents in old age.
- Illiteracy, lack of knowledge, superstitions unemployment and lack of means of entertainment, etc.
- Unavailability of the family welfare services in rural and remote areas.
- Low woman's status, gender insensitivity, etc.
- Use of contraception is forbidden in some religions.
- Medical termination of pregnancy (MTP) and sterilization are considered sin and it is against the will of God in some religions.
- Survival of child is not assured because of high mortality and accidental deaths, etc.
- Religious factors: Hindus want a son to perform religious rites and last rites of parents.
- Muslim considered birth control against religion and for some Christian termination of pregnancy is considered a sin.

How to Overcome the Barriers

This requires a lot of stress on education, information and motivation of people in general and eligible couple in particular.

- Woman's education and empowerment and status will give her freedom for decision on size of family, timing and spacing of births, etc.
- Meeting minimum needs of the people
- Provision of comprehensive package of maternal and child health (MCH) and family welfare services
- Seeking support of various development sectors
- Counseling on motivation of adopting small family norms of the couple in reproductive phase.

Factors Promoting Small Family

- Sociocultural background
- Socioeconomic status of the family
- Health center and health worker's involvement and participation
- Family health services or programs effectiveness
- Education background of the individual and family members
- Effective contraceptive delivery services
- Health education and mass media participation.
- Importance of Family Planning in India

Factors Drawing the Importance of Family Planning in India

India is the first country in the world to launch a nationwide Family Planning Program in 1952. It was Indian's top most priority to control population growth as per the resources and improve the quality of life of people. The following factors draw the importance of family planning in India.

- **Increased population:** The increased population has adverse effect on our per capita income. >40% of India's population lives below the "poverty line". Poverty leads to sickness and sickness to poverty. People suffer from serious illness and they cannot get adequate medication due to poverty.
- **Population explosion:** The uncontrolled population has created various social and unemployment problems, overcrowding, illiteracy, low standard of living, urban deterioration, inadequate housing, poor and inadequate nutrition.
  - **As the family size increase:** Parents will not be able to cope with the increased family demands because family income is not increased comparing to family size. This leads to family disturbance, unhappiness and insecurity, etc.
  - **Mother's general health:** Due to repeated pregnancies and deliveries, mother's health gets impaired and leads to the problems of anemia and low immunity and all types of infections.
  - **As there is no proper spacing of children:** The child gets very little attention. This causes malnutrition, negligence and other sibling problems of previous child.

To avoid all these problems, family planning is necessary and it has attracted greater attention of the Indian government. Family planning is the urgent need and demand of the time in this growing population to control the growth rate which is necessary to maintain health and happiness of the family which ultimately depends upon the size of family.

FAMILY WELFARE

Family welfare is broader term than family planning. It is basically related to raise the living standard of the people and to improve the quality of life. Family welfare includes the integrated package of the services provided to the family such as education, nutrition, health, employment, woman's empowerment, shelter, safe drinking water and environment health. It is the government policy to promote family planning through a total welfare of the family.

CONCEPTS OF FAMILY WELFARE

The concepts of family planning is to make people realize the need for family planning for better life and healthy living. It is a target-free approach and decision left to the couples. Family welfare services are provided to improve the quality of life of the people. Recognizing that the planning of families would enhance individual health and welfare, the Government of India was the first in the world to initiate a comprehensive family welfare during the first Five-Year Plan. The concept of family planning is very comprehensive and related to raise the living standard of the people through education, nutrition, employment basic health services. Woman's welfare and rights, shelter, environmental sanitation, safe drinking water, i.e., all vital factors associated with the concept of welfare. Family welfare services are provided as a complete healthcare of the people so that they understand the need of good health and to improve the living standard. Keeping in view the limited resources of the country and extensive population, family welfare is given the top priority so that through these services, the quality of life can be improved and make people realize voluntary choice for limiting the size of the family to lead a quality of life. In 1977, the Government of India designated the Family Planning Program as a Family Welfare Program and changed the name of the Ministry of Health and Family Planning as a Ministry of Health and Family Welfare (Fig. 7.6).

SERVICES INCLUDED IN THE FAMILY WELFARE PROGRAM

Through the success of family welfare only the target of family planning can be achieved. The services included in the Family Welfare Program are as follows:

- Maternal and child health services
- Family planning
- Family life education of parents
- Nutrition of the family
- Immunization services
- Healthy environment in the home
- Care of the sick, aged and handicapped in the home
- Prevention of communicable disease.

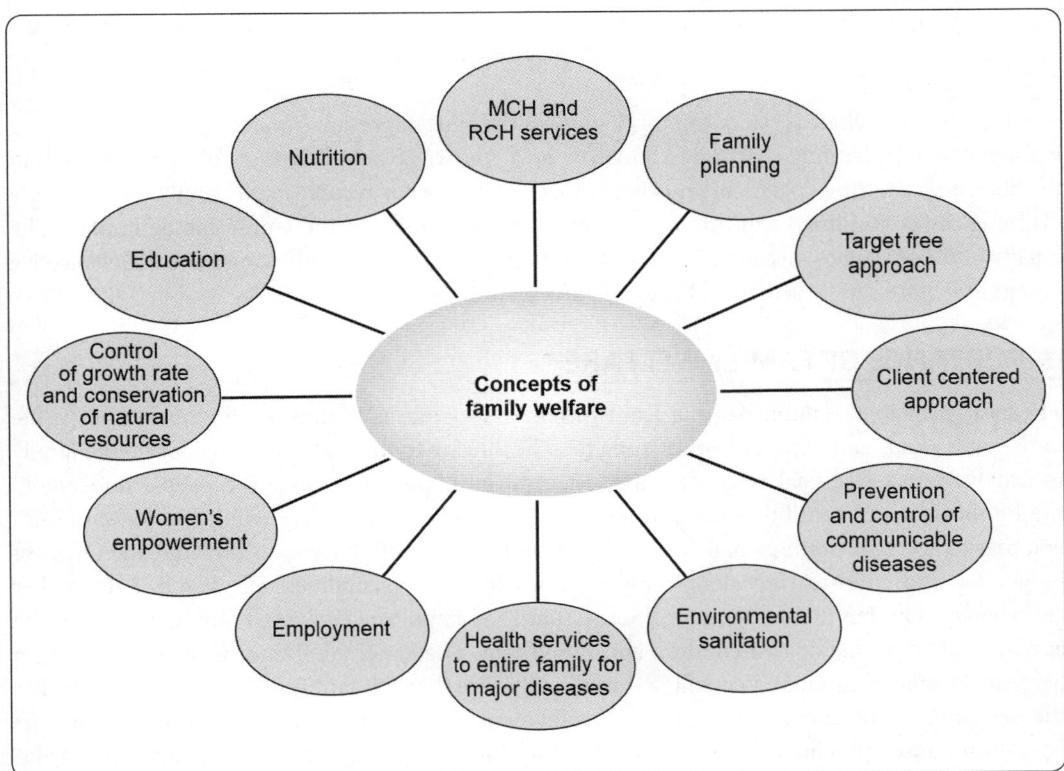

Figure 7.6: Concepts of family welfare

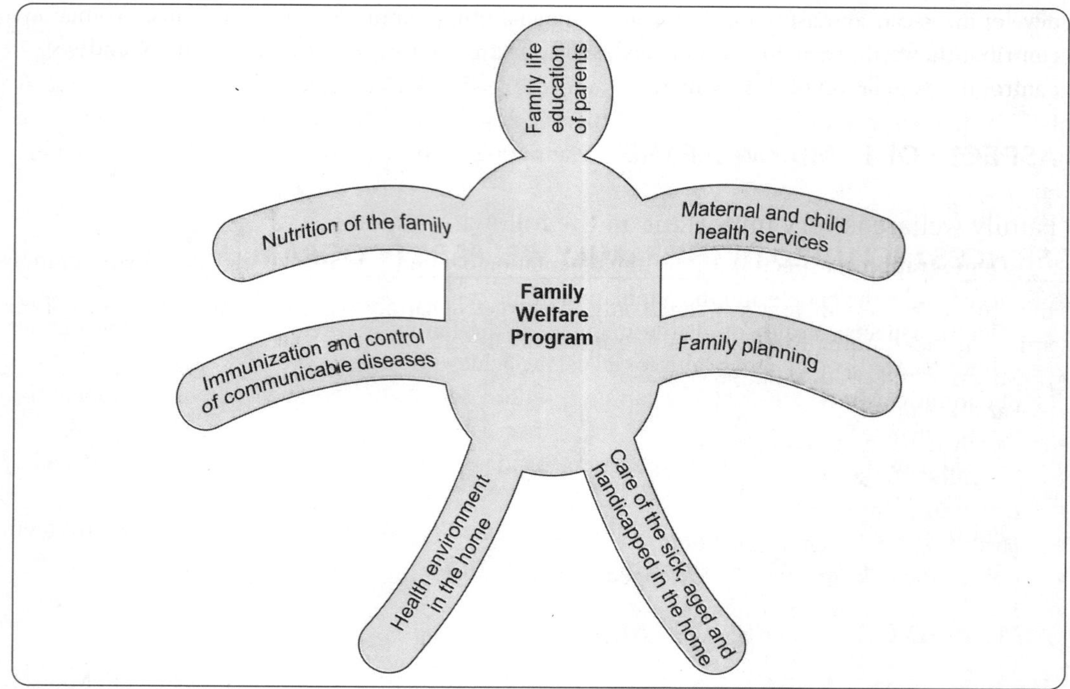

Figure 7.7: Family Welfare Program

For primary welfare services, family planning is the most important component. Family planning is the voluntary planning regarding childbirth by a couple, i.e., childbirth should be according to the choice and not by chance or in other words, "planning for responsible parenthood" is family planning. By controlling birth through family planning, the size of the family can be limited. The quality of life of the people can be improved and population growth can be controlled. The objective of family welfare can be achieved through family planning (Fig. 7.7).

IMPORTANCE OF FAMILY WELFARE

The basic principle of implementing Family Welfare Program is to improve the quality of the life of the individuals and families by providing total healthcare to the family and to educate the family to achieve target-free goal to control the fast growing population. Once the people understand the importance of healthful living and better status of healthy life, they will come forward with voluntary choice of opting small family size. It is the woman who has to undergo the stress of pregnancy and child-rearing along with her household responsibilities. She has to balance her employment and family life. If she will understand the importance of small family size, it will be easy to look after one or two children and raise them. The small family norms and spacing help her gain greater freedom and equality. This all will come through family welfare services only. For the development of any nation, woman's employment is essential to empower woman. Woman's education and employment is required to fight against poverty and solving economic problems. If both the parents are employed, they can give better social status and education to one or two children rather than having more children. So, the law and order, political system and economic development can be ensured only through implementing Family Welfare Programs. Women can contribute toward employment and raise social and economic status of the country and also to control the population of the country.

ASPECTS OF FAMILY WELFARE

Family welfare is very important on the following aspects:

- **Demographical aspect:** With the implementation of family welfare, family planning program is accepted by the people and the population of the country can be controlled.
- **Health aspects:** Health of all the member of the family is taken care specially the mother, children, aged and goal of health for all can be achieved.
- **Economic aspect:** Small family can give better education and nutrition to its members. Per capita income is increased.
- **Social aspect:** Good nutrition, education, good standard of living is the basis of good society and strong citizen.
- **Political aspect:** Family planning affects the density of population. It may bring improvement in resources and qualitative changes in political system.

AIMS AND OBJECTIVES OF FAMILY WELFARE

The aims and objectives of family planning as stated by the Government of India in the Ministry of Health and Family Welfare are given as follows:

Aims

- To provide adult education.
- To set up institutions, schools, colleges, trusts or societies in connection with the objectives of the society.
- To work for the promotion of education and to establish educational institutions in backward areas.
- To provide chances for higher and technical education for the scheduled tribes, scheduled castes and other backward classes (OBC) of rural background in India.
- To provide education for disabled children.
- To take all necessary steps to ensure the betterment and improvement of the economic and general conditions of living in the area of operation.
- To promote and encourage the practice and spirit of mutual help, cooperation and collaboration among the members.
- To amalgamate with other society or societies, organization or institutions in pursuit of all or any of its object.
- The society should work for the health and family welfare of the population, rural development through participatory approach, environment conservation and other related issues with the problems of our social and economical system.
- To promote health and medical problems preventive as well as curative, for the tribal rural and urban people and to establish dispensaries (mobile and stationary) maternity homes, hospitals, health centers, etc.

- Health, family welfare, and nutrition with education and awareness.
- Physical, mental and social well-being of the woman and children.
- Education and awareness about acquired immunodeficiency syndrome (AIDS), cancer, hepatitis, tuberculosis (TB) and other diseases and promote research in the area of medicine and general health.
- Prevention of substance abuse through education, awareness and rehabilitation.
- To create nutritional awareness in community for healthy motherhood and control of malnutrition.
- To collect, publish, disseminate and make available to the members of the society and public at large, literature, circular, books, bulletins, records and information in whatever manner to know the science or to arrange seminars on education program which are of use, interest and importance.
- Environment protection and local action for natural resource conservation, development and management:
  - Environmental awareness among rural/urban people
  - Industrial waste water/effluent management
- Pollution monitoring and management through vegetation.
- Joint forest management.
- The society may provide consultation services to other organization in the areas of health and environment with or without changes.
- To undertake roads, housing, electrification, sanitation and other activities for the benefit of tribal, rural and urban people.
- To improve, manage, develop, and grant rights or privileges or respect otherwise deal with all at any part of the property and rights of the society.

Objectives

- To adopt small family norms on the basis of voluntary choice
- To promote the use of spacing methods
- To ensure adequate supply of contraceptives to all eligible couples within easy reach
- To make provision for clinical and surgical services so as to achieve the set target
- To avoid unwanted births
- To bring about wanted births
- To keep spacing between the pregnancies
- To control the time at which birth occurs in relation to the age of the mother
- To determine the number of children in the family.

FAMILY PLANNING

Definitions of Family Planning

- Family planning is the voluntary planning regarding childbirth by a couple, i.e., childbirth should be according to their choice and not by chance or in other words "planning for responsible parenthood" is the family planning.
- An expert committee (1971) of the WHO defined family planning as "a way of thinking and living that is adopted voluntarily, upon the basis of knowledge, attitude and responsible decisions

by individuals and couples, in order to promote the health and welfare of the family group and thus contribute effectively to the social development of the country."

- Another expert committee defined and described family planning as follows: "family planning refers to practices that help individuals or couple to attain certain objectives":
  - To avoid unwanted births
  - To bring about wanted births
  - To regulate the interval between pregnancies
  - To control the time at which birth occur in relation to the age of parents and
  - To determine the number of children in the family

Objectives

- To plan pregnancy according to the choice
- To avoid unwanted births
- To limit the size of the family
- To keep spacing between the pregnancies

Goals

There are two main goals of family planning:

1. **Operational goal:**
   - To promote the voluntary acceptance of small family norms
   - To motivate people to adopt the use of spacing methods to control the interval between pregnancies
   - To ensure easy availability of contraceptives to all eligible couples
   - To arrange the medical and surgical services to achieve demographic targets
   - Some other programs are also included in the family planning program like:
     - Child survival
     - Status of woman
     - Employment
     - Female literacy and education
     - Poverty eradication
     - Socioeconomic growth programs.
     - Reproductive and child healthcare programs
2. **Demographic goals:** These are the part of National Population Policy and continue to change with a change in the policy.

Scopes

According to expert committee of WHO, family planning includes the following subject:

- Proper spacing between children
- Limited number of births
- Premarital counseling
- Pregnancy test
- Providing services to unmarried mother
- Preparing for the births
- Educating about nutrition and finances
- Sex education
- Genetic counseling
- Education about parenthood
- Marital guidance
- Adoption services

Aspects

Many aspects of life are affected by family planning. It affects the health services and controls populations. Some of the aspects of family planning are as follows:

- **Health aspects**
  - **Health of woman:** Pregnancy affects the health of woman. Anemia, pregnancy- induced hypertension; eclampsia, antepartum hemorrhage (APH), postpartum hemorrhage (PPH) and other abnormal conditions of pregnancy are dangerous to mothers. Maternal mortality and morbidity can be reduced to great extent by the use of family planning services. Mother can be protected from many health problems by reducing the number of pregnancies and by spacing between the pregnancies and children can be protected from many congenital disabilities.
  - **Health of children:** Planned pregnancy is important for better growth and development of the child. Health of the child is looked after right from intrauterine life. Children get better nourishment in small families resulting into better physical and mental development. Possibility of childhood diseases and communicable diseases are also reduced.
- **Economic aspects:** Philosophy of small family, happy family explains the economic attitude of this program. Parents can look after and provide better education to one or two children. So the growth of individuals, community and the economy of nation can be achieved through success of family planning.
- **Social aspects:** Better economy of the country results into better social status, i.e., good education, good standard of living and proper nutrition is the base of good society and strong nation. The social discrepancies are also narrow down and personality of the individuals develops due to growing awareness. Marital relation becomes stronger and mental health improves.
- **Political aspects:** Family affects the density of population. Success in family planning may bring improvement in the resources and qualitative change in the political system thus bringing transformation in the social, cultural, educational, economic and political perspective of individuals as well as countries.

METHOD OF FAMILY PLANNING

Contraceptive Methods or Fertility Regulating Methods

Contraceptive methods are by definition, preventive methods to help woman avoid unwanted pregnancies. They include all temporary and permanent measure to prevent pregnancy resulting from coitus.

Characteristics of Ideal Contraceptive

- It should be inexpensive and have long life.
- It should be effective in preventing pregnancy.
- It should be safe for health and free from any harmful effect.
- It should be simple and could be used without any consultation or supervision of doctor/medical personnel.
- It should be reversible and should not obstruct pregnancy when desired.

TYPES OF CONTRACEPTIVES

Contraceptive methods are broadly grouped into two (Table 7.17).
1.   Spacing methods
2.   Terminal methods

TABLE 7.17: Contraceptive methods

Spacing methods	Terminal methods

• Barrier methods
    ▪ Physical methods
    ▪ Chemical methods
    ▪ Combined methods
• Intrauterine devices
• Hormonal methods
• Postconceptional methods
• Miscellaneous
	• Male sterilization
	• Female sterilization

Spacing Methods

Spacing methods include the following:

Barrier Methods

The aim of barrier methods is to prevent live sperm from meeting the ovum. These methods are described as follows:

Physical Methods

Male condom

It is a thin latex or plastic sheath worn by men on erect penis before starting sexual act to trap sperms at ejaculation (Fig. 7.8). Male should wear the condom before any contact with the vagina. After ejaculation, it should be withdrawn carefully without spilling any semen. Condom serves as a barrier by preventing the contact of semen into the vagina.

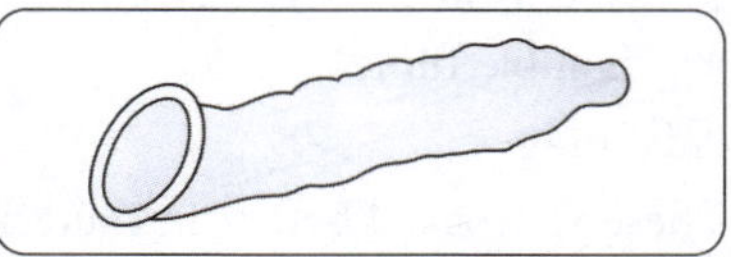

Figure 7.8: Male condom (Nirodh)

In addition to preventing pregnancy, condom protects both male and female from sexually transmitted diseases. Condom prevents the deposition of semen into vagina. The effectiveness of condom can be increased by using it in conjunction with a spermicidal jelly inserted in the vagina before intercourse.

Advantages of male condom:
- Easily available
- Inexpensive and safe
- Easy to use
- No side effects
- Protects not only against pregnancy but also against sexually transmitted diseases (STD)
- Light, compact and disposable.

Disadvantage of male condom:

May slip off or tear during coitus due to incorrect use.

Female condom

It is a pouch made up of polyurethane with an internal ring which covers the cervix and an external ring which remains outside the vagina (Fig. 7.9). It is prelubricated with silicon and spermicidal is not required. It is an effective barrier to STD infection. Due to high cost and failure rate 5%, it is not used.

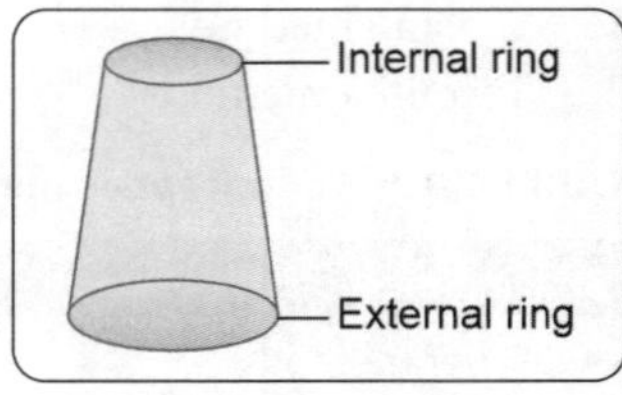

Figure 7.9: Female condom

Diaphragm

It is a shallow cup made of synthetic rubber or plastic material of 5–10 cm in diameter. It has got flexible rim made of spring or metal. It is used by the woman according to the size. It is held in position partly by the spring tension and partly by the vaginal muscle tone. A spermicidal jelly is used along with it. It is inserted into the vagina before sexual intercourse and remains in place for 6 hours after intercourse. Its side effects are nil but failure rate is 6–12%.

Vaginal Sponge

It is a small, polyurethane foam sponge measuring 5 × 2.5 cm, saturated with spermicidal nonoxynol-9. It is less effective than diaphragm and failure rate is also high.

Chemical Methods

These are the chemical contraceptives which are placed in vagina. The chemical presents in the devices destroy sperms. There are four categories of chemical devices:

1. Foam tablets, foam aerosols
2. Creams, jellies and pastes
3. Suppositories inserted manually
4. Soluble films

Advantages:

These were used before intrauterine devices (IUDs) and oral pills were invented. Nowadays their use is only recommended with condom for the sake of extra protection.

Disadvantages:

- Produce irritation and burning in the vagina.
- Failure rate is high.
- These are to be highly placed in vagina.

Combined Methods

Combined device: Using chemical contraception along with condom is known as combined devices. It provides double protection against pregnancy.

Intrauterine Devices

These are the devices which when placed in the uterus provide protection against pregnancy. Types of IUDs currently in use are given in Figure 7.10:

Advantages of IUDs:

- Cost-effective

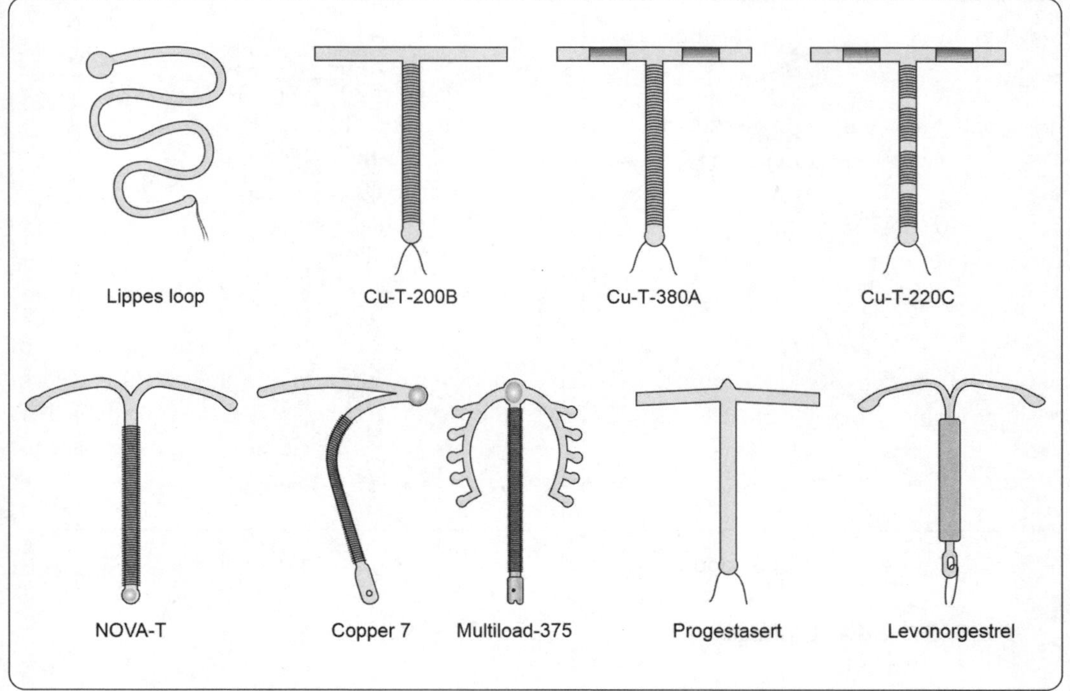

Figure 7.10: Types of IUDs currently in use

- Easy to use
- No interruption of intercourse
- Partners are mentally relaxed
- Can be removed immediately in case of any problem or on request
- Fertility returns with 1st ovulation cycle
- Contraceptive effect is reversible after removal of IUD
- Hormonal IUDs help in relieving heavy menstrual flow
- Copper IUDs can be used as an emergency contraceptive within 5 day of unprotected sex

Disadvantages of IUDs:
- IUDs do not protect against STDs
- Need clinician for insertion and removal
- Leads to some side effects such as nausea, acne, lower abdominal pain, backache, headache and mood swings
- The LNG-IUDs may increase risk of ovarian cyst
- 2–8% IUDs expelled from uterus within 1st year
    - **Absolute disadvantages**
        - Suspected pregnancy
        - Pelvic inflammatory disease
        - Vaginal bleeding of undiagnosed etiology
        - Cancer cervix, uterus or adnexa
        - Previous ectopic pregnancy

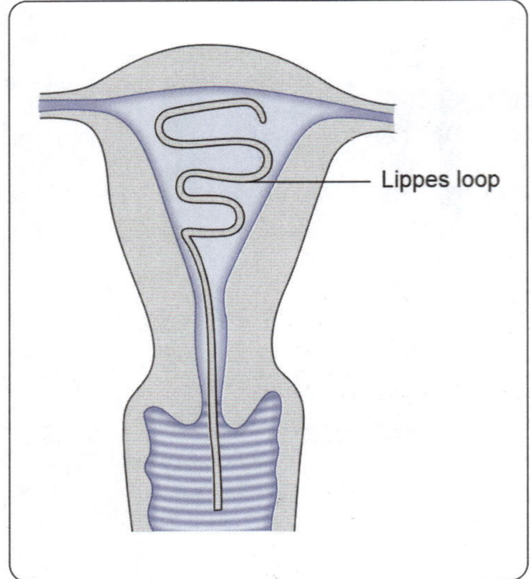

Figure 7.11: Lippes loop

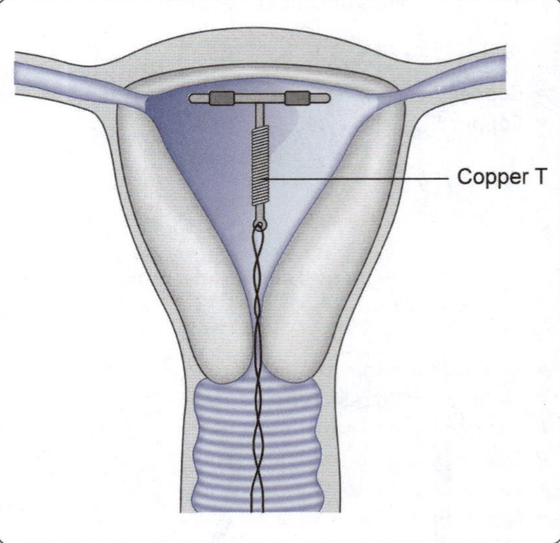

Figure 7.12: Copper-T

- **Relative disadvantages**
  - Anemia
  - Menorrhagia
  - History of PID
  - Fibroid uterus
  - Any abnormality of uterine cavity

These are available as:

- Nonmedicated, i.e., Lippes loop (Fig. 7.11)—First Generation IUDs.
- Medicated, i.e., copper-T (Fig. 7.12)—Second Generation IUDs.
- Hormone-releasing IUDs—Third Generation IUDs.

Lippes Loop

It is the first generation intrauterine device. It is made of polyethylene and has a shape of double S. It has a nylon thread attached to it which lies in the vagina and helps in pulling out the loop. It is available in four sizes A, B, C and D. It is nontoxic, reliable and stable. It may cause perforation of the uterus. It contains some amount of barium due to which it can be spotted on X-rays, nowadays it is not used.

Copper IUDs

The copper IUDs comprise the second generation IUDs

Copper T

It is the second generation IUDs. Copper reduces the fertility of a woman. Many types of copper T are made available with different amount of copper in each type. Types of Copper T available are given in Table 7.18. Copper T should be inserted within 10 days of beginning of menstruation or 6–8 weeks after delivery. Its advantages and disadvantages are given in Table 7.19.

TABLE 7.18: Types of copper T available

Earlier devices	New devices—variant of T device

• Copper 7
• Copper T$_{200}$
	• Cu-T220C
	• Cu-T380A or Ag
	  ▪ NOVA-T
	  ▪ Multiload devices-ML Cu250
	  ▪ ML Cu 375

TABLE 7.19: Advantages and disadvantages of Cu-T

Advantages	Disadvantages
• An effective contraceptive • Fertility can be restored • Inexpensive and easy to use • Does not require continuous supervision • Can be used up to 10 years • Free from any harmful effects	• Pain and bleeding • Ectopic pregnancy may occur • Spontaneous expulsion may take place • Infection of pelvis • Perforation of uterus

Currently used IUCD device in India in National Family Welfare Program is Cu-T380Ag which is distinguished by a silver core over which the copper wire is wrapped.

Multiload-375

It consists of a small plastic rod wound with copper wire and provided with two flexible arms and a nylon string. If measures 35 mm in length 20.5 mm in width. The plastic body of multiload contains barium sulfate to make it radiopaque. The flexible sidearm of multiload ensures that IUD remains in position (Fig. 7.13).

Hormone Releasing IUDS

These are Third Generation IUDs

Progestasert

It is T shaped device filled with 38 mg of progesterone the natural hormones. Hormone gets released slowly in the uterus at the rate of 60 mcg daily. It has higher failure rate and needs to be replaced yearly as the reservoir of progesterone can last for 12–18 months.

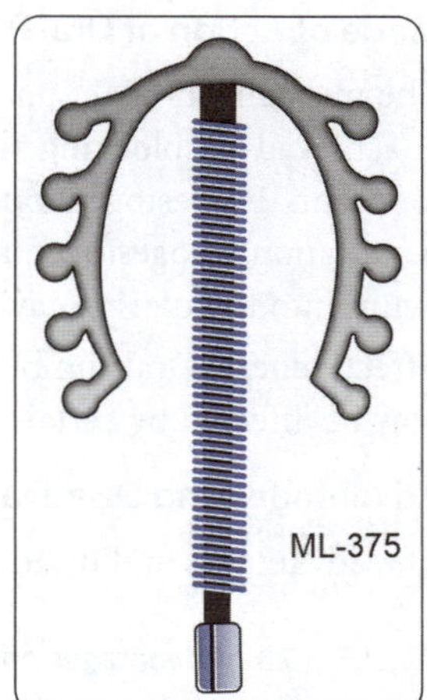

Figure 7.13: Multiload 375

Hormonal Device LNG-20 (Mirena)

It is T shaped IUD, releases 20 mcg of levonorgestrel which is a potent synthetic steroids. Pregnancy rate is 0.2 per woman and ectopic pregnancies are also few. It causes lower menstrual blood flow compared to copper devices. This is as effective as copper IUDs and can be used for 7–10 years.

Hormonal Methods

These are effective means of maintaining intervals between births. These are available in various combinations.

Oral Pills

- **Combined pills:** These are taken orally from 5th day of menstrual cycle to 21st day continuously after that there is a break of 7 days during which the cycle begins again. It should be taken regularly. The day bleeding starts, it is considered 1st day of menstruation cycle. In case if no bleeding, the day after 7th days should be considered the first day and course of pills starts again. Generally menstrual cycle begins at the end of second course.
    - Mala N, i.e., norethisterone acetate + ethinyl estradiol
    - Mala D, i.e., D-Norgestrel + ethinyl estradiol
- **Mini pills:** These contain only progestin, i.e., norethisterone + levonorgestrel.
    - **Progestogen-only pills (POP):** This is known as micropil pills or mini pills. It should be taken throughout the menstrual cycle. It contains only progestogen. It is not much popular because of high failure rate. However, recommended in older women where combined pills are contraindicated because of cardiovascular risks.
- **Long-acting pills (once in a month):** In this, a long-acting estrogen, i.e., quinestrol is given in combination with a short-acting progestogen. But the pregnancy rate is high so it is not recommended. Moreover bleeding occurs irregularly.
- **Nonsteroidal weekly oral pill:** These pills are famous by the brand name Saheli. It is free from side effects of nausea, vomiting, weight gain, dizziness, etc. The pill named as "centchroman" and to be taken once in a week.

Mode of Action of Oral Pills

The mechanism of action of combined pills is to prevent the release of ovum from the ovary. This is achieved by blocking the pituitary secretions of gonadotropin that is necessary for ovulation to occur. Progestogen only renders the cervical mucus thick and scanty and prevents sperm penetration. Progestogen also inhibits tubal motility and delays the transport of sperm and of the ovum into the uterine cavity.

Effectiveness: Oral combined pills are almost 100% effective in preventing pregnancy. Effectiveness may be affected by certain drugs like rifampicin, phenobarbital and ampicillin.

Advantages and Disadvantages of Oral Pills

The advantages and disadvantages of oral pills are given in Table 7.20.

TABLE 7.20: Advantages and disadvantages of oral pills

Advantages	Disadvantages
• Easy to use • Inexpensive and easily availab e • High rate of safety • Regularity in menstrual cycle • Reduction in breast cancer.	• Cannot be used in cardiovascular cases • Metabolic effects may result into weight gain, high blood pressure, clotting of blood and heart failure • Not suitable for woman above 40 years of age • May result in tenderness of breast, uneasiness, pain, headaches and irregularity of bleeding may occur • Other problems like liver disease, reduced lactation and ectopic pregnancy may occur.

Postcoital Contraception

Postcoital or ("morning after") contraception is recommended within 72 hours of an unprotected intercourse. There are two methods of postcoital contraception.

1. **IUD:** The simplest technique is to insert an IUD, (if accepted) especially a copper device within 5 days.
2. **Hormonal:** This method is preferable. Levonorgestrel 0.75 tablet is advised as an emergency contraceptive. One tablet of levonorgestrel 0.75 mg within 72 hours and second tablet is given after 12 hours of the first dose.
   - **Or two** oral contraceptive pills containing 50 mcg of ethinyl estradiol within 72 hours after intercourse and same dose is repeated after 12 hours.
   - **Or** four oral contraceptive pills containing 30–35 mcg of ethinyl-estradiol within 72 hours and four tablets after 12 hours.
   - **Or** mifepristone 10 mg once within 72 hours and 4 tablets after 12 hours.

Depot Formulation

These are effective, reversible, long-acting and estrogen-free devices used for spacing pregnancies in which a single administration is sufficient for months or years. These include.

Injectable Contraceptive

These are of two types:

1. **Progestogen-only injectable:** This includes:
   - **Depot medroxyprogesterone acetate (DMPA):** An intramuscular injection of 150 mg DMPA is administered every 3 months. It gives protection from pregnancy 3 months. It suppresses the ovulation, has indirect effect on endometrium, decreases the motility of fallopian tubes and decreases the thickness of the cervical mucus. All these factors help in reducing fertility. It does not affect lactation and can be safely given after postpartum period.
     - **Side effects:**
       - Weight increase
       - Irregular menstrual bleeding
       - Prolonged infertility after use.
   - **Norethisterone enanthate (NET-EN):** 200 mg NET-EN is given intramuscularly every 60 days. Contraception action is inhibition of ovulation and progestogen effects on cervical mucus. Its failure rates are higher than DMPA. Its initial dose is given during the first 5 days of menstrual period to rule out pregnancy. It is given deep IM and injection site should never be massaged.
   - **DMPA-SC 104 mg:** It contains 104 mg of depot medroxyprogesterone acetate and injected under the skin every 3 months.

Side effects of DMPA-SC-104 mg and NET-EN:

- Irregular menstrual bleeding
- Amenorrhea in some cases can cause anxiety.

Contraindications of DMPA-SC-104 mg and NET-EN:

- Hypertension
- Cardiovascular disease
- Cancer of breast and genital organs.

Advantages of DMPA-SC-104 mg and NET-EN:
- Highly effective
- Long lasting
- Reversible contraception

2. **Combined injectable contraception:** This combined injectable contains progestogen and estrogen. They are given every month, ± 3 days. They act by suppressing the ovulation and the progestogen makes the cervical mucus a thick obstacle to prevent the penetration of sperms. It also changes the endometrium, making it unsuitable for implantation of the fertilized ovum. These injectable contraceptives include cyclofem/cycloprovera and mesigyna.
   - **Side effects:** These are same as that of progestogen-only injectable.
   - **Failure rate:** 0.2–0.4%
   - **Contraindications**
     - Suspected pregnancy
     - Thromboembolic disorders
     - Cerebrovascular diseases
     - Coronary artery disease
     - Local migraine
     - Malignancy
     - Diabetes mellitus
     - Unsuitable for woman who are breastfeeding.

Subdermal Implants

These include norplant and norplant (R)-2.
- **Norplant:** It consists of 6 silastic (silicon rubber) capsules containing 35 mg each of Levonorgestrel .
- **Norplant (R)-2:** This is the fabrication of Levonorgestrel into two small rods which are comparatively easier to insert and remove. These silastic capsules or rods are inserted beneath the skin of forearm or upper arm. Effective contraception is provided for 5 years. The contraception effects are reversible on removal of the implant.

Disadvantages of implants:

Irregularities of menstrual cycle. Surgical procedure is needed to insert and remove the implants.

Vaginal Rings

It contains Levonorgestrel. These are effective. The hormone is slowly released through the vaginal mucosa. The ring is worn into the vagina for 3 weeks of cycle and removed on the 4th week.

Postconceptional Methods

Menstrual Regulations (MR)

In this method, the uterine contents are aspirated after 6–14 days of missed period. Before MR, it is ensured by all pregnancy tests whether the woman is pregnant or not. The cervical dilatation is indicated in nullipara or in an apprehensive woman. It is an OPD procedure.

Complications:
- The immediate complications are uterine perforation and trauma.

- Late complications are as follows:
  - Abortion
  - Premature labor
  - Infertility
  - Menstrual disorders
  - Increase in ectopic pregnancy
  - Rh-Immunization

Menstrual Induction

In this method, 1–5 mg solution of prostaglandin F2 alpha is introduced into the uterine cavity. It is based on disturbing the normal progesterone-prostaglandin balance. After few minutes of induction, the uterine contractions are started and continue for 3–4 hours. The bleeding starts and continues for 7–8 days. Prior to induction, pregnancy is confirmed by all pregnancy tests. The procedure is performed under sedation.

Oral Abortifacient

It is used to terminate pregnancy up to 9 weeks duration. The commonly used regimen is mifepristone 200 mg orally on day 1, followed by misoprostol 800 mcg vaginally either immediately or within 6–8 hours.

The other regimen is a dose of mifepristone 600 mg on day one, followed by 400 mcg orally of misoprostol on day three. Patient should visit the OPD after 2 weeks after administration of mifepristone to confirm by clinical examination or by ultrasonography to ensure complete termination has taken place.

Contraindication of mifepristone and misoprostol:

- History of allergy
- Suspected ectopic pregnancy
- Undiagnosed adnexal mass
- IUD in place
- Chronic adrenal failure
- Hemorrhagic disorders
- Patient on anticoagulant therapy
- Inherited porphyria

Abortion

Termination of pregnancy before the fetus becomes viable (capable of living independently) is termed abortion. This duration is of almost 24–28 weeks.

Medical Terminations of Pregnancy (MTP)

It is an important part of family planning. It is also performed for birth control. The induced abortion is deliberately performed. It may be legal or illegal. The illegal abortion is hazardous. In India two-thirds of the abortions take place outside authorized health services by unauthorized and unskilled persons.

- **The optimal time for termination of pregnancy:** Seventh and eighth weeks of pregnancy. If performed during the second trimester risk of maternal death is seven times more.
- **Early complications of MTP/abortion:**
  - Hemorrhage
  - Shock
  - Sepsis
  - Uterine perforation
  - Cervical injuries
  - Thromboembolism
  - Anesthetic and psychiatric complications
- **Late complications:**
  - Infertility
  - Ectopic gestation
  - Increased risk of spontaneous abortion
  - Reduced birth weight

Nursing Considerations

LEGALIZATION OF ABORTION

Until 1971, abortions in India were governed by Indian Penal Code (IPC) of 1860 the code of criminal procedure 1898, and were considered crime except when performed to save the life of a pregnant woman. The Medical Termination of Pregnancy Act was passed by the Indian Parliament in 1971 and came into force on April 1972 except from Jammu and Kashmir where it came into effect from November 1, 1976. Medical Termination of Pregnancy Act is a healthcare measure with objectives of reducing maternal mortality and morbidity rate resulting from illegal abortions, MTP is an important part of family planning program and is an important tool for termination of early pregnancy up to 7–9 weeks.

The Medical Termination of Pregnancy Act 1971

The Government of India passed Medical Termination of Pregnancy Act in 1971 and made amendment in it in 1975 and in 2003 to legalize the abortion following three points lie at the center of it:
1. Conditions due to which pregnancy can be terminated
2. Who is authorized to perform this kind of termination?
3. Place where MTP can be done

The conditions under which a pregnancy can be terminated under MTP Act 1971

- **Medical ground:** Where continuation of pregnancy may endanger mother's life or her physical or mental health likely to be harmed seriously
- **Eugenic:** Where the child is likely to be born with serious congenital disorders or abnormalities
- **Humanitarian:** Where the rape is the cause of pregnancy
- **Socioeconomic ground:** Where the life of the mother is threatened by social and economic conditions
- **Failure of contraceptives:** Where cause of pregnancy is the failure of contraceptives devices or resources.

The person or persons who can perform abortion/MTP

A registered medical practitioners who have experience in gynecology and obstetrics can perform abortion where the length of pregnancy does not exceed 12 weeks. However, where the pregnancy exceeds 12 weeks and is not >20 weeks the option of two registered medical practitioners is necessary to terminate pregnancy. According to amendment of 1975, chief medical officer of a district is authorized to certify a doctor who is capable of terminating pregnancy.

Place of MTP and consent

The Act stipulates that no termination of pregnancy shall be made at any place other than a hospital established and maintained by the government or place approved for the purpose of the Act by government.

Woman should be an adult and should sign the letter of consent. In case of minor <18 years of age or mentally ill, written consent of the parents or guardians are necessary. These services are a matter of extreme confidentiality.

MTP Rules (1975)

The rule and regulation were altered in October 1975
- **Approval by board:** The chief medical officer of the district is empowered to certify that a doctor has the necessary training in gynecology and obstetrics to do abortion.
- **Qualification required to do abortion:** The new rules allow for registered medical practitioner to qualify through on the spot training "If he/she has assisted a RMP in the performance of 25 cases of medical termination of pregnancy in an approved institution.

  The doctor may also qualify to do MTP under the new rules if he/she has one or more of the following qualifications which are similar to the old rules:
  - 6 months houseman ship in obstetrics and gynecology
  - Postgraduate qualification in OBG

Contd...

- 3 years of practice in OBG for the doctors registered before the 1971 MTP Act was passed
- One year of practice in OBG for the doctors registered on or after the date of commencement of the Act
- **The place where abortion is performed:** Under the new rule, nongovernment institutions may also take up abortions provided they obtain a license from the chief medical officer of the district thus, eliminating the requirement of private clinic obtaining a Board license.

MVA Technique

Manual vacuum aspiration (MVA) technique is a surgical technique has been introduced in MTP services. It is a less invasive, safe and comfortable method for client.

Complications of abortion

There are numerous hazards of abortions:

- Bleeding
- Shock
- Sepsis
- Uterine perforation or injuries
- Anxiety and mental disturbance
- Abortion can never be safe as efficient contraceptive

Miscellaneous Methods

These methods include the following:

Abstinence

The only method which is completely effective is complete sexual abstinence. It was postulated by Saints and Seers in India, i.e., extreme of patience and control. It is sound in theory and practice. But the repression of natural force is liable to manifest itself in other directions such as temperamental changes and even nervous breakdown. It is not practical and not possible for the young couples.

Coitus Interruptus

This is also the oldest method of avoiding pregnancy. During sexual intercourse the male pulls out his penis from the vagina and ejaculate outside it. Some couples are able to practice it successfully while others find it difficult to manage. The drawback of this method is that precoital secretion of male may contain sperms and even precoital semen can cause pregnancy. Secondly the slightest delay in timing of withdrawal may lead to deposition of certain amount of semen.

- **Failure rate:** Failure rate is 25%
- **Side effects**
    - Pelvic congestion
    - Vaginitis
    - Anxiety neurosis
    - Mental confusion

Safe Period (Rhythm Method)

This is also known as calendar method described by Ogino in 1930. This method is based on the fact that ovulation occurs from 12 to 16 days before the onset of menstruation. The days on which conception is likely to occur is calculated. The shortest cycle minus 18 days gives the first day of fertile period. The longest cycle minus 10 days gives the last day of the fertile period. If a woman is having menstrual cycle varying from 26 to 31 days, the fertile period during which she should not have intercourse is from 8 to 21 days of menstrual cycle. But such calculation is not possible (Fig. 7.14).

- **Drawbacks of the method**
    - The menstrual cycle is not always regular.
    - Possible for educated and responsible couples.
    - Not applicable for postnatal period
- **Failure rate:** High about 90%
- **Complications:**
    - Ectopic pregnancy results following conception late in the menstrual cycle and displacement of the ovum.
    - Embryonic abnormalities resulting from conception of over aged sperm or overage ovum

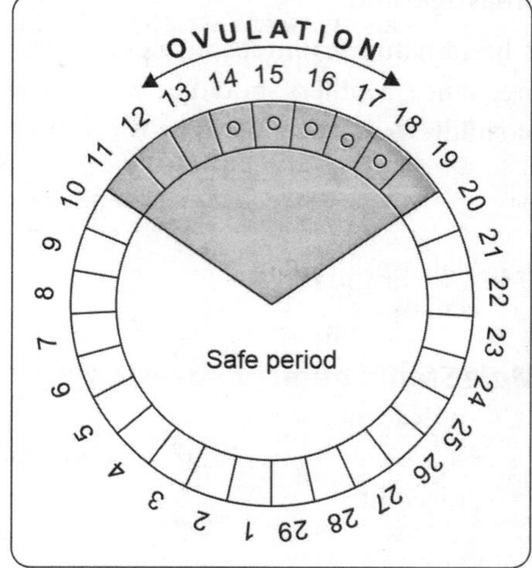

Figure 7.14: Safe period in 28 days cycle

Natural Family Planning Methods

Basal Body Temperature Method

There is slight increase in basal body temperature ranging from 0.3°C to 0.5°C as a result of increase in the production of progesterone. The temperature is measured before getting out of bed in the morning. Sexual intercourse is safe from the 3rd day of ovulation till the beginning of next menstrual cycle. This method is not popular because of total abstinence required before ovulation and skill required to record temperature.

Cervical Mucus Method

This is also known as Billings method or ovulation method. At the time of ovulation, cervical mucus becomes watery, clear resembling raw egg white, smooth, slippery and profuse. After ovulation under the influence of progesterone, the mucus becomes thick and scanty. The woman should use the tissue paper to judge the quantity and characteristics of mucus and should be able to distinguish between different types of mucus. Higher degree of skill and motivation is required to practice the method.

Symptothermal Method

This method combines the temperature, cervical mucus and calendar method for identifying fertile period. If the woman cannot clearly interpret one sign, she can double check interpretation with another this method is more effective than Billings method.

Birth Control Vaccine

The most advanced research involves immunization with a vaccine prepared from beta subunits of human chorionic gonadotropin (hCG), a hormone produced in early pregnancy, immunization with hCG would block continuation of pregnancy. Antibodies appeared in 4–6 weeks and reached maximum after about 5 months and slowly declined reaching zero level after a period ranging from 6 to 11 months. The immunity can be boosted by a second injection. Two types of pregnancy vaccines employing variants of beta subunits of hCG are now about to go into clinical trial.

Breastfeeding

It has a natural contraceptive effect. The release of oxytocin hormone during breastfeed prevents pregnancy. Mothers should be encouraged to breastfeed their babies for one year it helps in spacing of children.

Terminal Methods/Permanent Method

- Male sterilization
- Female sterilization

Male Sterilization or Vasectomy

Vasectomy is a simple operation performed under local anesthesia. In vasectomy, the vas deferens is cut one centimeter each after clamping and removed. The ends are ligated and then folded back on themselves and sutured into position so that the cut ends face away from each other. This will reduce the risk of recanalization of a later stage date. It should be explained to acceptor that he is not immediately sterile after operation until approximately 30 ejaculations have taken place. During this intermediate period another method of contraception must be used. If properly performed, vasectomies are almost 100% effective (Fig. 7.15).

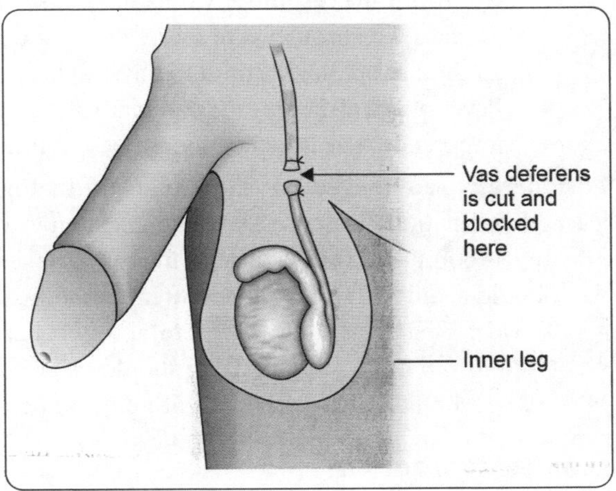

Figure 7.15: Vasectomy

No-Scalpel Vasectomy

It is the latest and most popular technique of male sterilization. It is popular among men and showing positive trends year by year.

Advantages

- No side effects on hormones
- Cheaper and simpler than tubectomy
- No hospitalization is required as it is an OPD procedure can be performed in primary health centers by trained doctors.
- Does not interface with normal working after the operation
- Recanalization is possible
- Permanent, safe and inexpensive technique
- Does not interfere with sexual pleasure

Complications

Very few complications may occur, these are as follows:
- **Operative complications:**
  - Pain
  - Scrotal hematoma
  - Local infection
  - Wound infection

Note: Good hemostasis and administration of antibiotics will reduce the risk of these complications.

- **Postoperative complications:**
  - **Sperm granules:** It is caused by accumulation of sperms, which is a local complication of vasectomy. It appears 10–14 days after the operation. Symptoms include pain and swelling. Clinically the mass is hard and 7 mm in size. Sperm granules eventually subside.
  - **Spontaneous recanalization:** The epithelial tubes will recanalize after damage. The incidence is 0.6%. Surgeon should explain the possibility of recanalization.
  - **Autoimmune response:** Vasectomy causes autoimmune response to sperm. Blocking of the vas causes reabsorption of spermatozoa and subsequent development of antibodies. But these antibodies are not harmful to physical health but causes reduction in subsequent fertility.
  - **Psychological:** Some men complain of headache, uneasiness, diminution of sexual vigor and impotence. The acceptor should be given sufficient time to make up his mind voluntarily.

Postoperative advice: Patient should be told that he is not sterile immediately after operation. At least 30 ejaculations are necessary before semen examination is negative.

- To use contraceptives until aspermia has been established.
- Should avoid bath for 24 hours after operation.
- To wear T bandage to provide scrotal support at least 48 hours.
- Cycling and heavy weight lifting should be avoided for 15 days.
- Stiches should be removed after 5th day of operation.

Female Sterilization

Tubectomy is a permanent method of female sterilization. It involves cutting and tying of fallopian tubes to block the passage of ovum (Fig. 7.16).

- **Postpartum sterilization:** When sterilization is performed 1–3 days after delivery it is known as postpartum sterilization.
- **Internal sterilization:** When the operation done at any time other than childbirth or abortion. It is called internal sterilization.

There are three main methods of female sterilization.

Traditional Tubectomy

This method is known as abdominal tubectomy. It is done under general anesthesia or spinal anesthesia. A lower abdominal incision is made and a part of fallopian tubes is cut and tied or clamped again and the abdomen is closed in layers. It works as a permanent contraceptive by

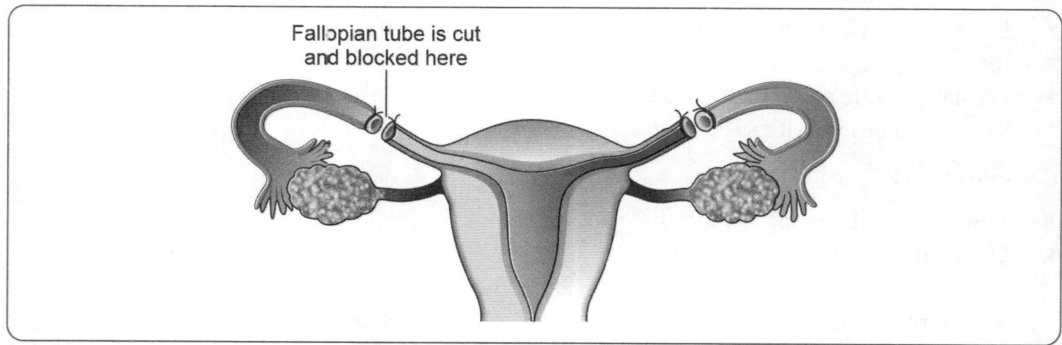

Figure 7.16: Tubectomy

blocking the path of ovum. Hospitalization is required for 5–6 days. Sutures are removed on 5th days of operation.

Postoperative advices

- Not to lift heavy weight for 6 weeks
- Heavy manual works to be avoided for 3 weeks
- Sexual relation can be assumed after 4 weeks of operation.

Minilap Operation

This is minor form of abdominal tubectomy in which under local anesthesia an incision of 2.5–3 cm is made in the lower abdomen. A part of fallopian tube is cut and clamped. Abdomen is sutured in layers. This is very safe and effective technique. This procedure can be performed at PHC level and mass campaigns. It is a good technique for postpartum sterilization.

Advantages:

- This technique is suitable for postpartum sterilization
- Less traumatic than abdominal tubectomy
- Safe technique
- Minimum complications

Laparoscopic Sterilization

This technique of female sterilization is very popular nowadays using laparoscope through the abdomen. Fallopian tubes are located and are blocked by a fallopian ring or rubber ring so that ovum cannot reach the uterus. Before inserting laparoscope, abdomen is expanded using carbon dioxide, nitrous oxide or air. The tubes are visualized after inserting the laparoscope. Once the tubes are visualized, accessible, the Falope rings or clips applied to occlude the tubes and the laparoscope is removed and incision is closed.

Advantages:

- The incision is very small, the scar is small.
- Very little time required for operation, the whole procedure completed in one attempt
- Less expensive
- Minimum complications
- 100% safe against pregnancy
- Shorter stay in the hospital for 48 hours.

Disadvantages

- Cannot be performed for postpartum patients. They have to wait for 6 week and hemoglobin should not be <8%.
- Not suitable for patients having medical disorders like heart diseases respiratory diseases, diabetes and hypertension.

Complications

- Pain and stretching
- Irregular menstruation
- Local infection
- But the serious complications like puncture of blood vessels and other potential complication are hazardous and an experienced surgical intervention is required.

Follow-up care: Patient should attend postpartum/postoperative OPD after 7–10 days of operation and once between 12 and 18 months of operation.

ELEMENTS OF SUCCESS IN FAMILY PLANNING

The success of family planning largely depends upon reaching the services to the consumer easily through multiple services delivery channel in a good quality and reliable manner.

The main points of success are as follows:
- To make services accessible through a variety of delivery points
- To make methods of family planning available to the potential users
- To provide client centered services
- To rely on evidence based technical guidance. Up to date services delivery guideline tools and job aids can help translate research finding into better practice
- Communicate effectively in simple language that client can understand
- Assure contraceptive security
- Work for supportive policies
- Good coordination
- High performing staff: Well-trained motivated staff, good working environment, matching skills and tasks can perform better success
- Secure adequate budget. Making proper use of the allocated budget, spending wisely doing more with less. Ensure financial sustainability
- Decision based on evidence, research monitoring and evaluation yield important information to guide decision-making.
- **Lead strongly:** Strong leadership goes a long way to implement the program successfully
- Integrate services appropriately, program can address a wider range of health needs by integrating services and providing referrals.

FAMILY PLANNING COUNSELING

Counseling plays a vital role in achieving the success of family planning program. It is in fact a part and parcel of the family welfare program. The health personnel providing services in family planning specially the community health nurse LHV, ANM and others make use of counseling process in helping their clients to find appropriate solution to their problems.

Counseling is a process that helps the client to recognize his/her problems and manage his/her stress by using problem solving technique when the help is provided by the counselor. The counselor helps her clients to recognize and understand their problems to be solved and implement the solution which are feasible, acceptable and evaluate the solution in terms of outcome. The counseling helps the client to achieve positive outcome and maximize the client's freedom to make right choice and act within the condition imposed by the environment.

Problems Faced by Couples that Require Family Planning Counseling

The community health nurse and other health personnel working in family planning come across with eligible and target couples require counseling services to deal with their individual problems which they may face during their entire period of reproductive phase due to lack of awareness, knowledge and facilities available. Their problems may be related to:
- Spacing of children
- Regarding sterilization operation

- Maybe suffering from reproductive tract infection or sexually transmitted infection
- Maybe requiring MTP
- Infertility problems and not having child
- Maybe having chromosomal defects and children born with severe congenital anomalies who die immediately after birth which may be incompatible with life.
- Problem may be related to physical, sexuality, lifestyle and behavior problem, etc.

Therefore, need-based counseling must be provided at subcenter, primary health centers and at family welfare clinic, hospitals and at home during the home visit.

Individual Family Planning Counseling

Individual counseling makes use of technical skill involving insight, persuasion, suggestion, re-assurance and instructions which help couples to perceive themselves and their problem more realistically. This in turn creates desire to find solution to their problems. Majority of the couples need help in spacing of children but due to lack of knowledge, they are unaware of the facility and services available. These couples are given education and information regarding the services available and select the best method appropriate to suit them for adoption.

The couples who have one or two healthy children are counseled to go for sterilization operation and be free from the tension of unwanted pregnancies. They are explained about the operation and its benefits. These couple are referred to the concerned doctor for the needful.

Those couples who are suffering from reproductive tract infection or sexually transmitted infection but they do not explore their problems because of social barriers. While taking history their problems should be brought out carefully without any social trauma to them. They should be counseled sympathetically and re-assured to get rid of their problem by proper investigations and treatment. They should be referred to the doctor for the management and follow-up care. The couples who are facing infertility problem and not having children should be counseled to undergo the investigation to rule out the cause of infertility. Once they are treated for the infertility, they may have children if the cause of infertility is curable. They are referred to infertility clinic and follow-up care.

The couples who require MTP are also counseled and advised after MTP to adopt spacing method to control pregnancy. It they have completed their family they are motivated and counseled to go for sterilization operation. The couples who have chromosomal or genetic defects having children born with severe congenital anomalies, the child died soon after birth or if survived with severe congenital malformations incompatible with life, are also counseled and advised not to have such children. They are given advice for adoption of a child. These issues are very sensitive. Such people require specialist's counseling (gynecologist, pediatrician and a specialist in counseling services).

Individual counseling may be required for a longer or shorter duration depending upon the nature of problems and the client's himself/herself confidentiality. In counseling on individual basis promotes sharing of problem and seeking information.

Errors to be Avoided during Family Planning Counseling

- The privacy and confidentiality should be ensured while providing counseling services.
- Biasness and judgment attitude can create critical barriers.

Requirements of Family Planning Counseling

Health personnel need to be specially trained in counseling services.

Services of professional counselor should be made available wherever possible.

Counseling helps to resolve the problem of individuals. There should be a separate cell for counseling in each health department for specialized counseling on sensitive issues in addition to the routine counseling. Benefits of Family Planning Counseling

So counseling in family planning is an ongoing process. It goes a long way to contribute toward achieving its goal and success depends upon the services and facilities made available in family planning and services. In addition counseling:

- Promotes Healthy lifestyle
- Develops appropriate information, education and communication regarding small family norms
- Provides education on sexuality and responsible parenthood
- Creates safe, secure and supportive environment
- Enables and empowers couples to solve their problems and become responsible citizen
- In the long run, it contributes toward the economy and development of the country
- Maintains its resources as per the requirement of the population of the country
- Helps in stabilization of population growth.

NATIONAL FAMILY WELFARE POLICY

The National Family Welfare Policy was implemented first in 1966 on the basis of target-free approach besides focus on National Welfare Policy. The term family welfare explains much broader scope than family planning. Family welfare is aimed at overall improvement in the quality of life. The services to be provided under family welfare are as follows:

- Education
- Nutrition
- Health services
- Family planning
- Employment
- Women's welfare and rights
- Shelter
- Environmental sanitation
- Safe drinking water, etc.

Family welfare includes the vital factors that are associated with the concept of welfare. In 1977, the Government of India redesigned the National Family Planning Program as the National Family Welfare Program and also changed the name of Ministry of Health and Family Planning to Ministry of Health and Family Welfare.

Objectives

- **The immediate objectives are as follows:**
  - To address the unmet needs for contraception, healthcare infrastructure and health personnel
  - To provide integrated services delivery for basic reproductive and child healthcare
- **The medium-term objective:**
  - To bring the TFR replacement levels by 2010 through implementation of various intersectoral operation strategies.

- **The long-term objective**
  - To achieve a stable population by 2045 at a level consistent with the requirement of sustainable socioeconomics growth and development and environment protection.

The National Socio-demographic Goals

- Address the unmet needs for basic reproductive and child health services, supplies and infrastructure
- Make school education up to the age 14 years free and compulsory and reduce the drop outs at primary and secondary school levels to below 20% both for boys and girls
- Reduce infant mortality rate below 100 per 100,000 live births
- Achieve universal immunization of children against all vaccine preventable diseases
- Promote delayed marriage for girls not earlier then the age of 18 years and preferable after 20-year age
- Achieve 80% institutional deliveries and 100% deliveries by trained personnel
- Achieve universal access to information, counseling and services to fertility regulation and contraception with a wide basket of choice
- Achieve 100% registration of births, deaths, marriages and pregnancy
- Control the spread of acquired immune-deficiency syndrome (AIDS) and promote greater integration between the management of reproductive tract infections (RTI) and sexually transmitted infection (STI) and the National AIDS Control Organization.
- Prevent and control communicable diseases
- Integrate Indian system of medicine (ISM) in the provision of reproductive and child health services and in the reaching out to household
- Promote vigorously the small family norm to achieve replacement level of TFR
- Bring about convergence in implementation of related social sector programs so that family welfare becomes a people centered program

Anticipated Targets of National Population Policy (NPP), 2000

- In the year 2010, the population will be 1,107 million instead of 1,162 million projected by the technical group of people projects.
- Crude birth rate will be 21 per 1000 population.
- Infant mortality rate 30 per 1000 live birth.
- Total fertility rate is 2.1.
- Population stabilization will be effective only if an integrated package of essential services is directed at village and household level.
- The NPP is to be largely implemented and managed at Panchayat and Nagar Palika levels in coordination with the concerned State/UT administration.

NATIONAL FAMILY WELFARE PROGRAM

Recognizing the need for population planning as a top priority, India launched a nationwide Family Planning Program in 1952. India was the first country in the world to do so. Though the records have been found that the birth control clinics functioning in the country since 1930. In 1977, the name of the program was changed to Family Welfare Program. National Family Welfare Program is completely sponsored by Union Government. At Central level, it is the duty of the central government to make policies and implement them whereas the State Governments are responsible for administration and implementation of the Family Welfare Program in their respective states.

National Family Welfare Program is run by family planning division of Ministry of Health and Family Welfare. The objectives, strategies and activities of the family planning division are designed and operated toward achieving the family welfare goals and objective and stated in the various policy documents. These include

- National Population Policy 2000
- National Health Policy 2002
- National Rural Health Mission

The objective of Family Welfare Program also honors the commitments of the Government of India which include international conference on population development (ICPD) and millennium development goals (MDG) and others.

Basic Principle of the Family Welfare Program

The basic principle of family welfare has remained the same from the very beginning.

- Family welfare services are voluntary.
- Family Welfare Program will provide comprehensive maternal and child health services and also family planning services.
- For creating awareness, information, education and communication will be effectively used.
- Popular and easily available family planning services will be provided free of cost.

Strategies of Family Welfare Program

- **Integration with health services**: Family Welfare Program has been integrated with other health services instead of being separate services.
- **Integration with maternity and child health:** Family planning program has been integrated with maternal and child health. People are motivated for postdelivery sterilization, MTP and use of contraceptives.
- **Concentration in rural area:** The program is concentrated at subcenter and primary health centers in addition to the hospital, district, state and central level.
- **Literacy:** There is a direct correlation between illiteracy and fertility. Stress and priority are given for girl's education. Fertility rate among educated female is low.
- **Breastfeeding:** It is encouraged at least for 1 year of age of child. It has been estimated that five million births per annum can be prevented through breastfeeding.
- **Raising the age for marriage:** Under the Child Marriage Restraint Bill (1978), the age of marriage has been raised for female 18 years and for males 21 years. This has some impact on fertility
- **Minimum needs program**: It was launched in the 5th Five-Year Plan with an aim to raise the economic standard. Fertility is low in higher income groups. Fertility rates can be reduced by raising economic standard.
- **Incentives:** Monetary incentives have been given in family planning program especially for poor classes but these are not very effective so the program must be on voluntary basis.
- **Mass media:** Motivation through radio, television, cinemas, newspaper, puppet shows and folk dances is an important aspect to this program.

- **Eligible couple, target couple and couple protection rate:** Family Welfare Program can be successful only when it reaches those who are eligible and also those who are the targets,
  - **Eligible couple:** It is a married couple the wife being in the reproductive age group, i.e., 15–45 years. It is estimated that there are 150–180 eligible couples per 1000 population in India. These couples are in need of family planning services. Eligible couples can be approached during home visits by ANMs and other health workers or at subcenter and PHC area. They can also be motivated at clinics, hospital and dispensaries. They are given contraceptives free of cost. Sterilization also done free of cost.
  - **Target couples:** These are the couples who have had 2–3 children. They have to be motivated for family planning as it is largely directed to such couples. The definition of target couples has been gradually enlarged to include families with one child or newly married couples. The aim is to develop acceptance of the idea of family planning from the earliest possible stage.
  - **Couple protection rate:** It is defined as the percentage of eligible couples effectively protected against childbirth by one or other method of family planning. CPR is an indicator of the prevalence of contraceptive practice in the community. The long-term demographic goal is to achieve couple protection rate of 60 percent by the year 2000 AD.

Aims of Family Welfare Program

- The Family Welfare Program aims at small family norms through family planning and total welfare of the families. The family planning that aims at small family will serve the welfare of the individual, family and community and country. The Family Welfare Program has the following components:
  - Educational material
  - Services
  - Training
  - Research
- Family planning is a Family Welfare Program and its aim is to create a social welfare state. Family planning is the responsibility of men and women. While population control is a government policy to reduce birth rate, motivated by social and economic interest with the help of community health services
- The family welfare program aims at achieving the highest objective and that is to improve in conjunction with other development programs and to improve the quality of life
- To reduce birth rate from 29/1000 (1992) to 21/1000 population
- To reduce the death rate from 10 (1992) to 9/1000
- Reduction in average family size from 4.2 (1992) to 2.1
- To reduce infant mortality rate from 79 (14.42) to <30/1000 live birth.
- Reduction in net reproduction rate from 1.48 (1981) to 1.
- To provide basic health services to the family and community, i.e., integrated preventive, promotive and curative health services with high priority for improving education and health status of mothers and children.
- The overall aim to stabilize population growth and improve the quality of life through education, information, communication, improved health services, basic facilities, employment, women's empowerment so that every individual is responsible and recognize the need of small family, norm.

The Planning Commission of India has given top priority for stabilizing population and has recommended:

- Wide spread education to create necessary social background for the success of family planning program
- Integration of family planning with the normal health services
- Provision of family planning services, even sterilization through medical and health centers
- Development training program and teaching in hospitals and medical colleges
- Stimulation and utilization of the voluntary leadership

Historical Development of Family Welfare Program

- The first family planning clinic opened by Prof Karve at Pune in 1923. In 1946, a Health Survey and Development Committee, chaired by Sir Joseph Bhore, advised for deliberate limitation of family size and recommended the provision of integrated preventive promotive and curative primary healthcare services with high priority for improving nutritional and health status of mother and child.
- National Family Planning Program was launched during the first Five-Year Plan in 1952 with the establishment of a few clinics, contraceptive supplies and educational material were distributed as required. Training and research was conducted as necessary.
- During the second Five-Year Plan (1956–1961), it was suggested to integrate family planning and health education with community development to systematize the program.
- During the third Five-Year Plan (1961–1966), there was a shift from clinic approach to extension education approach. The services were extended to community level in the villages and urban areas both through extension education to motivate people for small family norm and provide contraceptives.
- In 1965, Lippes Loop was introduced and a separate department of family planning was set up in 1966 in the Ministry of Health.
- During the period of 1966–1969, there were annual plans as fourth Five-Year-Plan was delayed due to political reasons. Specific targets were fixed for different fertility regulating methods. The family planning infrastructure which included urban family planning centers, district and state bureaus were strengthened.
- During the fourth Five-Year Plan (1969–1974), Family Planning Program was given top priority by the Government of India. Family planning services were rendered through subcenters, primary health centers, MCH and family welfare centers as an integral part of MCH services.
- All India Postpartum Program was started in 1970 to motivate mothers for family planning soon after delivery.
- In 1972, Medical Termination of Pregnancy Act 1971 was implemented.
- During fifth Five-Year Plan (1974–1979), the Family Planning Program suffered a major set-back during this period because of rigid implementation of target approach and forcible sterilization campaign during emergency. However, the program got further boosting since 1977 from Rural Health Scheme and from involvement of village health guides, indigenous trained dais and local opinion leaders, etc.
- During the sixth Five-Year Plan (1980–1985), as a result of commitment of health for all by 2000 AD, The National Health Policy 1983, laid emphasis on reorganizations and strengthening of healthcare delivery system to achieve the demographic goals by 2000 AD. These goals were:

- Net reproduction rate—1(2 child norm)
- Crude birth rate—21/1000 live births
- Crude death rate—9/1000 populations
- Couple protection rate—60%
- During seventh Five-Year Plan (1985–1990), the various maternal and child related programs were started during this period for effectively tackling the issue of population stabilization
- These programs included universal immunization therapy, oral rehydration therapy and various MCH programs were brought under the child survival and safe motherhood (CSSM) program
- During the eighth Five-Year Plan (1992–1997), achieving a slower rate of growth considered one of the most important priority. The Reproductive and Child Health Program was widened and scope of Family Welfare Program was widened. RCH Program included safe motherhood program, reproductive tract infections/sexually transmitted diseases all the components of child survival, fertility regulation with a focus on quality care.

RCH Program

- Aims to improve management of services at the center, state, district and block level
- To seek holistic approach in implementation of program
- Focus on neglected geographical areas, i.e., area projects in poorly performing states and districts
- Integrated projects in remote border or districts
- Focus on previously neglected segment of population such as urban slums, men and adolescent, etc.

During the ninth Five-Year Plan (1997–2002) reduction in population growth has been recognized as one of the priority objective. Target free approach has been renamed as community need assessment approach. A comprehensive population policy 2000 was formulated to promote Family Welfare Program and achieve the set goals and objectives

In the year 2005, India launched National Rural Health Mission for seven years (2005–2012) and extended for another 5 years up to 2017. Then came National Urban Health Plan and merging both these plans as National Health Mission.

In the year 2013, RMNCH+A strategy was launched which was based on continuum of care approach and defines integrated package of services for different stages of life.

In 2014, India Newborn Action Plan (INAP) came with the goal to attain single digit neonatal mortality rate by 2030 and single digit stillbirth rate by 2030.

Organization of National Family Welfare Program

The main components of National Family Welfare Program are as follows:
- Administration
- Training
- Information, education and communication (IEC)
- Supplies and services

The functionaries of NFWP at center level are: Ministry of Health and Family Welfare, Family Planning Division, Central Family Welfare Council, National Population Commission, DGHS, National Institute of Health and Family Welfare (NIHFW) all departments concerned with the human resources and development.

Contraceptive Services Under NFWP

- Counseling services, access to the provision of good quality services, follow-up care are emphasized in all contraceptive services
- Government of India is promoting fixed day static services (CFDSI) approach in sterilization services within the public health system with the aim of increasing access to sterilization services
- Increasing male participation in Planned Parenthood, including nonscalpel vasectomy (NSV)
- Camp approach for male sterilization
- Providing wide range of contraceptive services at various levels of health system

National Institute of Health and Family Welfare

National Institute of Health and Family Welfare (NIHFW) is the apex institute as well as a "Think Tank" for the promotion of Health and Family Welfare Program in the country. It is an autonomous organization which was constituted in 1977 by the merger of two national level institutes, i.e., National Institute of Health Administration and Education (NIHAE) and the National Institute of Family Planning (NIFP)

Functions of NIHFW

- Preparing modules for training
  - Training of trainers (TOT)
  - Midterm evaluation of ASHA, JSY, IPHS
  - Development of curriculum
  - **At the state level:** State Ministry of Health and Family Welfare, Directorate of State Health and family welfare/State Family Welfare Bureau, State Institute of Health and Family Welfare and other concerning department
  - **State Institute of Health and Family Welfare (SIHFW):** It is the main organ of family welfare program at state level. It is also coordinating body with the NIHFW. It runs the following programs:
    - Education activities
    - Training for health personnel at state level
  - **At district level:** Chief Medical and Health Officer, District Family Welfare Bureau, DyCM and health officer (FP)/District Family Welfare Officer, Urban Family Welfare Centers, urban health posts, etc.
  - **At block and village level:** Block CMO, medical officer incharge of CHC/PHC, subcenters ANM/FHW, MPW (male), TBAs, village health guide (VHG) and ASHA, etc.

NATIONAL FAMILY PLANNING INSURANCE SCHEME

Government of India launched the National Family Planning Insurance Scheme (NFPIS) in November 2005 to take care of case of failure of sterilization, medical complications or death resulting from sterilization and also provided indemnity cover to doctors and health facilities performing sterilization procedures, with effect from 01-04-2013. It has been decided that States/ UTs would process and make payment of claims to acceptors of sterilization in the event of death/ failure/complications/indemnity cover to doctors/health facilities. Problem Implementation Plans

(PIPs) under the NRHM and the scheme is renamed as "Family Planning Indemnity Scheme" claims arising out of sterilization operation as follows:

1. Death at hospital/within 7 days of discharge ₹2,00,000
2. Death following sterilization after 8th day to 30th day ₹50,000
3. In case of medical complications ₹25,000
4. Failure of sterilization ₹30,000
5. Doctors/facilities covered for litigation up to 4 cases per years including defense cost ₹200000

The scheme also provides for indemnity insurance cover to the medical officers and the health facilities for up to 4 cases of litigations per year that the healthcare provider or the facility may face as a consequence of performing sterilization operations. According to new clause a compensation of ₹50,000 will be paid to the sufferer from Rogi Kalyan Samiti (RKS) immediately after an unlike event and it will be recouped from the insurance company.

Compensation schemes for acceptors of sterilization: Government of India has been providing compensation to the acceptors of sterilization for their loss of wages for availing the services as per the revised rates since September 2007. All states are covered under this scheme.

Funding of Family Welfare Program: It is a centrally sponsored program. The funding is done by the central government in addition to central government funding, RCH Program financed by World Bank, UNICEF and European Commission, etc. United Nations fund for population activities, WHO, United States Agency for International Development (USAID), etc. These agencies also provide technical and financial help for Family Welfare Program.

Evaluation of family planning: Evaluation is defined as the "process of judging about selected objectives and events by comparing with them with specified value standards for the purpose of deciding alternative course of action" in other words it is to know that whether the desired objectives have been achieved or to what extent by comparing them with the set standards.

Purposes of evaluation:

- To improve the design and delivery of family planning services WHO expert committee in 1975, has defined five types of evaluation
- **Evaluation of need:** That is health demographic and socioeconomic needs for family planning. For example, the current status of maternal mortality in a given area is an indicator of the need for family planning

Evaluation of plans: That is an assessment of the feasibility and adequacy of program plans

Evaluation of performance:

- **Services:** Clinic services, mobile services, postpartum services, contraceptive distribution, follow-up services, education and motivation activities
- **Response:** Number of new acceptors, characteristic of acceptors
- Cost analysis
- **Other activities:** Administration, manpower data system, etc.

Evaluation of effects: Changes in knowledge, attitudes, motivation and behavior

Evaluation of impact: Change in birth rate and growth rate. A WHO study group in 1976 prepared the following indices for impact:

- Family size, i.e., number of living children
- Desired number of additional children
- Birth interval

- Age of mother at the birth of first child and last child
- Birth order
- Number of abortions

Evaluation is a technical activity that requires trained personnel, statistical facilities and adequate flow of data and information

ROLE OF NURSE IN FAMILY WELFARE PROGRAM

The role of nurse in Family Welfare Program is diverse and multifaceted. A nurse plays different roles in different settings of family welfare services. However, it depends upon his/her post and in what capacity he/she is employed. It may be governed by the policies of the government or health institute employing him/her. Policies may vary from those that require nurse to participate in family welfare activities to those that forbid them to do so or that limit their participation to giving advice to high-risk mothers because of specific health reasons. Some of the important functions carried by a nurse in Family Welfare Program are described as follows:

Survey work:
- Collects demographic facts.
- Makes list of number of houses and finding out their location
- Collects information about pregnant mothers, eligible couples, contraceptive users, children and infants below the school going age
- Classifies couples into low, medium and high priority groups
- Review couples not using and using contraceptives to plan further action

Health educator:
- Educates the individuals, family and community regarding health and family planning
- Makes people aware of the family planning services available
- Places different choice of contraceptives to adopt for spacing
- Teaches mothers to breastfeed their babies for at least one year. It works as natural contraceptives
- Teaches about immunization, nutrition, first aid and personal and environmental hygiene

Coordinator and provider of family welfare services:
- Makes provision of different types of contraceptives available to the eligible couples
- Arranges family planning clinics, camps and campaigns to make people aware of the need and services available
- Provides direct services within the legal and professional limits of the state government and state's rules and regulations
- Coordinates the services of the gynecologist and other personnel of family welfare services team

Motivational function:
- Motivates eligible couples about the use of contraceptives and adopting small family norms
- Explains the necessity and importance of family planning
- Identifies women requiring MTP and refers them to the doctor
- Maintains adequate supplies and distribution depots establishing of each village to ensure continuous supply of contraceptives

Administrative role:
- Deciding the date and place of family planning clinics
- Arranging equipment and supplies and other resources of clinics

- Supervising and guiding multipurpose health workers at clinics
- Arranging and distributing contraceptives and insertion and removal of IUDs
- Assisting medical officers in conducting clinics
- Organizing family planning camps and assisting the doctors in cases of operation, i.e., male and female sterilization operation
- Following aseptic technique during operation
- Providing follow-up services for those couples who have accepted family planning methods
- Conducting and evaluating health education program

Consultant: Being a coordinator and direct care provider in family welfare services, advice is taken from him/her before starting any healthcare program in the community.

Counselor: He/She conducts the counseling of eligible couples and target couples on various contraceptive methods and provides opportunity to them to select the best suitable method for spacing.

Supervisory role: As a supervisor, the nurse working in family welfare department should encourage their staff to participate actively in Family Welfare Program. The nurse should organize in service education program for other health workers, professionals and auxiliary nursing personnel.

Domiciliary services: Home visits form an important part of Family Welfare Program. The multipurpose health workers and health assistants perform these services. These services comprise:

- Education and motivation of eligible couples
- Follow-up of IUDs and pill users and postoperative follow-up vasectomy, tubectomy and MTP cases
- Domiciliary care of antenatal, postnatal, newborn and toddler care
- Referral services-for those having special problems of postoperative complications

Record maintenance: He/She is responsible for maintaining all records pertaining to family welfare program through all the subcenters, primary health centers, family welfare clinics and hospitals. These records include:

- Eligible couple records
- Target couple records
- Intrauterine devices records
- Sterilization operation records
- Clinic and camp records
- Health education activity records
- Training records
- Medical records

Nurse is responsible for preparing monthly reports and making it available to the concerned authorities

Role in research: Community health nurse is a primary member of the multidisciplinary research team. He/She has to extend directly or indirectly his/her cooperation, participation and motivation in all research activities on family welfare services.

Evaluation role: He/She assesses or evaluates the work done in Family Welfare Programs and prepares a report about it. On the basis of evaluation, further necessary changes are made in the implementation of the programs so as to achieve the desired targets. He/She also evaluates the work of ANMs, Anganwadi workers and other paramedical staff.

Collaborator: Community health nurse works in collaboration with other health teachers of government or nongovernment organizations in the community.

Nurse works with doctors, dispensers, vaccinators, TBA, midwives and lady health visitors in the community on family welfare services

Identification of community leaders: The community health nurse always finds opportunity to meet the influential community leaders and political leaders of the area to strengthen the family welfare services and makes these services universally available to all for the long-term effect on small family norms.

Summary

- Demography is the study of population in terms of its size, composition, behavior and distribution. Demography had been studied over the centuries, the demographic cycle passes through five stages. The first stage is high stationary stage.
- The ten most populous States of India include Uttar Pradesh, Maharashtra, Bihar, West Bengal, Andhra Pradesh, Madhya Pradesh, Tamil Nadu, Rajasthan, Karnataka, and Gujarat. India is very densely populated country.
- The reason of high birth rate is child marriage, illiteracy, poverty, lack of recreation, unavailability of family planning services, and religious superstitions, dependency of women, preference for male child, etc.
- The impact of population explosion includes poverty, inadequate food production, energy utilization, unemployment, antisocial activities, pollution, global warming and accidents, etc.
- The higher fertility rate in India is due to low age at marriage, low level of literary, poor standards of living and limited use of contraceptives Family planning is a key factor in declining fertility.
- Infertility may be due to problem of conception in male or female or both. Treatment includes psychological support to the couple.
- Small family norm has several advantages. Basic human needs can be better fulfilled. Better nutrition, education, employment and better health facilities. It contributes to stabilize population and development of the country.
- Large family has several hazards like illness, low birth weight babies, abortion, increased maternal and infant's mortality, difficulties in meeting basic human needs, malnutrition, illiteracy, poverty, unhappiness disharmony in the family.
- Family welfare concept is much broader in scope than "family planning" and in addition to family planning, it includes MCH and RCH services.
- Family planning methods for female include intrauterine devices, hormonal contraceptives, female condom, diaphragm, foam tablets jelly and cream, rhythm method and tubectomy (or laparoscopic tubectomy).
- Family planning methods for male include condom (Nirodh), withdrawal and vasectomy.
- Nurse's role in family welfare program includes survey work, health educator, coordination and provider of family welfare services, motivator, administrative role, consultant, counselor, supervisor, domiciliary services, record maintenance, researcher, evaluator, collaborator and identification of community leaders for strengthening the family welfare services.

STUDENT ASSIGNMENT

LONG ANSWER TYPE QUESTIONS

1. Define demography. Describe demographic trends in the world.
2. Explain the causes of over population in India and its impact.
3. Discuss the factors affecting fertility in India.
4. Enumerate the advantages of small family size and importance of family planning in India.
5. Describe the methods of family planning.
6. Describe the nurse's role in Family Welfare Program.
7. Explain the stages of demographic cycle.
8. Describe the concept of family planning.

SHORT ANSWER TYPE QUESTIONS

1. Write short notes on the following:
    a. Sex ratio
    b. Dependency ratio
    c. Density of population
    d. Life expectancy
    e. Literacy and education
    f. Determinants of fertility
    g. Principles of fertility regulation
    h. Benefits of fertility regulation
    i. Condom/Nirodh
    j. Vasectomy
    k. Oral contraceptives
2. Enlist the hazards of large family.
3. Enlist aim of family welfare.
4. Write notes on any two of the following:
    a. National sociodemographic goals of family welfare policy.
    b. National Family Welfare Program.
    c. Family planning services during Five-Year Plans.

MULTIPLE CHOICE QUESTIONS

1. **Population count is taken on:**
    a. 1st January
    b. 1st April
    c. 1st July
    d. 1st December

2. **Which of the following goal was set by the Planning Commission working group, 1980 for all states of India on net reproduction rate (NRR)?**
    a. NRR of 1
    b. NRR of 2
    c. NRR of 3
    d. NRR of 4

3. **Which is the denomination in general fertility rate?**
   a. Married women
   b. Women in reproductive age group (15–44 years)
   c. Married women in the age group of 15–44 years
   d. All women

4. **The national policy is to bring the couple protection rate to:**
   a. 60%
   b. 50%
   c. 70%
   d. 80%

5. **The expected growth rate by 2000 AD is:**
   a. 1.2
   b. 2.2
   c. 2.3
   d. 2.4

6. **Mortality experience is taken into consideration when defining:**
   a. General fertility rate
   b. Total fertility rate
   c. Net reproduction rate
   d. Gross reproduction rate

7. **The National Family Planning Program in India was started in:**
   a. 1950
   b. 1951
   c. 1952
   d. 1953

8. **A stage of declining death rate and more declining of birth rate is known as:**
   a. Late expanding
   b. Early expanding
   c. High stationary
   d. Declining

9. **The lowest cut-off age for literary rate in Indian census is:**
   a. 7 years
   b. 4 years
   c. 5 years
   d. 10 years

10. **The death rate as reported in India:**
    a. 8
    b. 10
    c. 7
    d. 6.5

11. **Under the National Population Policy, family size should be brought down to:**
    a. 1
    b. 2.3
    c. 3.2
    d. 4.2

12. **In demographic study of population, a country with low birth rate and a low death rate is in which stage of the demographic cycle?**
    a. 1st stage
    b. 2nd stage
    c. 3rd stage
    d. 4th stage

13. **Net reproduction rate by 2000 AD:**
    a. 1 to 1.2
    b. 2.5 to 2
    c. 2.5 to 3
    d. 3 to 5

14. **All are the true indications for "Health for All" by 2000 AD; except:**
    a. Family size
    b. Annual growth rate 1.2
    c. Life expectancy 64
    d. IMR <60

15. **Net reproduction rate of 1 implies a couple protection rates:**
    a. 60
    b. 50
    c. 70
    d. 80

16. **The denominator to calculate literacy rate is:**
    a. Entire population
    b. Population above 7 years
    c. Population above 14 years
    d. All males

17. **At what stage of demographic cycle is India today?**
    a. Low stationary
    b. High stationary
    c. Early stationary
    d. Late stationary

18. **The best method of postcoital contraception is:**
    a. IUCD
    b. High estrogen pill
    c. Menstrual regulation
    d. Androgens

19. **Best method for spacing is:**
    a. Condom
    b. Pessary
    c. IUCD
    d. Tubectomy

20. **The MTP Act was passed in:**
    a. 1951
    b. 1963
    c. 1971
    d. 1974

21. **Which of the following is the natural means of contraception?**
    a. Condom
    b. Skin patch
    c. Lactational amenorrhea
    d. Hormonal pills

22. **Loop is the example of:**
    a. First generation IUDs
    b. Second generation IUDs
    c. Third generation IUDs
    d. Medicated IUDs

23. **By 2000 AD, the crude birth rate is to be brought down to:**
    a. 20
    b. 21
    c. 22
    d. 25

24. **DMPA is an injectable contraceptives given every:**
    a. Three weeks
    b. Four weeks
    c. Three months
    d. 6 months

25. **Which of the following is suitable for emergency contraceptives?**
    a. Copper bearing IUD
    b. Progesterone-only pill
    c. Skin patch
    d. Diaphragm

26. **Which of the following is at most priority while advising a postvasectomy patient who is discharged from the hospital?**
    a. Wear scrotal support
    b. Take well-balanced diet
    c. Maintain personal hygiene
    d. He is not sterile until semen shows negative reports

27. **The following are the terminal methods of sterilization; except:**
    a. Vasectomy
    b. Dermal implant
    c. Minilap sterilization
    d. Laparoscopic sterilization

28. **The risk of pregnancy in IUCD acceptor is highest in:**
    a. First year
    b. Second year
    c. Third year
    d. Fourth year

29. **The male contraceptive method is:**
    a. Vasectomy
    b. Tubectomy
    c. Copper-T
    d. Oral pills

30. **The proportion of school age children in India's population is approximately:**
    a. 15%
    b. 25%
    c. 40%
    d. 50%

31. **In commercial sex worker the best contraception is:**
    a. IUCD
    b. Oral contraceptive pills
    c. Barrier method
    d. Permanent sterilization

32. **The Indian MTP Act allows abortion up to:**
    a. 16 weeks
    b. 20 weeks
    c. 24 weeks
    d. 28 weeks

33. **Copper-T 200 needs to be replaced after:**
    a. 1 year
    b. 2 years
    c. 3 years
    d. 5 years

34. **In demography, estimated family size is given by:**
    a. NRR
    b. GFR
    c. TFR
    d. GMFR

35. **Consent from guardian for MTP required, if the female is:**
    a. Below 17 years of age
    b. Below 25 years of age
    c. Female is divorcee
    d. Below 28 years of age

36. **Fertility rate can be reduced by the following methods:**
    a. Early marriage
    b. Female literacy
    c. Spacing of pregnancy
    d. Compulsory sterilization

37. **Which of the following would say no for laparoscopic sterilization?**
    a. Hemoglobin 12 g
    b. Has 6 days old baby
    c. Had normal delivery
    d. Medically fit

38. **A women forgets to take her oral contraceptive pill at her regular time. Which of the following would be a correct advice?**
    a. Consult the doctor
    b. No problem
    c. Take it immediately
    d. Use another methods

39. **The Minimum Needs Program was launched during:**
    a. First Five-Year Plan
    b. Second Five-Year Plan
    c. Fifth Five-Year Plan
    d. Seventh Five-Year Plan

40. **The postoperative complication of vasectomy includes:**
    a. Pain and scrotal hematoma
    b. Local infection
    c. Wound infection
    d. All of these

41. **Multiload device refers to:**
    a. First generation IUCD
    b. Second generation IUCD
    c. Oral contraceptive pills
    d. Barrier contraceptive

42. **Minipill contains:**
   a. Only progesterone in small quantity
   b. Progesterone and estrogen in small quantity
   c. Only estrogen in small quantity
   d. None of these

43. **Multiload device contains:**
   a. Zinc
   b. Copper
   c. Silver
   d. Progesterone

44. **World Health Organization (WHO) South East region covers; all except:**
   a. Indonesia
   b. Afghanistan
   c. Thailand
   d. India

45. **Calendar method was discovered by:**
   a. Hermann Knaus and Kyusaku Ogino
   b. Young and Marry
   c. Wallace & Gromit
   d. None of these

46. **In census, literacy rate is assessed by:**
   a. Ability to write signature
   b. Ability to read and write
   c. Ability to read newspaper
   d. Attended literacy classes for one year

ANSWER KEY

1. c	2. a	3. b	4. a	5. a	6. d	7. c	8. d
9. a	10. c	11. b	12. d	13. a	14. a	15. a	16. b
17. d	18. a	19. c	20. c	21. c	22. a	23. b	24. c
25. a	26. d	27. b	28. a	29. a	30. b	31. d	32. b
33. c	34. c	35. a	36. b	37. b	38. c	39. c	40. d
41. b	42. a	43. b	44. b	45. a	46. b		

Note

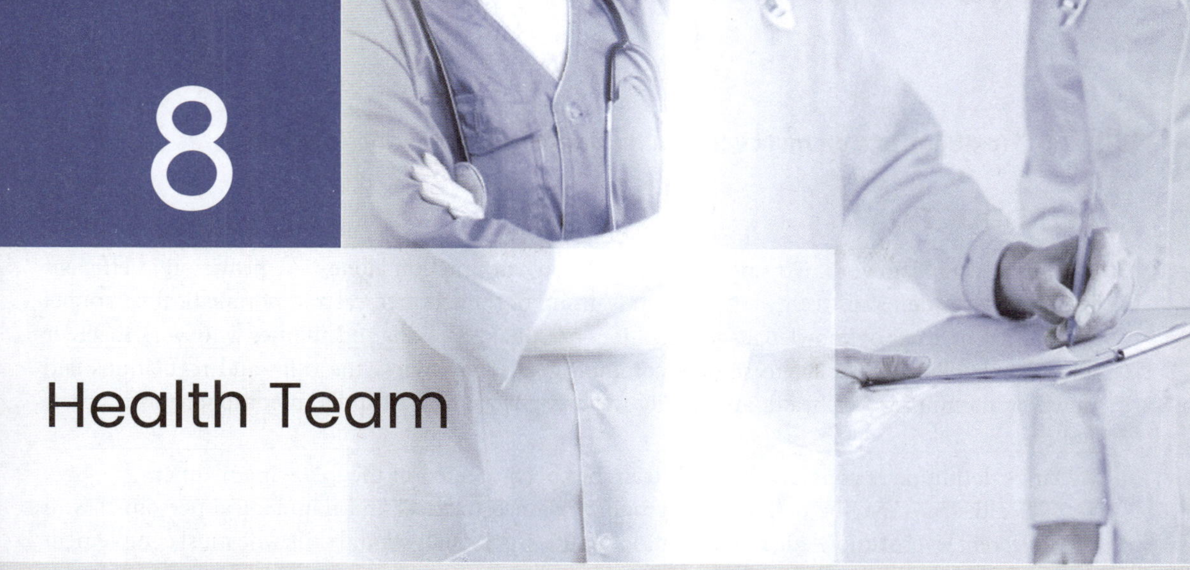

8

Health Team

LEARNING OBJECTIVES

After the completion of the unit, the readers will be able to:
- Describe the concept and composition of health team at various levels.
- Explain the functions of health team.
- Discuss the role of public health nurse at various levels.

UNIT OUTLINE

- Introduction
- Concepts of Health Team
- Medical and Nonmedical Health Team
- Community Health Nursing Team
- Role of Nursing Personnel at Various Levels

KEY TERMS

Health team: Group of trained people working together for achieving common goal to improve health services.

Public health nurse: The person who is working with the individuals, family and community.

Role: Role is the activity done by a particular person according to his/her position.

Abbreviations

DHO: District Health Officer	**NBCP:** National Blindness Control Program
DPHNO: District Public Health Nursing Officer	**NLEP:** National Leprosy Control Program
LHV: Lady Health Visitor	**NVBDCP:** National Vector-Borne Disease Control Program
MDA: Mass Drug Administration	**UIP:** Universal Immunization Program

INTRODUCTION

Healthcare is a teamwork. No single medical person can function alone. The provision of efficient health services demands teamwork. A team is group of trained medical and nonmedical personnel with different levels of knowledge, qualification, personalities, skills and abilities who work together and complement each other to share a common goal. They follow the rules and regulations laid down by the ministry of health and family welfare, government of India in consonance with their policies.

As far as definition is concerned, health team has been defined in the following manner:

- "Health team may be defined as a group of trained medical and nonmedical personnel with different level of knowledge, qualification, abilities, personalities and skill, who must complement each other and who share a common goal."
- Health team is a group of persons who work together to protect the health of the community and hospital. The members of the team differ in their level of knowledge, qualifications, skills, abilities and personalities. Health team includes medical and nonmedical personnel who are complementary to each other. They follow the rules laid down by the Ministry of Health and Family Welfare, Government of India.

CONCEPTS OF HEALTH TEAM

The concept of modern medicine has become joint effort of many groups of personnel. They include specialists, super specialists, medical and paramedical branches of medicine. The concept of health team includes joint efforts of different categories of medical, paramedical and nonmedical personnel who are trained in different branches of medicine to contribute different types of services directed towards healthcare delivery to achieve the objectives. The members of health team work within the framework of policies and rules and regulations laid down by the health department of union or state government. The role of health workers is very important in health team.

MEDICAL AND NONMEDICAL HEALTH TEAM

In government health agency, all the persons working in the organization form a health teams.

The medical personnel of health team include:
- Physician/medical officer
- Nursing officers/staff nurses
- Physiotherapist
- Laboratory technicians
- National social workers
- Health assistants include, *dais*, accredited social health activist (ASHA), and Anganwadi workers.

The nonmedical members of health team are:
- Panchayat leaders
- Teachers
- Postmasters
- Woman health leaders

The characteristics of health team are as under:
- Team has an objective
- Team follows rules
- Team organizes themselves to achieve their objectives
- The team members have unity and team spirit to achieve the goal.

Health Team Members

The health team at primary health center consists of the following members:
- Medical officer who is team leader
  - Staff nurse
  - Pharmacist
  - Laboratory technician
- Block extension educator
- Health assistant male and female
- Health workers male and female

COMMUNITY HEALTH NURSING TEAM

In community, the community health nurse has to take the leadership of community health nursing team. The community health nursing team consists of the following members:

Members Directly Related to Health

- Male and female health workers
- Male and female health assistants
- Dai/Anganwadi worker
- Depot holder ASHA
- Voluntary health associations
- Public Health Nurse (PHN)/District Public Health Nursing Officer (DPHNO)

Members Indirectly Related to Health

- Teachers
- Pradhan community leader/women leader
- Gram Sevak
- Ayurvedic doctors
- Elected representatives

Thus, health team is a group of people working together for common goal in order to provide preventive, promotive, curative, rehabilitative and restorative health services to the individual, family and community.

Composition of Health Team

Health personnel of different units of the health administration, the social workers and local workers working for health constitute the health team. Composition of the health team depends upon the type of organization. In government health agency, all the persons working in the organization form a health team, which is headed by the supreme authority of the health agency, whereas in NGOs, it may be of different shape. At local level, all persons related to health together form health team, for example, all health workers, health assistants and the nursing and other officers employed at the primary health center together form the health team of the primary health center. The teamwork under the leadership of the medical officer is to achieve their objectives. In the local level team, some members are directly engaged in health work, whereas some may be related to health field indirectly or when there is a need. Composition of the health team at primary health center for a population of 20,000 at hilly and tribal area and 30,000 at plains in rural area constitutes the members as listed in Table 8.1.

Composition of Health Team at Primary Health Center

TABLE 8.1: Composition of health team at primary health center

Staff	Number	Indian Public Health Standards (IPHS) recommended numbers
Medical offices-MBBS	1	3 lady MO + 1 from AYUSH
Nurse midwife (staff nurse)	1	5 for 24 hours
Pharmacist	1	2
Health worker (female) ANM	1	1
Block extension educator	1	1
Health assistant (male)	1	1
Health assistant (female) LHV	1	1
Upper divisional clerk (UDC)	1	1
Lower divisional clerk (LDC)	1	1
Lab technician	1	2
Driver	1	Optional
Class IV employees	4	4
Accountant-cum data entry operator	–	1
Total	**15**	**24/25**

Composition of Health Team at Subcenter

Population at:

Hilly, tribal and backward area—3000

Rural area plains—5000

1. Multipurpose health worker female (ANM)	1	(If the deliveries at the
2. Multipurpose health worker male	1	subcenter are 20 or
3. Safai Karamchari (part-time worker)	1	more another ANM to
Total	**3**	be outsourced)

In addition to the above staff, the subcenter will have support from ASHA/TBA/AWW.

Composition of Health Team at Community Health Center

Composition of health team at community health center is given in Table 8.2.

TABLE 8.2: Composition of health team at community health center

Existing Position	Number	As per IPHS recommendation Position	Number
Medical officers (Physician, Surgeon, Pediatrician, Gynecologist)	4	Block health officer	Senior most specialist among physician, surgeon, pediatrician, anesthetist, obstetric and gynecologist, ophthalmologist
Nurse midwives	7	General surgeon	1 MS/DNB (General Surgeon)
Dresser	1	Physician	1 MD/DNB (General physician)
Pharmacist	1	Obstetrician gynecologist	1 MD/DNB/DGO (OBG)
Lab technician	1	Pediatrician	1 MD/DNB/DCH
Radiographer	1	Anesthetist	1 MD/DNB anesthesia
Ward boys	2	Public health manager	1 MD (PSM), MD Community Medicine a postgraduate degree with MBA
Dhobi	1	Eye surgeon	1 MD/MS (one for every 5 CHC)
Safai karamchari	3	Dental surgeon	1 BDS
Mali	1	General duty MO	6 MBBS at least 2 female doctors
Chowkidar	1	Specialist of AYUSH	1 Postgraduate in AYUSH
Aya	1	General duty MO AYUSH	1 Graduate in AYUSH
Peon	1	**Total**	15/16
Total	25	**Supporting manpower**	
		Staff nurses	19
		Public health nurse	1
		ANM	1
		Pharmacist/compounder	3
		Pharmacist AYUSH	1
		Lab technician	3
		Radiographer	2
		Ophthalmic assistant	1
		Dresser	2
		Ward boys	5
		Safai Karamchari	5
		Chowkidar	5
		Dhobi	1
		Mali	1
		Aya	5
		Peon	2
		OPD attendant	1
		Registration clerk	2
		Data entry operator	2

Contd...

Existing	Number	As per IPHS recommendation	
Position		Position	Number
		Accountant/Admin assistant	1
		OT technician	1
		Total	**64**

Functions of Health Team

The functions of health team members depend upon their status in health team, qualification or work assigned to them by the team leader. The work of the members of health team is determined either by their post or according to their job description.

Other members of the health team who are not directly related to the health services fulfil the responsibilities entrusted to them in achieving the objectives of the health team.

Functions of the Team Leader

- The work of the team leader is to keep the group organized in order to achieve objectives
- Maintaining team spirit among team members and boosting the moral of the group
- Maintaining cooperation and coordination among the members at all times
- Providing opportunity to each member of the team to utilize his/her knowledge, skill and qualification
- Making proper decision according to the needs
- Maintaining the dignity and respect of team and its members
- Solving the problems
- Reporting to higher officials or institutions in proper time

General Functions of the Team

- Maternal and child health services
- Family planning
- Immunization services
- Control of communicable diseases
- To provide preventive, promotive and curatives services
- Provision of school health services
- Education on nutrition
- Provide education on environmental sanitation
- Maintaining records and reports
- Conducting laboratory investigations and procedures, e.g. HB%, VDRL, malaria, TB and leprosy test, etc.
- Registration of vital events
- Field visits and conduct surveys
- Preparing reports about communicable diseases
- To provide control services
- Follow-up and referral services
- Guiding health workers for planning programs and organizing the programs
- Conducting group meeting

- Maintaining supplies and equipment
- Cooperate activities between the team and village persons
- Training of health workers, i.e., *dais* and student nurses
- Administration at subcenter, PHC and district level

Relationship among Health Team Members

Good relationship among the workers of health team is important for smooth functioning of health units and to achieve the desired objectives. Strong relations should be built among the members with a positive attitude toward the duties and responsibilities assigned to them. The relationship among them are as follows:

Functional or Working Relationship

The relationship which exists among the members according to their post or job description is called working relationship. This type of relations initially is formal in nature but as the time passes, there is a possibility of developing personal relationship.

Personal Relationship

Personal relationship develop among the members of the health team due to mutual contacts, common objectives, common interests and team spirit. In this type of relations, informality is more frequently observed. Good interpersonal relationship among the members increases the strength of health team.

The members of health team should have the following qualities to establish good relationship among them:

- Members should have complete faith and confidence in leader
- Members should have right knowledge as to when, where and how to make proper use of their skills and knowledge
- They should have complete knowledge about the objectives of the team
- They should have qualification to achieve the objectives
- They should have the understanding to speak honestly and openly
- They should be bound by the rules of the team and also by time
- Members should have the qualities of cooperation and coordination.

Method of Solving the Problems of Team Members which May Occur During Working

Many problems may be encountered by the team members while the work is going on. The problems may be due to insufficient equipment and supplies or equipment may not be working properly, too much of work, lack of cooperation and coordination among the workers. These problems can be solved by problem solving method (Fig. 8.1) as mentioned here:

- Identify the problem
- Collecting data related to problems
- Analyze the problem on the basis of data collected
- Make action plan to remove the hindrance and ways to overcome them
- Implementation of the work plan
- Evaluation

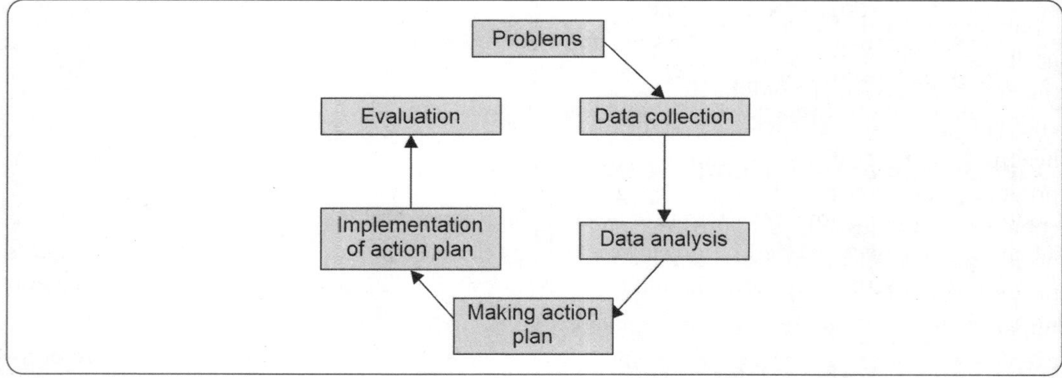

Figure 8.1: Steps of problem solving

Characteristics of Effective Health Team

- Team leader should have administrative qualities.
- Members should have confidence in the leader.
- Health targets should be clear to all the members.
- Objectives should be achievable and measurable.
- Members of the health team should have clear knowledge of their work and role.
- There should be maximum possible utilization of skill and knowledge of members.
- There should be open and effective communication.
- Conflicts and problems should be resolved by problem-solving method.
- There should be definite work schedule.
- Members should be qualified enough to achieve the objectives.
- There should be clear standing orders of the priorities.
- There should be periodical meeting and discussion of the team for further improvement and smooth functioning..

ROLE OF NURSING PERSONNEL AT VARIOUS LEVELS

One of the fundamental principles of delivering quality health services for all is a solid workforce of well-trained and adequately supported community health workers at all levels. Nurses are on the frontlines of the battle to tackle all types of health problems in the community. They are always at the heart of every national health system and are the silent heroes of the healthcare system. The role of nursing personnel depends upon the qualification and post in the health team. The role of various categories of nursing personnel is discussed here:

Role of District Public Health Nursing Officer

The District Public Health Nursing Officer (DPHNO) is an important person responsible for looking after the work of all nursing staff employed in the district. His/her area of work is the entire district. In most of the states the appointment of district public health nursing officer is made on the basis of merit cum seniority. He/she must be highly qualified in community health. He/she is attached to the district health officer (DHO) and is directly responsible to the district health officer and gets guidance from the joint/deputy/director of nursing with the directorate/secretariat of health department of the concerned state. All the nursing personnel working in the cities and villages of the district, i.e., in primary health centers, subcenter, family welfare program, tuberculosis and other programs come under the jurisdiction of district public health nursing officer. From the nursing point of view, the post of district public health nursing officer is very important. He/she must exercise her powers to improve the standard of health services in the district. The main role of the district public health nursing officer (Fig. 8.2) is classified under the following headings:

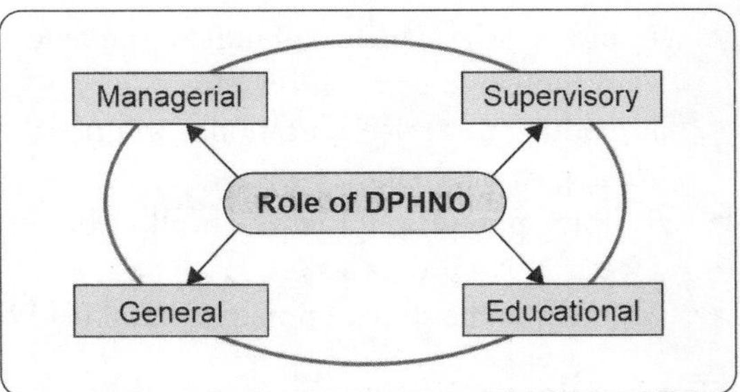

Figure 8.2: Role of district public health nursing officer

Managerial Role

- He/she is responsible for implementing the policies and programs related to nursing in the district.
- **Nursing administration:** He/she is an important member of the selection and recruitment committee, he/she is also responsible for in-service training, promotion, leave and retirement as she sends recommendation related to the abovementioned tasks to the district medical officer.
- He/she participates in preparing budget for nursing services, material and equipment.
- He/she is responsible for forwarding annual reports, work reports, etc. received from nursing personnel.
- He/she evaluates the work of nursing personnel working in the district.
- He/she organizes, directs and develops all community health nursing and midwifery services within the district.
- He/she takes part in all relevant discussions of health services in the district.
- He/she will interpret the needs of the nursing and midwifery services to the district health officer and to the Zila Parishad.

Supervisory Role

- Supervising the work of nursing personnel, health workers from time to time by making visits.
- Taking disciplinary action.
- Passing instructions to different nursing departments in the district to develop good cooperation, coordination and qualities among nursing services.
- Putting emphasis to improve the standard of patient care in the district and achieve the high quality of services.
- Taking the responsibility of nursing audit

Educational Role

- Observe the nursing educational institutes (nursing colleges, schools and clinical area) of the district by making visits from time to time to ensure the quality of training of students in theory and practical.

- Improving the standard of nursing students and nursing education by arranging health-related workshops and conferences, etc.
- Providing in-service educational programs
- Arranging orientation programs
- Training programs for female health workers
- *Dais* training programs
- Training of the student nurses in rural field health centers

General Role

- Participation at state level as a nursing representative of the district
- Getting cooperation from other institutions, organizations to improve the quality of nursing care.
- Organizing nursing workshops, seminars, discussions, etc.
- Encouraging nursing researches

Role of Block Health Nurse/Public Health Nurse Supervisor

There is one post of block health nurse in the block. He/she is responsible for the nursing administration of health services in the block. The block covers a population of 80,000 in hilly, tribal and backward area and 120,000 population at plain rural area. The block has one community health center, four public health centers and 24 subcenters. The roles of block health nurse are explained as under:

- The block health nurse is responsible to the district public health nursing officer for the provision, supervision and improvement of community health services.
- He/she guides and supervises the functions of public health nurses, health workers working in her assigned field.
- Assisting in determination of the philosophy and objectives of the community health programs
- Providing leadership in the planning of total healthcare to all individuals, families and community in her assigned area
- Carrying out preventive, promotive, curative and rehabilitative care
- Assisting in development of the standard of healthcare with the accepted philosophy, objectives and health policies
- Assisting in the preparation of budget for the community health department
- Utilizing the budget allotted to the department (community health)
- Supervision and guidance of public health nurse (PHN), lady health visitor (LHV), female health worker (FHW), male health worker (MHW) working in her field.
- Supervision of records and reports prepared by health workers working under her jurisdiction.
- Training of health personnel and community level workers, educates the community about health guide scheme and takes necessary steps to train the health guides from the primary health center (PHC) area
- Responsible for continuing education of health guides, primary school teachers, RCH group, trained *dais*
- He/she is actively involved in the field training components of basic and refresher training programs, conducted by the institutes for basic training of various categories of health personnel.

- Maintains a close liaison with the block development officer and his staff and with the other developmental program workers such as under National Adult Education Program, the national programs and the program for safe water supply and environmental sanitation.
- Works closely with community leaders and community organizations such as Mahila Mandals, Farmers clubs and other voluntary organizations, etc.
- Organizes camps, meetings, health education talks, demonstrations, display of posters, exhibitions and films and involves the health assistants, health workers and health guides in these activities
- Participates in the village health committee, village panchayat meeting to assess the health needs of the community to discuss the health programs with the community and enlist their cooperation in the programs
- Assisting the DPHNO for the preparation of job description and assignment of responsibilities for other community health program
- Ensures the proper implementation of the following health programs:
  - Control of communicable diseases
  - Maternal and child health
  - Universal immunization program
  - School health
  - Family planning
  - Environmental sanitation

Role of Public Health Nurse

The essential qualification for public health nurse is BSc nursing degree from any recognized university or certificate in public health nursing from any recognized institution. He/she should have working experience in rural community. Her important roles are:
- Assisting in the organization and implementation of national health programs such as:
  - Maternal and child health program
  - Immunization program
  - Prophylaxis against nutritional deficiency diseases
  - Family planning programs
  - Training of *dais* and their active involvement in maternal and child health (MCH) and family planning (FP) work
  - Providing healthcare, i.e., preventive, promotive, curative and rehabilitative services to the individuals, families and community
  - Assists the district medical officer/district family welfare officer in planning, implementing, evaluating maternal and child health and nutrition program
  - Training, supervising and guiding the health workers in the delivery of healthcare services to the community
  - Planning RCH including family planning program with health workers
- **Reporting MCH activities:** Helps the statistical officer in the district family welfare bureau in compiling the periodical progress reports of MCH activities
  - Reviews the periodical program on MCH/FP work done by the LHVs and auxiliary nurse midwife (ANMs), multipurpose worker (MPW), etc. and puts up to the district medical officer/DTFW officer the points requiring attention and further action

- Gives technical guidance, supervision and support to ANM, MPW, LHVs and PHN working in MCH/FP program in the district and reviews the annual confidential reports in respect of those functionaries
- Investigates into complaints against female paramedical personnel in the district and submits reports to the district medical officer/family welfare officer
- Provides continuing education to health team by short in-service training courses
- Promotes health and nutrition education activities through the lady health visitors
- Assisting in conducting school health records
- Carrying out supervisory functions of the home nursing. guiding the home visits in the area covered by the health workers
- Coordinating the work of male and female health workers and other personnel
- **Distribution of supplies:** Ensures regular supply of equipment, records, registers, drugs, vaccines and other supplies necessary for MCH work in PHC and subcenters by assisting storekeeper in procuring and distributing the supplies
- **Maintenance of records:** Ensures the maintenance of prescribed records and submission of periodical program report of MCH/FP and nutritional activities
- Follow-up services in school health, family health and family welfare programs

Role of Lady Health Visitor/Health Supervisor (Female) or Health Assistant (Female)

A lady health visitor or female health assistance or health supervisor (female) is expected to cover a population of 20,000 in hilly, tribal and backward area and 30,000 in rural plain areas in which there are six subcenters. Each subcenter is manned with one female health worker. The LHV will carry out the following duties:

- **Supervision and guidance:** Supervise and guides the health worker (female), *dais* in the delivery of healthcare services in the community
- Strengthening the knowledge and skill of the health workers (female)
  - Helps the health worker (female) in planning and organizing her program of activities
  - Visits each subcenter at least once a week on a fixed day to observe and guide the health worker (female) in her day-to-day work
  - Assess fortnightly the progress of work of HW (F)
  - Carry out supervisory home visits in the area of HW (F)
  - Supervises referral of all pregnant women for VDRL testing to CHC/Sub-divisional hospital
- **Teamwork:**
  - Helps the health workers to work as part of the health team
  - Coordinate her activities with those of the health assistant (male) and other health personnel including the *dais*
  - Coordinates the health activities in her area with the activities of workers of other departments and agencies
  - Conducts regular staff meeting with the health workers in coordination with the health assistant (male)
  - Attends staff meetings at the primary health center
  - Assists the medical officer of the primary health center in the organization of the different health services in the area

- **Supplies, equipment and maintenance of subcenter:** In coordination with the health assistant (male), checks at regular intervals the stores available at the subcenter and help in the procurement of supplies and equipment
    - Checks at the subcenter the drugs are properly stored and the equipment are well maintained
    - Ensures that the health worker (female) maintains her general kit, midwifery kit and dai kit in the proper way
    - Ensures proper maintenance of the subcenter
- **Records and reports:**
    - Scrutinizes the records maintained by the HW (F) and guides her in their proper maintenance
    - Reviews reports received from HW (F), consolidates them and submit monthly reports to the medical officer of the PHC
- **Training**
    - Organizes and conducts training for *dais*/ASHA with the help of female health worker
    - Assists the medical officer of the primary health center in conducting training program for various categories of health personnel
- **Maternal and child health:**
    - Conducts weekly MCH clinics at each subcenter with the assistance of female health worker and *dais*
    - Responds to the calls of female health worker, male health worker, health guide and ASHA and render necessary help to them
    - Conduct deliveries when required at PHC level and provide domiciliary and midwifery services
- **Family planning and medical termination of pregnancy:**
    - She will ensure that female health worker maintains up to date records of eligible couple registers all the time
    - Conducts weekly family planning clinics at each subcenter with the help of female health worker
    - Provides information on the available services for medical termination of pregnancy and sterilization
    - Refer suitable cases for medical termination of pregnancy (MTP) to the approved institutions
    - Guide the female health worker in establishing female depot holder for the distribution of conventional contraceptives with the help of female health worker
    - Provide intrauterine device (IUD) services and their follow up
    - Assists medical officer (MO), primary health center (PHC) in organization of family planning camps and drives
- **Nutrition:**
    - Ensures that all cases of malnutrition among infants and young children (0–5) years are given necessary treatment and advice and refer serious cases to the primary health center
    - Ensures that iron, folic acid and vitamin A are distributed to the beneficiaries as prescribed
    - Educate the expectant mother regarding breastfeeding and weaning food
- **Universal immunization program:**
    - Supervises the immunization of all pregnant mothers and children 0–5 years
    - He/she will also guide the multipurpose health worker (male and female) to procure supplies, organize immunization camp

- Provides guidance for maintaining cold chain, storage of vaccines, health education and immunization
- **School health:**
  - Helps medical officers in school health services
- **Acute respiratory infections (ARI):**
  - Ensures early diagnosis of pneumonia cases
  - Provides suitable treatment to mild/moderate cases of ARI
  - Ensures early reference if doubtful or severe cases
- **Primary medical care:**
  - Ensures treatment for minor ailments
  - Provides ORS for diarrhea and first aid treatment for accidents and emergencies
  - Refer cases beyond her competence to the primary health center or nearest hospital
- **Health education:**
  - Carries out the educational activities for MCH, family planning, nutrition and immunization, control of blindness, dental care and other national health programs like leprosy and tuberculosis with the assistance of the health worker female
  - Arranges group meetings with leaders and involves them in spreading the messages for various health programs
  - Organizes and utilizes Mahila Mandal, teachers and other women in the community in the family welfare program including integrated child development services (ICDS) personnel

Role of Health Assistant (Male)/Health Supervisor (Male)

Health assistant (male) will also cover a population 20,000 in hilly/tribal or backward area and 30,000 in rural plains. The area having six subcenters each subcenter having one male health workers. The duties of health assistant (male) are mentioned as under:

- **Supervision and guidance:** Health assistant male will supervise and guide male health worker in the delivery of healthcare services to the community
  - He helps to strengthen the knowledge and skills of male health workers and improving his skills in working in community
  - Helps the male health worker to plan and organize his program of activities
  - Visits male health worker at least once in a week on fixed day
  - Assess the program of male health worker monthly and submit the report to medical officer primary health center
  - Carry out supervisory home visits in the area of the health worker male
- **Teamwork:**
  - Helps the health workers as a part of the health team
  - Coordinate his activities with the health assistant female and other health personnel
  - Coordinate health activities in his area with the activities of workers of other departments and agencies and attend meeting at PHC level
  - Assist the medical officer of PHC in the organization of the different health services including training program
- **Supplies equipment and maintenance of subcenters:**
  - In collaboration of female health assistant, checks the stores at regular intervals and ensure timely placement of indent and procure the supplies and equipment in time. Ensures that health worker male maintains his general kit in a proper way.

- **Records and reports:**
  - Scrutinize the records maintained by the health worker (male) and guide him in their proper maintenance
  - Review the records received from health worker (male) and submit reports to the medical officer of the primary health center
- **Additional duties:**
  - **Malaria:** He will supervise the work of health worker (male) during concurrent visits and checks that the worker is performing his duties as laid down in the schedule:
    - He should check minimum of 100 houses in the village to verify the work of the health worker
    - He will carry with him a kit for collection of thick and thin blood smear in case if comes across a fever case and will administer presumptive treatment of prescribed doses of antimalaria drug
    - He is also responsible for prompt radical treatment of positive cases of malaria in his area
    - Supervise the spraying of insecticides during local spraying along with health worker (male)
  - **Kala-azar:** Where kala-azar is endemic, his additional duties include:
    - He should check minimum of 10% of the houses in a village to verify that health worker (male) has really visited those houses and carried out his job properly
    - Identify suspected cases of kala-azar and ensure proper treatment
    - Carry with him proper record forms, diary and guidelines for identifying suspected kala-azar cases
    - He is responsible for ensuring complete coverage treatment of kala-azar patients in his area and spray activities, search operations and health education activities related to kala-azar.
  - **Japanese encephalitis:** If Japanese encephalitis is endemic, his special duties are:
    - Check minimum 10% of houses to ensure the health worker (male) has visited those houses and carried out his job properly
    - Identify suspected cases of encephalitis and motivation of the community
    - Carry with him proper records, forms, diary and guidelines for identifying suspected cases of Japanese encephalitis
    - Ensuring proper treatment of suspected cases and health education related to Japanese encephalitis
  - **Lymphatic filariasis:** Where lymphatic filariasis is endemic, his additional duties are:
    - Visit minimum 10% of the houses to ensure that, health worker male has visited those houses and carried out his duties properly
    - He will carry with him proper record forms, diary and guidelines for mass drug administration (MDA) and drug distribution
    - Responsible for ensuring coverage and compliance of drug above 80% during MDA and health education activities related to filariasis
- **Communicable diseases:** He should be alert to the sudden outbreak of communicable diseases such as diarrhea, fever with rash, whooping cough, tetanus, diphtheria, poliomyelitis, acute eye infections, tetanus, neonatorum, jaundice and encephalitis, etc., and take necessary control

measures if any noticeable disease is reported to him, carry out the eradication of stray dogs with the help of health worker (male).

- **Noncommunicable diseases:** Health promotion and IEC activities to be carried out.
- **Leprosy:** He should ensure that all the leprosy cases take regular and complete treatment and ensure retrieval of defaulter.
- **Tuberculosis:** To check whether all the cases under treatment of tuberculosis are taking regular treatment. Motivate the defaulters to take regular treatment and bring them to the notice of medical officer PHC.
- **Environment sanitation:** Helps the community sanitation and motivate them for:
  - Safe water sources
  - Motivating kitchen gardens
  - Soakage pits
  - Compost pits
  - Sanitary latrines
  - Smokeless chullahs

  He supervises the chlorination of water sources including wells.
- **Universal Immunization Program:** Conducts immunization of all school-going children with the help of health worker (female).
- **Family planning:** Guides the health worker (male) in establishing female depot holder with the assistance of health worker (female) and supervise the functions:
  - Assists MO, PHC in organization of family planning camps and drives
  - Provides information on the availability of services for medical termination of pregnancy (MTP) and refer suitable cases to the approved institutions
  - Ensure follow up of all cases of vasectomy, IUD and other family planning acceptors

Role of Health Worker (Female)

The health worker (female) has a key role in delivering health services at subcenter level. She is in direct contact with the village community and is peripheral worker. She is a frontline fighter with community health problems. She caters a population of 5000 at rural plains and 3000 at hilly, tribal and backward areas. She plays the following role in the delivery of healthcare services:

- **Maternal and child health:**
  - Register and provide care to pregnant women throughout the period of pregnancy. Ensure that all registered cases make at least four visits to antenatal clinic for checkup including registration. The schedule of visits is explained to them:
    - **First visit:** Within 12 weeks or as soon as she misses her period
    - **Second visit:** Between 14 and 26 weeks
    - **Third visit:** Between 28 and 34 weeks
    - **Fourth visit:** Between 36 week and term
      She can make visit at any time if she gets any problem.
  - Testing urine for albumin and sugar and estimation of hemoglobin level during her home visit or at the clinic
  - Refers cases of abnormal pregnancy and cases with medical and gynecological problems to PHC
  - Refers all primigravida and high-risk cases to LHV at PHC
  - Conduct deliveries at subcenter if facilities of labor room are available in her area.
  - Supervise deliveries conducted by *dais* and assist them whenever called for

- Refer cases of difficult deliveries and newborn with abnormalities and help them to get institutional care and provide follow up care to patients referred to or discharged from hospital.
- Make postnatal home visits at 0, 3, 7 and 42 days of deliveries at home and on 3, 7, 42 days for institutional deliveries and provide care to newborn and help mother in feeding the newborn
- Assess the growth and development of newborn and take necessary action where required
- Help the LHV and MO in conducting MCH and family planning clinics at subcenters
- Provide health education on personal care, family health, family planning and immunization
- Control of communicable diseases, personal and environmental hygiene and care of minor ailments

- **Family planning:**
  - Utilizes the information from the eligible couple and child register for the family planning programs
  - Responsible for maintaining eligible couple register
  - Responsible for spreading the message of family planning to the couples and motivating them for family planning individually and in groups
  - Distributes conventional contraceptives to the couples, provides facilities and helps the prospective acceptors in getting family planning services by accompanying them or arranges for *dais*/ASHA to accompany them to the hospital
  - Provides follow up care to the family planning acceptors, identifies side effects, gives treatment on the spot for side effects and minor complaints and refers cases to PHC/hospital requiring attention of the physician.
  - Establishes female depot holder and provides continuous supply of conventional contraceptives to the depot holders
  - Builds rapport with the acceptors, village leaders, ASHA, *dais* and others and utilize them for promoting family welfare program
  - Identifies women leaders and trains them with help of the health assistant female
  - Participates in Mahila Mandal Meetings and utilizes such gatherings for educating women in family welfare program

- **Medical termination of pregnancy:**
  - Identify the women requiring help for medical termination of pregnancy and refer them to nearest approved institutions
  - Educate the community for the consequences of septic abortion and inform them about the availability of services for medical termination of pregnancy (MTP)

- **Nutrition:**
  - Identify cases of low birth weight, malnutrition among infants and young children of 0–5 years age, give the necessary treatment and advice and refer serious cases to the PHC
  - Distribute iron and folic acid tablets as prescribed to pregnant and nursing mothers, infants and young children (0–5 years age) and family planning acceptors
  - Administer vitamin A solutions as prescribed to children of 1–5 years
  - Educate community for nutritional diet for mothers and children
  - Coordinate with Anganwadi workers

- **Universal Immunization Program (UIP):**
  - Immunize pregnant woman with tetanus toxoid
  - Administer BCG vaccination, oral polio, DPT, ROTA virus, measles and hepatitis B and pentavalent as per the immunization schedule
  - Ensure injection safety, safe disposal, record, report and manage minor and serious adverse events following immunization (AEFI) monthly UIP reports, weekly surveillance reports
  - Responsible for cold chain maintenance of vaccination during fixed and outreach sessions
  - Utilize posters/paintings on key message, immunization schedule
- **Communicable diseases:** Identify cases of communicable diseases such as cholera, plague, poliomyelitis and persons with continued fever, prolonged cough or spitting of blood when she comes across during her home visit and notifies health worker (male) about them.
- **Dais training:** Lists *dais* in the intensive and twilight areas and involves them in promoting family welfare.
- **Vital events:**
  - Record births and deaths in the birth and death register and inform to health authority particularly of mothers and infants
  - Maintenance of all the relevant records concerning mothers, children and eligible couples in the area
- **Recordkeeping:** She registers the following records:
  - Pregnant woman at the earliest contact
  - Infants 0–1 year of age
  - Women aged 15–44 years through systematic home visits and clinics
  - Maintenance of prenatal and maternity records and child care records
  - Prepares the eligible couple and child register and keeps it up-to-date
  - Maintains the records of contraceptive distribution, IUD insertion, couples sterilized, clinics held at the subcenter and supplies received and issued
  - Prepares and maintains the maps and charts for her area, utilizes them for planning her work
  - Prepares and submits the prescribed weekly/monthly reports in time and submits to health assistant female (LHV)
  - While maintaining passive surveillance register for malaria cases, she will record:
    - Number of fever cases
    - Number of blood slides prepared
    - Number of malaria positive cases reported
    - Number of cases given radical treatment
- **Primary medical care:**
  - Provides treatment for minor ailments
  - Provides first aid for accidents and emergencies
  - Refers cases beyond her competence to the primary health center or nearest hospital
- **Team activities:**
  - Attends and participates in staff meetings at primary health center/community development block or both
  - Coordinates her activities with the health worker male and other workers including the health guides and *dais*

- Meets the LHV each week and seeks her advice and guidance wherever necessary
- Maintains the cleanliness of the subcenter
- Participates as a member of the team in camps and campaigns
- **House to house survey:** These surveys would be done once in the month of April annually. Some of the diseases require special surveys but not more than one survey per month would be expected.
- **Health education:** Provides health education on the following:
  - Awareness on communicable diseases
  - Utilization of local health services
  - Involvement in mid-day meal program
  - Environmental hygiene
  - Identification of health problems
  - Information about rich and nutritious diet
- **Role of health worker (female)/ANM as facilitator of ASHA:**
  - Holds weekly/fortnightly meetings with ASHA and discuss the activities undertaken during that period or any problem encountered during the performance of her activities
  - Acts as a resource person for the training of ASHA
  - ANM will inform ASHA regarding date and time of outreach session and will also guide her for bringing the beneficiaries to the outreach session
  - ANM will participate and guide in organizing health days at Anganwadi center
  - She will utilize ASHA in motivating the pregnant women for coming to the subcenter for initial antenatal checkups. ASHA will also help ANM in bringing married couples to subcenter for adopting family planning
  - ANM will guide ASHA in motivating pregnant women to take full course of iron and folic acid tablets
  - ANM will educate ASHA on the dose schedule and side effects of oral pills. She will also educate her on dangerous signs of pregnancy and labor so that she can timely identify and help beneficiaries in getting further treatment
  - ANM will inform ASHA about time and date for initial and periodic training schedule
  - She will also ensure that during the training ASHA gets the compensation for performance and also TA/DA for attending the meeting.

Role of Multipurpose Health Worker (Male)

He will carry out the activities related to different national health programs and other functions described here:

- **National Vector-Borne Disease Control Program (NVBDCP)**
  - **Malaria**
    - Early diagnosis and complete treatment:
      - To conduct fortnight domiciliary house to house visit
      - To collect thick and thin blood smears in fever cases and perform radical treatment of suspected cases of malaria
      - To refer seriously ill cases to PHC
      - To contact ASHA/fever treatment depots (FTDs) of the area during visit to the village and collect blood smears for transmission to the laboratory

- ▲ To keep records of blood smears taken and treatment of malaria given to patients
- ▲ To ensure early diagnosis and radical treatment of positive cases (Pv and Pf) compliance of RT, etc.
  - ◆ **Integrated vector control program**
    - ▲ To decide dumping sites for insecticides.
    - ▲ Supervise the work of spray squads.
    - ▲ Male health worker will ensure the quality of spray in the human dwellings.
    - ▲ Spray should be uniform.
    - ▲ Deposits should be in small discreet droplets.
    - ▲ All sprayable surfaces like walls, ceilings should be covered.
    - ▲ All false ceilings and attics should be sprayed.
    - ▲ If the houses are built on platforms, the under surface of platform, should be sprayed.
    - ▲ To ensure all precautions are taken by spray man to avoid contamination of food material, cooked food and drinking water in the house.
  - ◆ **Information, education and communication:** To educate the community about signs and symptoms of malaria, its treatment, prevention and vector control.
  - ◆ **Recording or reporting:** To maintain records of all fever cases diagnosed by blood slides, radical treatment and prepare subcenter report, minutes of Village Health Sanitation Committee (VHSC) decision
  - ◆ **VHSC:** Male health worker is expected to be the member of VHSC. He should take part in meetings actively and lead the discussions.
- ■ **Where filaria is endemic:**
  - ◆ Identification of cases of lymphedema, elephantiasis and hydrocele and their referrals to PHC/CHC for appropriate management
  - ◆ Identification and training of drug distributor including ASHA and community health guides for mass drug administration (MDA)
- ■ **Where kala-azar is endemic:** To enquire any fever cases having fever >15 days duration and refer them to nearest PHC for clinical examination by medical officer and adequate treatment.
- ■ **Where acute encephalitis syndrome/Japanese encephalitis is endemic:** During home visit to enquire each family about fever cases with encephalitis presentation and refer them to nearest PHC for diagnosis and treatment by the medical officer.
- ■ Where dengue/chikungunya is endemic
  - ◆ To guide the suspected cases to the nearest PHC/CHC for diagnosis and proper treatment by medical officer
  - ◆ Coordinates the activities carried out by VHSC
- ● **National Leprosy Eradication Program (NLEP)**
  - ■ He imparts health education on leprosy and its treatment
  - ■ Refers suspected cases with complication to PHC
  - ■ Provides subsequent doses of MDT
- ● **National blindness control programs**
  - ■ Identify and refer all cases of blindness including suspected cases of cataract to medical officer PHC

- **Revised national tuberculosis control program (RNTCP)**
  - Identify cases having fever for 15 days or more with prolonged cough or presence of blood in sputum. Take sputum smear from those cases. Refer these cases to MO with PHC. To check all cases of tuberculosis, take regular treatment
- **Universal immunization programs**
  - Administer DPT vaccine OPV, BCG oral polio-vaccine, measles, hepatitis-B to all infants and children in his area
  - Assist health worker (female) in administering TT to all pregnant women
  - Assist the health assistant males in the school immunization program
- **Reproductive and child health programs**
  - Utilize the information from the eligible couple and child register for the family planning program
  - Spread the message of family planning to all the couples and motivate them for family planning individually and in groups
  - Distribute conventional contraceptives and oral contraceptives to the couples
  - Provide follow up services to male family planning acceptor and refer those cases that need attention by the physician/hospital
  - Identify the women requiring help for medical termination of pregnancy and refer them to the nearest approved institution and inform health worker female
  - Provide care for diarrhea, ARI and other common newborn and childhood illness
- **Communicable diseases**
  - Counseling of HIV/STI cases
  - Screening of HIV/STI after receiving training
  - Identify cases of diarrhea, dysentery, fever with rash, jaundice, encephalitis, diphtheria, whooping cough and tetanus, poliomyelitis, neonatal tetanus and acute eye infections, and notify the health supervisor male and MO, PHC immediately about these cases
  - Carry out control measures according to the guidelines
- **Noncommunicable diseases**
  - IEC activities for prevention and early detection of hearing impairment, for harmful effects of tobacco use, mental illness, IDD, diabetes, CVD and strokes
  - House to house surveys to detect cases of hearing and visual impairment and maintain records
  - Motivation for quitting and referral to tobacco cessation center at district hospital
  - Sensitize ASHA/Anganwadi about the noncommunicable diseases
  - Identification and referral for common mental illness for treatment and follow up in the community
  - Ensuring regular testing of salt for iodine through salt testing kits by ASHA
  - Provide IEC to affected districts for prevention of fluorosis
  - Promoting self-healthcare of elderly persons
  - Oral health education to school children, adolescent, antenatal or lactating mothers, first aid and referral for cases of oral health problems
  - Health message on disability, identification of disabled persons and their appropriate referral
- **House to house survey:** These surveys are done once in the month of April annually and once more after six months. Some diseases require special survey, but not more than one survey per month is expected.

- **Environmental sanitation**
  - Chlorinate the public water sources at regular intervals
  - Educate community on method of disposal of liquid waste and solid waste
  - Home sanitation, smokeless chullah
  - Motivate the community to construct sanitary type of latrines
  - Coordination with village health and sanitation committee
- **Primary medical care**
  - Provide treatment for minor ailments
  - First aid for accidents or emergency cases
  - Refer cases beyond his competence to nearest PHC/CHC
- **Health education**
  - Educate people about awareness of health facilities available
  - Treat minor ailments at home
  - Personal hygiene
  - Nutrition
  - Environmental sanitation
- **Nutrition**
  - Identify cases of low birth weight and malnutrition among infants and children 0–5 years in the area
  - Give necessary treatment and advice
  - Refer them to Anganwadi for supplementary foods
  - Refer serious cases to PHC, MO
  - Educate the community about importance of nutritious diet of family from locally available foods.
- **Vital events**
  - Maintain birth and death register
  - Sharing the information of vital events with ANM and report them to health supervisor (male) and health supervisor (female)
  - Educate community on the importance of registration of birth and deaths
- **Recordkeeping**
  - Survey all the facilities in the area and prepare maps and charts for the village
  - Prepare family and village records
  - Assist ANM and LHV to maintain eligible couple and MCH register
  - Maintain record of TB, leprosy cases who are under treatment in his area
  - Prepare and submit monthly report to health supervisor (male)
  - While maintaining record of malaria cases the following points to be noted carefully:
    - Number of fever cases
    - Number of blood slides prepared
    - Number of malaria positive cases reported
    - Number of cases given radical treatment

Summary

- Healthcare is a teamwork. No single medical person can function alone. The provision of efficient health services demands teamwork.
- The composition of the health team varies according to the setting of healthcare services and the population to be covered.
- The members of the health team carry out their responsibility according to their qualification, job description and position held.
- Block health nurse is responsible for nursing administration of health services in the block.
- She ensures proper implementation of all national health programs, maintains close liaison with the block development officer, MO, PHC, community leaders, community organizations, Mahila Mandal, Farmer's club and other voluntary organizations.
- Public health nurse assists district medical officer, district family welfare officer, helps in organization of health programs, reports MCH activities, provides nutritional education, provides education to the team members.
- LHV/health supervisor (female) covers one PHC with six subcenters. She organizes health programs in the community. Supervises and guides health workers.
- Health supervisor (male) covers one PHC with six subcenters. He supervises and guides the male health workers in carrying out national health programs. Counterchecks the work of male health worker by home visiting. Conducts survey of communicable and noncommunicable diseases.
- Female health worker, at subcenters, provides MCH, family planning, MTP, nutrition immunization services. Provides training to dais. Maintains records of vital events. Provides primary medical care.
- Health worker (male), at subcenters conducts survey of his area and maintains records of all vital events. Participates in all national health programs and family planning services. Reports communicable diseases, coordinates female health workers, ASHA and village health guide in the delivery of healthcare services.

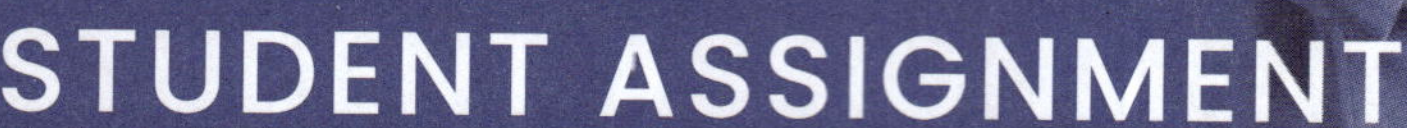

STUDENT ASSIGNMENT

LONG ANSWER TYPE QUESTIONS

1. Define health team. Explain the functions of health team.
2. Enlist the team members at different levels of health system.
3. Describe the functions of health worker (female).
4. Explain the role of public health nurse in the delivery of health services.
5. Enumerate the duties of lady health visitor.
6. Explain the role and responsibilities of district public health nursing officer.

SHORT ANSWER TYPE QUESTIONS

1. Write short notes on the following:
   a. Medical and nonmedical health workers
   b. Characteristics of a team
   c. Composition of health team at PHC
2. State the role of any one of the following:
   a. Health assistant (male)
   b. Public health nurse
   c. Health worker (female)
   d. ASHA

MULTIPLE CHOICE QUESTIONS

1. **Which of the following is the team leader at primary health center?**
   a. LHV
   b. PHN
   c. MO
   d. DPHNO

2. **Which of the following is nonmedical health worker?**
   a. Health supervisor
   b. Woman health leader
   c. National social worker
   d. Dai

3. **Which of the following is not true about LHV?**
   a. Expected to cover a population of 30,000
   b. Supervision and guidance of female health worker and dai
   c. Survey work
   d. Family planning, MTP and UIP

4. **Which of the following is not true about PHN?**
   a. She should possess BSc degree in nursing or certificate in public health nursing
   b. Management and supervisory services
   c. Working experience in rural community
   d. Assists district medical officer/district family welfare officer

5. **The role of block health nurse includes:**
   a. Assisting DPHNO for preparation of job description
   b. Supervision and guidance of PHN/LHV/FHW
   c. Supervision of records and reports prepared by health workers working under her jurisdiction
   d. All of the above

6. **A female health worker is expected to cover a population of:**
   a. 5000
   b. 10,000
   c. 50,000
   d. 80,000

7. **One community health center provides referral services to:**
   a. Two PHC
   b. Four PHC
   c. Six PHC
   d. Three PHC

8. **The role of health worker male includes:**
   a. Survey work
   b. Carry out national health programs
   c. Primary medical care
   d. All of the above

ANSWER KEY

1. c	2. b	3. c	4. b	5. d	6. a	7. b	8. d

Note

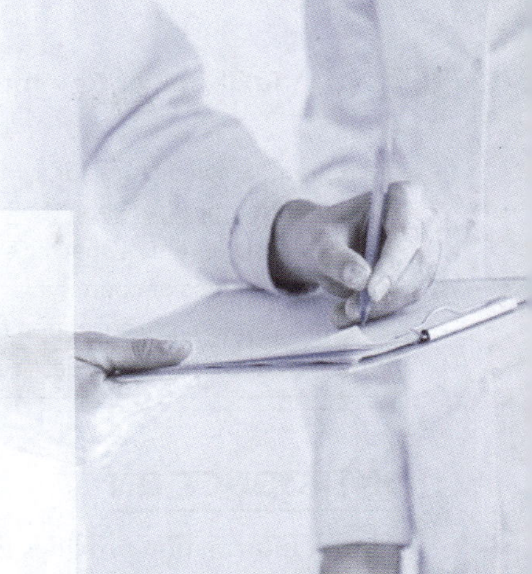

9

Health Information System

LEARNING OBJECTIVES

After the completion of the unit, the readers will be able to:
- Explain the concepts of health information system.
- Discuss the uses of health information system.
- Explain the vital statistics, its importance.
- Appreciate the role of community health nurse in health information system.

UNIT OUTLINE

- Introduction
- Health Management Information System Planners
- Sources of Health Information System
- Vital Statistics
- Important Rates and Indicators
- Useful Rates and Indicators
- Vital Health Record
- Basic Statistical Methods
- Statistic Average
- Measures of Dispersion or Variability
- Descriptive Statistics
- Responsibility of Community Health Nurse in Vital Statistic

KEY TERMS

Biostatistics: A branch of statistic concerned with mathematical facts and data relating to biological events.

Data: Discrete observation of the event.

Frequency: The rate at which an event is repeated.

Frequency polygon: Diagrammatical representation obtained by joining the mid-points of the histogram blocks.

Health information system (HIS): A system in which collection, utilization, analysis and transmission of information is done for conducting health services, training and research.

Health statistics: Statistical information regarding health and diseases.

Histogram: Pictorial diagram of frequency distribution.

Information: When the data is processed by reducing, summarizing and adjusting for variations and transformation into information.

Information system: A system that provides information support to the decision-making process.

Mean: A measure obtained by summing up all the observations and dividing by the total number of observations

Median: The middle observation obtained by arranging all observations in ascending or descending order.

Mode: Most frequently occurring observation in a series.

Pictogram: Small pictures or symbols used to present the data.

Range: Difference between the highest and lowest figure in a given sample.

Rate: Measurement of specific event, condition or disease in a given population within a specific time period.

Statistics: Science of counting.

System: A system is a collection of components that work together to achieve a common objective.

Vital statistics: Numerical data regarding important incidents in a community and analysis of this data.

INTRODUCTION

Health information provides the state of health of the population. The information regarding health can be assessed and monitored from the people. But in this present era of information technology an effective health information system is an essential requirement. A well developed and modern information system can help to furnish the required information about health problems and needs which can help the policy makers and managers to plan their health services adequately.

HEALTH MANAGEMENT INFORMATION SYSTEM PLANNERS

The health management information system incorporates all the data needed by policy maker, clinicians and health services planners to improve and protect the health of the population. Thus, the health management information system may be defined as **"An information system specially designed by WHO 2004** to assist in the management and planning of health program as opposed to delivery of care".** Let us discuss the important elements of Health Information System:

Definition of Health Information System

"A mechanism for the collection, processing analysis and transmission of information required for organizing and operating health services, and also for research and training". Therefore, health information system is a process whereby health data (input) are recorded, stored, retrieved and processed for decision making (output). Decision making broadly includes two aspects, which are:

- **Managerial aspect:** Managerial aspects include planning, organization and control of healthcare facilities at the national, state and district level.
- **Clinical aspect:** Clinical aspect can be subdivided into:
  1. Providing operational care
  2. Training of medical personnel to generate appropriate human resources and facilitate research and development activities in various fields of health and medicine.

Must Know

Distinction between data and information

Data and information are two different aspects. Data is the discrete observations of the attributes or events. It has got very little meaning when considered alone. Data collected from operating healthcare system or institutions are inadequate for planning. Data has to be processed or transformed into information by reducing them, summarizing them and adjusting them for variations such as age and sex composition of the population so that comparisons over time and place are possible. It is the transformation of information through integration and processing with experience and perception based on social and political value that produces intelligence. Data that are not transformed into information and information that are not transformed into intelligence to guide decision makers, policy makers, planners, administrators and healthcare personnel themselves are of little value.

Concepts of Health Information System

Health information system is a basic tool of management for planning health services. It is an integral part of the national health system. Health management information incorporates all the data needed by policy makers, clinicians and health services users to improve and protect the health of the population. The concepts of health information is to provide reliable, relevant, up to date, adequate timely and reasonably complete information to the health managers at all levels, i.e., central, state and district. It includes sharing of technical and scientific information by all health personnel participating in the health services of a country and also to provide at periodic intervals, data that will show the general performance of the health services and to assist planners in studying their current functioning and trends in demands and work load. However, it is very difficult to get the information at the community level. But it is true that no country at present has constructed system of health information in operation; however, this concept is receiving much attention. In the past few decades, the whole science of health has undergone a considerable change. In 1973, the World Health Assembly stressed the need for complete reconstruction of health information system.

Objectives of Health Information System

- To provide reliable, latest and useful health information to all levels of health officer and administrators.
- To create electronic medical records.
- To improve clinical and diagnostic services.
- To amend health policies and working system on the basis of feedback received from health information system.
- To provide information about periodical and time bound programs and for mid-term evaluation.
- To provide early alerts on disease trend and cause of death as per international codes for disease surveillance and rapid action.
- To monitor identified indicators and to get comparison of efficiency and performance among hospitals.
- To provide evidence-based effective and responsive hospital management.
- To provide tools for effective health policy making and planning.

Characteristics of Health Information System

A World Health Organization (WHO) expert committee identified the characteristics shown in Figure 9.1 to be satisfied by the health information system:
- The system should be problem oriented.
- Information should be based on population.
- The system should express information in short and in imaginative form (e.g., tables, graphs, charts and percentage).
- The system should employ functional and operational terms (e.g., episode of illness, treatment regimens and laboratory test).
- Facility for data feedback must be present in the system.
- Latest technology should be used in information system.
- Unnecessary data and figures should not be present in the system.

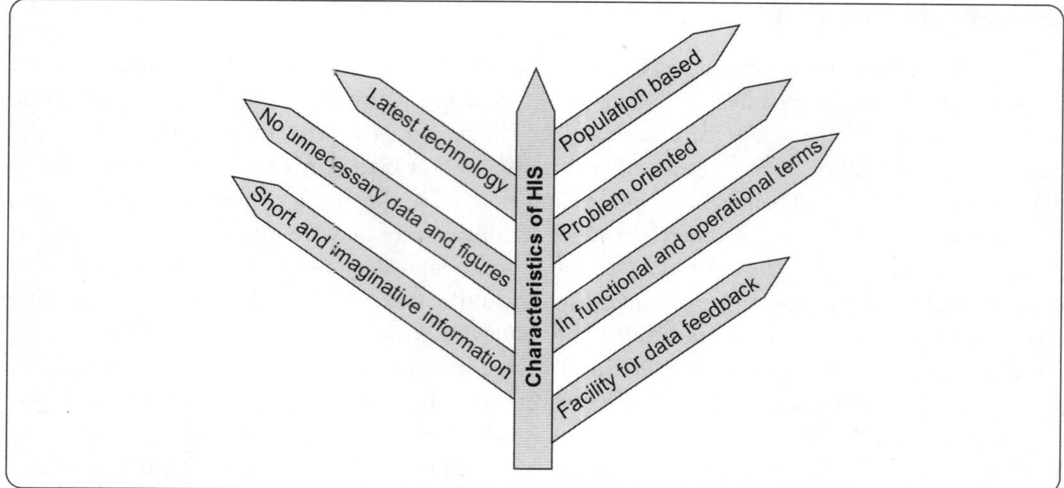

Figure 9.1: Characteristics of health information system

Fields of Health Information System

Health information system is multifaceted. It includes demography, vital statistics, health system input, output, health determinants, health economics, health statistics, health infrastructures resources and the outcomes, financial statistics and environmental health statistic, etc.

Components of Health Information System

The health information system is composed of several related systems (Fig. 9.2). According to WHO, A comprehensive health information system requires information and indicators on the following subjects.

- Demography and vital statistics
- Environmental health statistics
- Health status, i.e., mortality, morbidity, disability and quality of life
- Health resources: Facilities, beds and manpower
- Utilization and nonutilization of health services, attendance, admissions, waiting lists
- Indices of outcome of medical care
- Financial statistics and cost expenditures related to particular subjects.

Uses of Health Information System

- Used to measure the health status of the people and to quantify their health problems and medical care needs.
- Used to utilize for planning, administration and effective management of health services and health programs.
- Used to assess whether the health services provided are fulfilling their objectives in terms of their effectiveness and efficiency.
- Used to compare local national and international health status. For such comparisons data needs to be subjected to rigorous standardization and quality control.

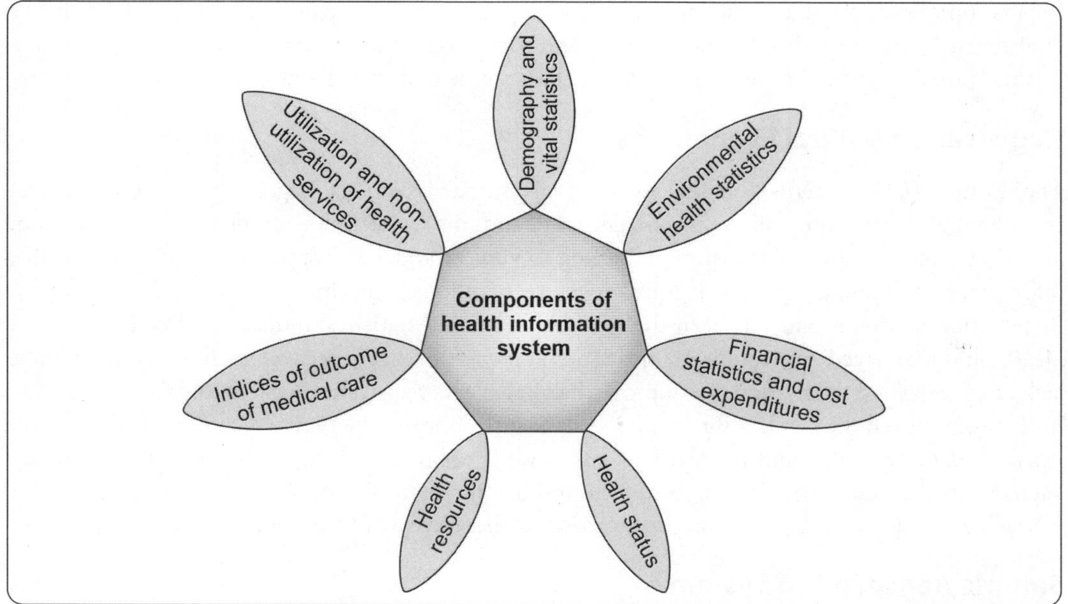

Figure 9.2: Components of health information system

- Used for assessing the attitudes and degree of satisfaction of the beneficiaries with the health system
- Used to research into particular problems of health and diseases
- Used to coordinate the efforts of partners and countries in the field of health indictor measurements and use, health data management and evaluation of health information system.

SOURCES OF HEALTH INFORMATION SYSTEM

The main sources of health information are the central government and state government agencies. The lifeblood of a health information system is the routine health statistics. Information requirement will vary according to the administrative level at which planning is envisaged. The information requirement of public health administrator will differ from hospital administrator. The main sources discussed are as follows:

Census

Census is defined by the United Nations as "the total process of collecting, compiling and publishing demographic, economics and social data pertaining at a specified time or times, to all people in a country or delimited territory." In most of the countries of the world it is taken at regular intervals of 10 years. The first census in India was conducted in 1881 and the last was held in 2011. Census provides demographic information, i.e., total count of population and its breakdown into groups and subgroups such as age, sex distribution. It also provides social and economic characteristics of the people and the conditions under which they live, work and their income. These data provide a framework of reference and baseline information for planning action and research not only in the field of medicine, human ecology and social science but also in the entire government system.

Population census provides baseline data (such as population by age and sex) needed to compute vital statistics and other health demographic and socioeconomics indicators. Without census data, it is not possible to obtain quantified health demographic and socioeconomic indicators.

Registration of Vital Events

The United Nations defines a vital events registration system as "legal registration statistical recording and reporting of the occurrence of, and the collection, compilation, presentation, analysis and distribution of statistics pertaining to **vital events,** i.e., live births, deaths, fetal deaths, marriages, divorces, adoptions, legitimations, recognitions, annulments and legal separation." Registration of vital events has been the foundation of vital statistics. India had passed the Births, Deaths and Marriage Registration Act in 1886. But it was unreliable because of illiteracy, ignorance, lack of concern and motivation. To improve the vital events registration system, the Government of India promulgated the Central Birth and Death Registration Act in 1969 which came into force on April 1, 1970. The time limit for registering the events of birth is 21 days uniformly all over India. Vital events provide information of birth rate and death rate in the population. The primary health workers are responsible in collecting and recording these events in the community.

Sample Registration System

Sample registration system (SRS) is major sources of health information. It was started in India in the mid-1960s to provide reliable estimates of birth and death rate at the national and state level. SRS is more reliable information of birth and death rate, age-specific fertility and mortality rates, infant under five and adult mortality rate, etc. SRS is dual record system consisting of continuous enumeration of birth and death by an enumerator and an independent survey every 6 months by an investigator supervisor.

Notification of Diseases

Notification of diseases provides valuable information about fluctuation in disease frequency. It also provides early warning about new occurrence or outbreaks of diseases. The primary function of notification is to effect prevention and control of the diseases. Notification is also an important source of morbidity data, i.e., incidence and distribution of certain specified diseases which are notified. List of notifiable diseases vary from country to country and even in the same country, from state to state and between urban and rural area. The notification system is linked up with the vital statistics machinery. Earlier the notification was the responsibility of village chowkidar but now the responsibility is shifted to multipurpose health workers.

Hospital Records

The hospital records provide a basic and primary source of information about diseases prevalent in the community. It provides information about age, sex, diagnosis, time interval between occurrence and hospital admission. The main drawback of hospital data are:
- They provide information on only those patients who seek medical advice.
- Mild cases may not report to hospital.
- Subclinical cases are always missed.
- Population served by hospital cannot be defined.

Disease Register

Morbidity registers are valuable source of information. These registers contain not only the certain diseases and conditions but also provide information about duration of illness, case fatality and survival. These registers allow follow-up of patients and provide a continuous account of the frequency of diseases in the community. Even in the absence of a defined population base, useful information may be obtained from registers on the natural course of diseases, especially chronic diseases in different parts of the world. If the reporting system is effective, the registers can provide useful data on morbidity from a particular disease, treatment given and diseases-specific mortality.

Record Linkage

The term "record linkage" refers to describe the process of bringing together record related to one individual (or the family), the records originating in different times or places. Medical record linkage implies the assembly and maintenance for each individual in a population of a file of the more important records relating to his health. The events commonly recorded are birth, marriage, death, hospital admission and discharge. The main problem of record linkage is the volume of data that can accumulate. Record linkage has been applied on a limited scale, e.g., twin studies, measurement of morbidity, chronic epidemiology.

Epidemiological Surveillance

Epidemiological surveillance is carried out in countries where particular diseases are endemic and where special controls eradication programs have been instituted, such as national diseases control programs against malaria, tuberculosis, leprosy, filariasis, etc. As a part of these programs surveillance system are conducted to report on the occurrence of new cases and on efforts to control the disease, e.g., immunization program has brought considerable decline in morbidity and mortality rate.

Other Health Service Records

A lot of information can be obtained in the records of hospital outpatient department, primary health centers, subcenters, polyclinic, private practitioners, child health center, school health records, diabetic and hypertension clinic, etc. The drawback of these records is that they relate only to a certain segment of general population.

Environmental Health Data

The environmental data is also very important source for the identification and quantification of factors causative of diseases. The health statistics are sought to provide data on various aspects of air, water, noise pollution, harmful food additives, industrial toxicants, inadequate waste disposal and population explosion with increased production and consumption of goods. Collection of environmental data remains major problem in the future.

Health Manpower Statistics

Health manpower statistics is the information about the number of physicians, dentist, pharmacists, veterinarians, hospital nurses, medical technicians, and others. Their records are maintained by the state medical/dental/nursing councils and the directorates of the medical education.

Population Survey

The routine statistics collected from the above sources do not provide all information about health and diseases in the population. Therefore, population survey is supplement to the routinely collected statistics. The statistics available for cholera, malaria, plague, respiratory diseases, fever and diarrhea are extremely useful for public health administration. The term health survey is applied to any aspects of health, i.e., morbidity, mortality, nutritional, status, etc. The types of surveys to be covered under health survey are:

- **Surveys for evaluating the health status of a population** that is community diagnosis of problem of health and diseases. It is information about the distribution of these problems over time and space that provide fundamental basis for planning and developing the needed services.
- **Surveys for investigation of factors affecting health and diseases.** It includes environment, occupation, income and circumstances associated with the onset of illness, etc. These surveys are helpful for studying natural history of the disease and obtaining more information about etiology and risk factors of diseases.
- **Surveys relating to administration of health services:** In this survey health services expenditure on health, evaluation of population health needs and unmet needs, evaluation of medical care, etc., are used. Population survey can be conducted in any setting. Population health survey may be cross-sectional, longitudinal, descriptive or analytic or both. Survey methods are classified into four types:
  - Health interview (face-to-face) survey
  - Health examination survey
  - Health records survey
  - Mailed questionnaire survey

Other Routine Statistics Related to Health

- **Demography survey** includes population density, movement and educational level.
- **Economic survey:** Consumption of consumer goods as tobacco, dietary fats and domestic coal, sales of drugs and remedies, information concerning per capita income, employment and unemployment data.
- **Social security survey:** Scheme and medical insurance schemes make it possible to study the occurrence of diseases in the insured population. Other useful data include sickness absences, sickness and disability benefits rates.

Nonquantifiable Information

Health planners and decision makers require lots of nonquantifiable information on health policies, health legislation public attitudes, program costs, procedure and technology. Health information system has multi-disciplinary inputs. There should be proper storage, processing and dissemination of information.

VITAL STATISTICS

Vital statistics have been used to denote facts systematically collected and complied in numerical forms relating to or derived from records of vital events, namely live birth, death, fetal death, marriage, divorce adoption, legitimating, recognition, annulment or legal separation. Vital statistics are derived from legally registrable events without including population data or a morbidity statistic.

Meaning of Statistics

The word statistics is derived from the Italian word "statista" which means statesman or a German word "statistic" which means a political state.

Definition of Statistics

It is a science and art of dealing with variation in such a way as to obtain reliable **statistics** may be called the science of counting.

Meaning of Vital Statistics

Vital statistics is concerned with the study of human population. Vital statistics means numerical data regarding important incidents occurring in a community and the method of analysis of this data. The important incidence means birth, marriage, diseases and death, etc.

Some Definitions Used in

- **Vital statistics:**
  - Vital statistics is data/record regarding marriage, birth, diseases and death on the basis of which community health and development are studied.   **—Benjamin**
  - Vital statistic is the numerical description of birth, death, abortion, marriage, divorce and adoption and judicial separation.   **—UNO**
  - Vital statistic is a part of demography and collective study of mankind. It deals with the data related to vital events.
  - Vital statistic is a branch of biometry that deals with data and law of human morbidity, mortality and demography. Vital statistics include birth, death, fetal death, marriage divorces and separation, and are considered primarily from the point of view of physical, mental and social wellbeing of the total community and of the individual. The health status cannot be judged simply by decline in mortality rate but it should also include the morbidity statistics.
- **Biostatistics:** It is the branch of statistics which is concerned with mathematical facts and data relating to biological events.
- **Health statistics:** It includes all statistics information required for the administration of health agency and would comprise not only vital statistics but also a good deal of other numerical information. Usually it is limited to health data and includes the data on all matter of sickness like morbidity, illness and ill health.
  - **Health statistics measurement:**
    - Measurement related to the state of health which includes sickness and death.
    - Measurement affecting health, i.e., nutrition, housing and environmental factors.
    - Items of services: Preventive, promotive and curative. Sources of vital health statistic are same as that of health information system.

Function of Vital Statistics

- It represents facts in a definite form.
- It converts the mass of numbers into useful information.
- It is used as machinery in health information system.
- It helps in formulating and testing hypothesis.
- It helps in planning effective strategy for future.
- It helps in production.
- It facilitates comparison.

Purpose of Vital Statistics

- **Administrative purpose:** It provides clues for administrative action and create administrative standard of health activities.
- **Health program organization:** It determines success or failure of specific health program or undertakes overall evaluation of public health work.
- **Legislative purpose:** To promote health legislation at local, state and national level.
- **Government purpose:** To develop policies and procedures at state and national level.
- Basis of social reform.

IMPORTANT RATES AND INDICATORS

- **Rate:** The rate is the primary measurement in descriptive epidemiology.
- **Definition of rates:** Rate may be defined as measurement of a specific event, condition or disease in a given population within a specific time period.

  Rate can be expressed in a formula as:

$$\text{Rate} = \frac{\text{Number of people affected in given time period}}{\text{Total population in a same area}}$$

Rates may be used for the comparison between groups. Specific rates have concern with specific events, time period, causes or specific group. By using rates, it is possible to compare events that occur at different time and place and different people. Rates present demographic data and morbidity data.

- **Demographic rates:** When the demographic data are converted into rates, they become very meaningful for the assessment of community health status. The rate consists of two parts, a numerator and denominator. The numerator is composed of the number of conditions or events of interest occurred within specified period of time. Denominator is the total population at risk during the same period of time. If the time period is long the population at risk is estimated at mid period such as mid-year.

General Principles of Calculation

- Numerator must include all of the events that are being measured such as deaths of cases and each of those must be in the denominator.
- Everyone in the denominator must be at risk for the events in the numerator because rate is a fraction or proportion.

- It is necessary to multiply by a base which is usually a multiple of ten. The procedure removes the decimal point and makes composition of the rates easier.
- Any base multiple of ten may be chosen that results in the rate above the volume of one. The rate should be reasonable size not a factor.

$$\text{Rate} = \frac{\text{Number of events occurring in a period of time}}{\text{Population at risk during the same period of time}} \times 1000$$

USEFUL RATES AND INDICATORS

Rates are calculated from the total number of events which occur in a defined geographical area during a calendar year. Rates include:

- Annual rate
  - Crude rate
  - Specific rate

$$\text{Crude rate} = \frac{\text{Number of total events in an area during the year}}{\text{Estimated mid-year population of the same area during the same year}} \times 1000$$

$$\text{Specific rate} = \frac{\text{Number of total events in specific population in an area during the year}}{\text{Estimated mid-year population of the same area during the same year}} \times 1000$$

- **General marital fertility rate (GMFR):** It is the "number of live births per 1000 married women in the reproductive age group (15–44 or 49 years) in a given year."

$$\text{GMFR} = \frac{\text{Number of live birth in a year}}{\text{Mid-year married female population in the age group of 15–49 year}} \times 1000$$

- **Age-specific fertility rate (ASFR):** Age-specific fertility rate is "defined as the number of live births in a year to 1000 women of any specific age group." The ASFR throws light on the fertility pattern. They are the sensitive indicators of family planning achievement.

$$\text{ASFR} = \frac{\text{Number of live birth in a particular age group}}{\text{Mid-year female population of the same age group}} \times 1000$$

- **Birth rate:** Birth rate is defined as "the number of live births during a year per thousand estimated mid-year population." It is represented by the formula.

$$\text{Birth rate} = \frac{\text{Number of live births during the year}}{\text{Estimated mid-year population}} \times 1000$$

- **Death rate:** The death rate "is defined as the number of deaths per 1000 estimated mid-year population in one year." It is given by the formula.

$$\text{Death rate} = \frac{\text{Number of deaths occurred during the year}}{\text{Estimated mid-year population}} \times 1000$$

- **Specific death rate:** The death rate due to specific cause, e.g., cholera in specific group, age, sex, occupation, social class and specific period annual, half yearly, monthly are called specific death rate.

  - Diseases-specific death rate $= \dfrac{\text{Number of deaths among males during the year}}{\text{Estimated mid-year population}} \times 1000$

  - Sex-specific death rate of males $= \dfrac{\text{Number of deaths among males during the year}}{\text{Estimated mid-year population}} \times 1000$

  - Time-specific death rate $= \dfrac{\text{Number of death in 2014}}{\text{Estimated mid-year population}} \times 1000$

  - Age-specific death rate $= \dfrac{\text{Number of death of specific age group during the year}}{\text{Estimated mid-year population}} \times 1000$

- **Infant mortality rate:** It is the number of infant deaths under one year of age per 1000 live births in one year. It is represented by the formula.

  $$\text{Infant mortality rate} = \dfrac{\text{Number of deaths under one year of age}}{\text{Total live birth in the year}} \times 1000$$

- **Neonatal mortality rate:** Deaths occurring within 28 days of birth are called neonatal deaths.

  $$\text{Neonatal mortality rate} = \dfrac{\text{Number of death under 28 days of age}}{\text{Total live birth}} \times 1000$$

- **Perinatal mortality rate:** It is the mortality of infants occurring during the period from 28 weeks of gestation to 7 days after birth per 1000 total births. It includes total stillbirths and deaths under 1 week.

  $$\text{Perinatal mortality rate} = \dfrac{\text{Fetal death of 28 weeks gestation + deaths under 7 days after birth}}{\text{Total live birth + still birth}} \times 1000$$

- **Maternal mortality rate:** According to WHO "Maternal mortality rate expresses the death of a woman while pregnant or within 42 days of termination of pregnancy, irrespective of the duration and site of pregnancy from any cause related or aggravated by the pregnancy or its management not from accidental or incidental cause."

$$\text{Maternal mortality rate (MMR)} = \frac{\begin{array}{c}\text{Total number of female deaths due to} \\ \text{complications of pregnancy, child birth of} \\ \text{within 42 days of delivery from puerperal} \\ \text{causes during the given year}\end{array}}{\text{Total number of live birth in the same year}} \times 100{,}000$$

- The multiplying factor can also be 1000, 10,000 and 100,000 if no deaths decline considerably
- **General fertility rate (GFR):** It is better measure of fertility than the crude birth rate because the denominator is restricted to the number of women in the child-bearing age, rather than the whole population.

$$\text{General fertility rate (GFR)} = \frac{\text{Number of live birth in an area during the year}}{\begin{array}{c}\text{Mid-year female population of age 15–45 years} \\ \text{in the same area in the same year}\end{array}} \times 1000$$

- **General marriage rate (GMR):** It is defined as the number of marriages during a year per thousand persons of age 15–45 years.

$$\text{GMR} = \frac{\text{Number of marriages within one year}}{\text{Number of unmarried persons of age 15–49 years}} \times 1000$$

- **Pregnancy rate (PR):** It is the ratio of number of pregnancies in a year to married women in the age group of 15–45 years. The number of pregnancies includes all pregnancies whether these had termination as live birth, stillbirth or abortions or had not yet terminated.

$$\text{PR} = \frac{\text{Number of pregnancies within one year}}{\begin{array}{c}\text{Number of women of reproductive age} \\ \text{(15–45 years) in the same year}\end{array}} \times 1000$$

- **Abortion rate:** The annual number of all types of abortions usually per 1000 women of childbearing age (usually defined as age 15–44 years).
- **Age-specific marital fertility rate:** It is the number of live birth in a year to 1000 married women in any specific age group.

$$\text{ASMFR} = \frac{\text{Number of live births in a particular age group}}{\begin{array}{c}\text{Mid-year married female population} \\ \text{of the same age group}\end{array}} \times 1000$$

- **Total fertility rate (TFR):** Total fertility rate represents the average number of children a woman would have if she were to pass through her reproductive years in each age group. It is computed by summing the age specific fertility rate for all ages, if 5 years of age groups are used the sum of the rates is multiplied by 5. This measure gives the appropriate magnitude of "completed family size".

$$TFR = 5 \times \sum_{15-19}^{45-49} \frac{ASFR}{1000}$$

- **Total marital fertility rate (TMFR):** Average number of children that would be born to a married woman if she experiences the current fertility pattern throughout her reproductive span

$$TMFR = 5 \times \sum_{15-19}^{45-40} \frac{ASMFR}{1000}$$

- **Gross reproduction rate (GRR):** Average number of girls that would be born to a woman if she experiences the current fertility pattern through her reproductive span (15–44 or 49 year) assuming no mortality

$$GRR = 5 \times \sum_{15-19}^{45-49} \frac{ASMFR}{1000}$$

- **Net reproductive rate (NRR):** NRR is defined as the number of daughters a newborn girl will bear during her lifetime assuming fixed age specific fertility and mortality rates.

$$NRR = Women \xrightarrow{\text{gave birth}} Daughter \xrightarrow{\text{birth given to}} girl\ born$$

  NRR is similar to GRR but takes in to account that some females will die before completing their productive lifespan

- **Marriage rate:** It is the number of marriages in the year per 1000 population.

$$Crude\ marriage\ rate = \frac{Number\ of\ marriage\ in\ the\ year}{Mid\ year\ population} \times 1000$$

- **Expectation of life or life expectancy:** Expectation of life or life expectancy at a given age is the average number of years which a person of that age may expect to live according to the mortality pattern prevalent in that country. Demographers consider it as one of the best indicators of a country's level of development and of the overall health status of its population.

- **Proportional mortality rate (PMR):** It is commonly used to study diseases pattern by cause in settings where population denominators are not available. The proportional mortality can be calculated by sex, age, group or any other appropriate subdivision of the population. Proportional mortality rate is simple and potentially useful way of portraying the burden of a specific disease within a population and PMR provides a way to compare population.

- **Morbidity indicators:** Morbidity is the state of departure from physiological well-being. The various morbidity indicators are incidence rate, prevalence rate, notification rate hospital attendance, admission and discharge rate, etc.

- **Incidence rate:** It indicates the number of new cases of a particular disease in a defined population during a specific period of time. Incidence rates provide a direct measure of the rate at which new cases occur in a given population. It serves as a valuable tool for the study of the causes of diseases, incidence rates are more useful in assessing the risk of acute diseases. Examples of incidence rates are hospital admission rate, case attack rate, secondary attack rates, etc.

$$\text{Incidence rate} = \frac{\text{Number of new cases of a disease starting illness in a defined period}}{\text{Mid-year population at risk during the same year}} \times 1000$$

- **Attack rate:** It is similar to the incidence rate and represents the incidence of illness among the exposed population during the specified time period and expressed as a percent.

$$\text{Attack rate} = \frac{\text{Number of new cases of a specified disease occurring in a particular place during the specified time interval}}{\text{Total populations at risk during the same time interval}} \times 100$$

- **Prevalence rate:** It indicates the number of existing cases (new and old) of a disease in the total population at a particular point of time. Prevalence rate is a ratio rather than rate. It is of two types:
  1. **Point prevalence:** It is defined as the number of all current cases (new and old) of a disease at one point of time in relation to a defined population

$$\text{Point prevalence} = \frac{\text{Number of all current cases (new and old) of a specified disease during a particular period of time interval}}{\text{Total population at the same point of time}} \times 100$$

  2. **Period prevalence:** It is defined as the number of cases (old and new) existing during a defined period of time expressed in relation to a defined population

$$\text{Period prevalence} = \frac{\text{Number of all existing cases (old and new) of a specified disease during a particular period of time interval}}{\text{Estimated mid interval population at risk}} \times 100$$

Prevalence rate may be affected by treatment. As the diseases is cured prevalence rate may be decreased. Prevalence rates are useful in:
- Planning the disease control program
- Administration of hospital
- For treatment and rehabilitation
- **Disability rate:** A disability is an umbrella term converging impairments, activity limitations and participation of restrictions. These include days of restricted activity, bed disability day, and work loss day. A disability may be present at birth or occur during a person's lifetime.
- **Healthcare delivery indicators:** They are doctor population ratio, doctor nurse ratio, population bed ratio, etc. These indicators show the availability and distribution of health services.
- **Environmental indicators:** These indicators represent the quality of physical and biological environment. They include the proportion of population who get safe water and also indication relating to pollution of air, light and water.
- **Social and mental indicators:** These indicators include suicides, homicides, smoking, alcoholism, violence and drug abuse.

- **Utilization rates:** Health usually investigated by this indicator to provide additional information on health status in use of health services. The percentage of children and mothers immunized, bed occupancy rate, length of hospital stay, percentage of people using family planning method, etc.
- **Socioeconomic indicators:** These include the rate of population growth, family size, housing, literacy rate, unemployment rate and per capita income, etc.
- **Others:** The health policy indicators, social indictors, basic needs indicators and health for all indicators.

VITAL HEALTH RECORD

The United Nations define a vital events registration system as including legal registration statistical recording and reporting of the occurrence of and the collection, compilation, presentation and distribution of statistics relating to vital events such as:

- Birth registers
- Death registers
- Fetal death registers
- Marriage registers
- Divorce registers
- Adoption registers
- Judicial separation registers

Therefore, the vital health records include the following records:

- Birth records
- Death records
- Fetal death records
- Marriage records
- Divorce records
- Adoption records
- MTP and abortion records
- **Morbidity records:** These records provide valuable information about the course of diseases, its duration, case fatality and survival. Natural cases of disease can be obtained from registers:
- Antenatal records
- Postnatal records
- **K sheets:** K sheets are maintained in the hospital setting and these give information about geographical area, age, sex duration of the hospital stay, distribution of diagnosis, association between diseases and hospital staff, period between diseases and hospital stay.

The distribution of patients according to social and geographical characteristics and cost of the hospital case, such information can be of great value in the planning and healthcare services.

Central Birth and Death Registration Act 1969

For the compulsory registration of birth and death, the Government of India promulgated a "Central Birth and Death Registration Act" which came into force on April 1, 1970. The Act makes registration of births and deaths compulsory throughout India. The time limit in registration of birth and death is 21 days uniformly all over India. In case of default, a fine up to ₹50 can be imposed. The parents or institution such as hospitals, nursing homes, hostels, jails or Dharamshalas where an indication of birth and death has happened, will register it with the concerned register.

Uses of Vital Health Records

- Vital health records help to determine the status of health of individual, family and community.
- Help in investigating the health problems and needs of the people so that health planning can be done to solve these problems.
- Help in making improvement in the administration.
- Help in evaluating the health program.
- Useful in health offices and institution in collecting data.
- Provide basis in formulating plans in the health service. These are the symbols of future plans.
- Useful for analysis of the trends of health statistics.
- Useful for making health programs.
- Useful in comparing the health status of one nation with another.
- Serve as an important tool for research related to health.
- The vital health records are of legal necessity.
- These are the basis of social reforms.
- These are the important tools for the epidemiologists.

BASIC STATISTICAL METHODS

Statistical data once collected must be arranged purposively in order to bring out the important points clearly and strikingly. The data is classified, analyzed and tested for accuracy by statistical methods. The data which is obtained directly from the individual is called primary data. The data which is obtained from records is called secondary data. The method of presenting statistical data is:

- Tables
- Charts
- Diagrams
- Graphs
- Picture
- Special curves

Tabulation

This is the first step before the data is used for analysis and interpretation. It can be simple or complex depending upon the number of measurements of a single set or a multiple set of items (Tables 9.1 and 9.2).

General Principle of Tabulation

- Tables should be numbered, e.g., Tables 9.1 and 9.2, etc.
- Title must be given to each table and the title should be brief and self-explanatory.
- Heading of rows or columns should be clear and concise.

TABLE 9.1: Simple table showing population of India in different years

Year	Population
1901	238,396,000
1921	251,321,000
1981	685,185,000
1991	843,930,000
2001	1027,015,247
2011	1210,193,422

Source: Census of India, 2011.

TABLE 9.2: Complex table showing population of India in different years with percentage of tuberculosis infection and annual mortality rate per 100 cases.

Year	Population in millions	Infection per 100 population	Annual mortality per 100 cases
1961	439.23	1.75	0.36
1981	685.18	2.74	0.57
2001	1052.50	4.21	0.88

Central Tuberculosis Division Government of India
Source: ADGH (TB) Government of India, New Delhi.

- The data must be presented according to the size or importance, chronologically, alphabetically or geographically.
- If the percentages or averages are to be compared they should be placed as close as possible.
- Table should not be very large.
- No abbreviation should be written.
- Total and grand total should be shown at the end of the table.
- Vertical arrangement is better than horizontal one because it is easier to scan data from top to bottom than from left to right.
- Footnotes should be given.
- Frequency distribution table: (Table 9.3) In the frequency distribution table the data is first split up into convenient groups (class intervals) and the number of items (frequency) which occur in each group is shown in the adjacent column.

TABLE 9.3: Frequency distribution table showing the percentage of diastolic blood pressure of males and females

Blood pressure	Number of males	Percentage	Number of females	Percentage
70–75	6	6.3	8	14.5
76–80	18	19.0	12	21.9
81–85	46	48.4	25	45.5
86–90	17	17.9	8	14.5
91–95	6	6.3	2	3.6
96–100	2	2.1	–	–
Total	95	100.0	55	100.0

Diagrammatic Representation of Data

Charts and Diagram

The statistical data becomes interesting when it is presented diagrammatically. People will understand it easily and would accept it with greater interest. The impact of picture depends on the way it is drawn.

The following are the rules for constructing diagram and charts:

- Diagrams presented should be attractive and of proper size.
- The data presented by diagram should be simple.
- Measurements should be easy and useful.
- The facts should be clearly classified in a diagram.
- Every diagram or chart should have a heading.
- Symbolic presentation and its explanation is essential.
- Minimum use of words and figures.
- Diagram should be meaningful and should present reality.

Bar Chart

In bar charts a set of numbers is exhibited by the length of a bar. The length of bar is proportional to the magnitude to be represented. Bar charts are popular media of presenting statistical data because they are easy to prepare and enable values to be compared visually. The bars are usually separated by appropriate spaces for neat and clear presentation. A suitable scale must be chosen to present the length of the bar. A simple bar chart is shown in the Figure 9.3.

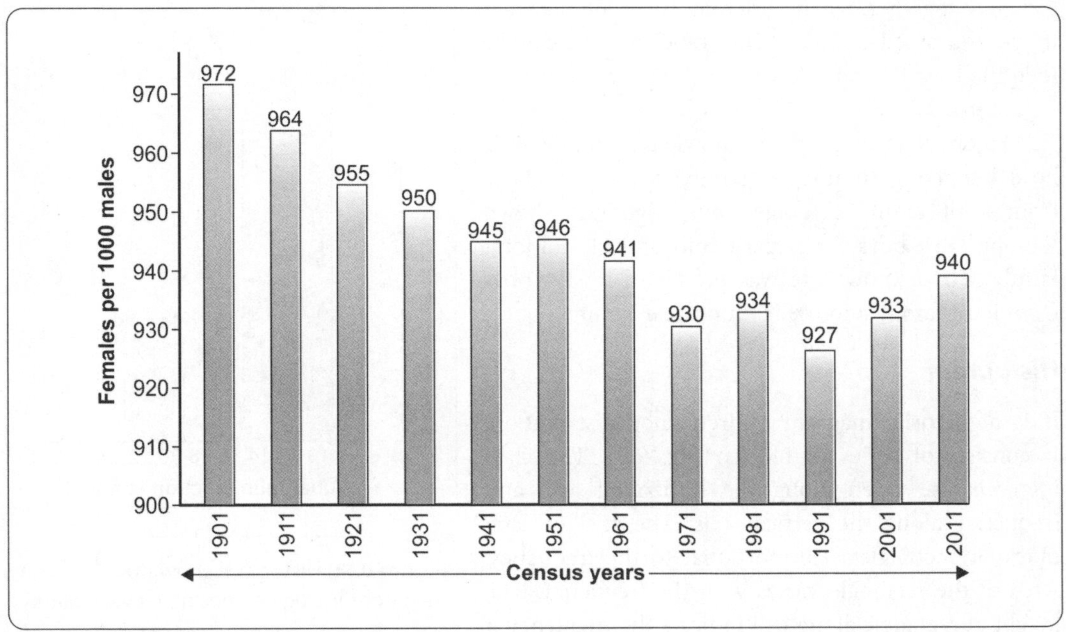

Figure 9.3: Bar chart showing females per 1000 males in subsequent census years

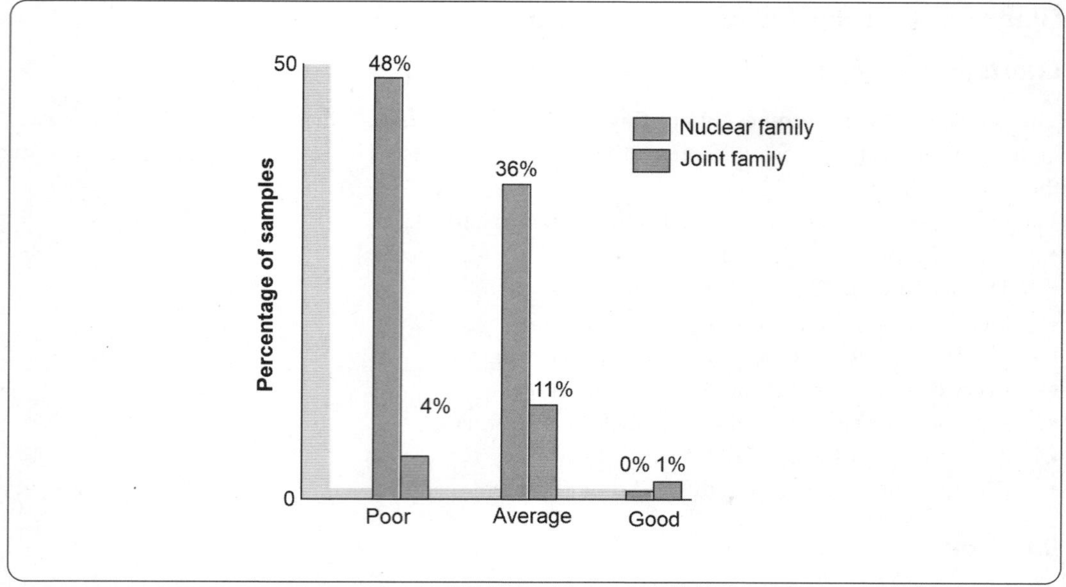

Figure 9.4: Multiple bar chart showing the percentage distribution of level of knowledge about ill effects of smoking among 13–19 years age in nuclear and joint familiar

Multiple Bar Charts or Compound Bar Chart

In this type of bar charts two or more bars can be grouped together when different types of data are to be compared at once. One type of data can be identified by the same color or design as shown in Figure 9.4.

Figure 9.4 shows poor knowledge among 48% boys belonging to nuclear family against 4% boys from joint family. Average knowledge was shown "among" 36% boys of nuclear family and 11% of joint family. Good knowledge was presented by 1% boys from joint family and 0% from nuclear family.

Histogram

It is a pictorial diagram of frequency distribution. It consists of series of blocks (Fig. 9.5). The class intervals are given along the horizontal axis and frequency along the vertical axis. The area of each block or rectangle is proportional to the frequency. Area of the rectangle varies with the frequency. The height of rectangle alone will indicate the frequency if the class interval is uniform.

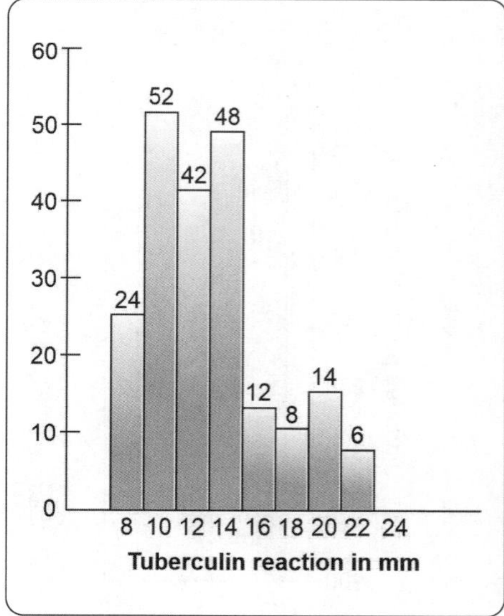

Figure 9.5: Histogram showing tuberculin reactions in 206 persons never vaccinated

Frequency Polygon

It is also a diagram of frequency distribution developed over a histogram. It is obtained by joining the mid-points of class intervals at the height of frequencies by straight lines (Fig. 9.6). It gives a polygon, i.e., figure with many angles.

Tuberculin reaction in 206 persons has been given in Table 9.4.

Line Diagram

This is a frequency polygon presenting variations by lines. It is used to show the trend of events with the passage of time. Figure 9.7 shows the population trends in India from 1901 to 2011. Here the class interval is 10 years.

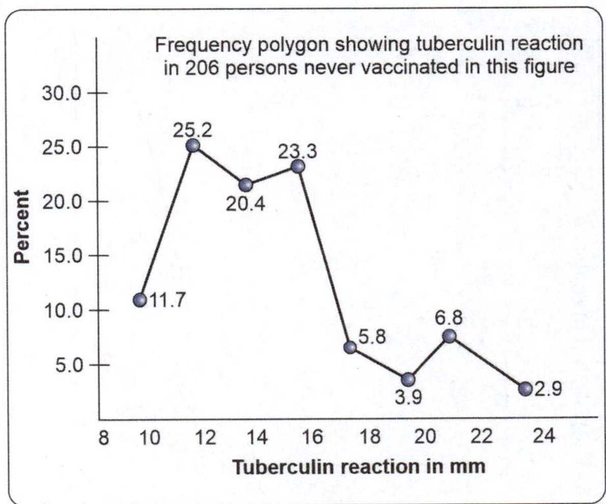

Figure 9.6: Frequency polygon

Pie Charts or Sector Diagram

This is another way of presenting discrete data of qualitative characters (Fig. 9.8). Instead of comparing the length of a bar, the area of segment of a circle is compared. The area of each segment depends upon the angle. The degree of angle shows the frequency and area of the sector. It gives comparative difference at a glance. Size of each angle is calculated by multiplying the class percentage with 3.6, i.e., or by the formula

$$\text{Class percentage with } 3.6, \text{ i.e } \frac{360}{100} \text{ of by the formula}$$

$$\frac{\text{Class frequency}}{\text{Total observation}} \times 360°$$

TABLE 9.4: Tuberculin reaction in 206 persons

Reaction in mm	Frequency	Percentage
8–10	24	11.7
10–12	52	25.2
12–14	42	20.4
14–16	48	23.3
16–18	12	5.8
18–20	8	3.9
20–22	14	6.8
22–24	6	2.9
Total	206	100.0

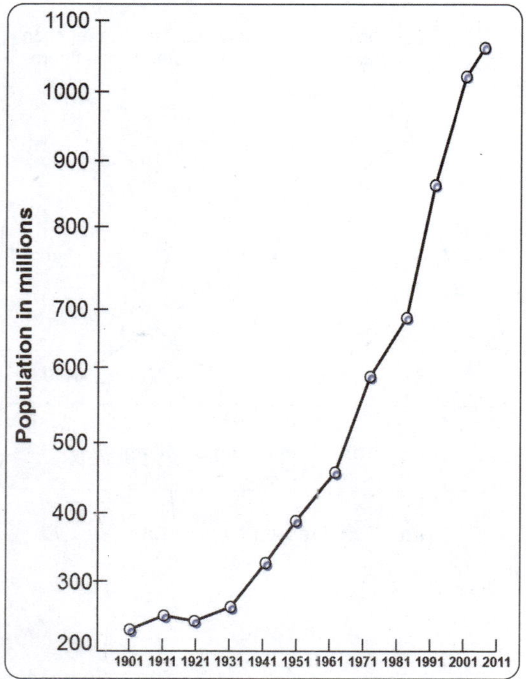

Figure 9.7: Line diagram showing population trends in India

Figure 9.8: Pie diagram showing percentage distribution of samples according to religion

One hundred samples were selected of 13–19 years boys to assess the knowledge on ill effects of smoking to find out association between different variables.

The percentage of samples according to religion—in a description study to assess the knowledge and attitude on ill effect of smoking, the 66% of samples were Hindus, 16% of the samples were Muslims where as 18% of the samples practiced other religion (Fig. 9.8).

Pictograms

In pictogram in spite of presenting traditional charts, data are made clear with the help of picture or symbols. It is a popular method to impress the frequency if the occurrence of events to common man such as number of patients admitted, discharged, accidents, deaths, number of operations, etc. Figure 9.9 shows the population per physician in different countries.

Statistic Maps

When the statistical data refer to geographical or administrative area, it is presented either as "shaded maps or dot maps" according to suitability. The shaded maps are used to present data of varying sizes. The areas are shaded with different colors or different intensities of the same color which is indicated in the key. Figure 9.9 shows the doctor's population ratio in different countries.

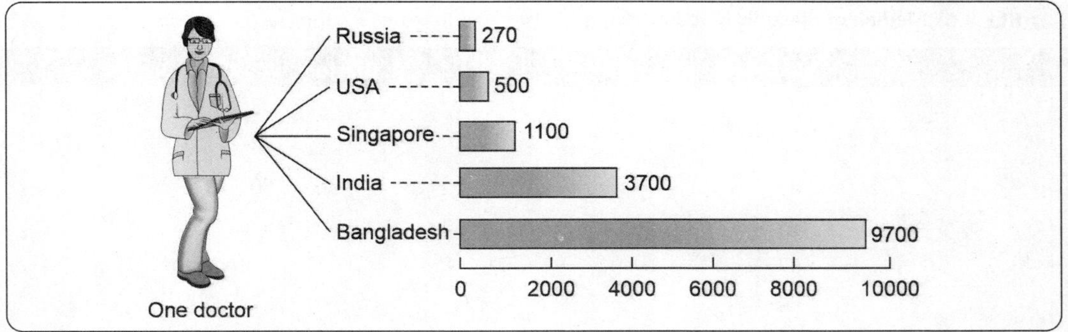

Figure 9.9: Population per physician in different countries

STATISTIC AVERAGE

Average is a general term which describes the center of services. There are three common types of averages or measures of central position or a central tendency, i.e.,

- Mean
- Median
- Mode

Mean

This measure implies arithmetic average or with arithmetic mean which is obtained by summing up all the observations and dividing the total by the number of observations.

The operation of adding is called summation and denoted by the sign Σ.

The individual observation is denoted by the sign η. and the mean is denoted by the sign $\overline{X}$ (called 'x' bar)

The mean is calculated as: $\overline{X} = \dfrac{\Sigma}{\eta}$

Example: The hemoglobin level of six subjects of same age and same sex are 13, 14, 12, 13, 11, 12 Calculate the mean hemoglobin.

Solution:

The mean hemoglobin $= \dfrac{13 + 14 + 12 + 13 + 11 + 12}{6} = 12.5$

by applying the formula,

$$\overline{X} = \frac{\Sigma}{\eta}$$

where X is mean hemoglobin, Σ is the sum of number of observations added and η is number of observations.

Hence, Mean hemoglobin is 12.5.

Mean is the one central value which is most commonly used in statistic methods.

TABLE 9.5: Median of diastolic blood pressure

Diastolic blood pressure	Diastolic blood pressure
80	72
72	76
83	80
85	83
87	85 medians
90	87
76	90
95	92
92	95

Median

When all the observations of a variable are arranged in either ascending or descending order, the middle observation is known as median.

To obtain the median the data is first arranged in an ascending or descending order of magnitude and then the value of the middle observation is located which is called median. For example, the diastolic blood pressure of nine subjects is shown in Table 9.5. The data is arranged in ascending order in the right column of Table 9.5. It shows the median is 85 which is the value of middle observation.

Mode

Mode is the most frequently occurring observation in a series. It is the most frequently item or the most fashionable value in a series of observations. For example, the diastolic blood pressure of 20 subjects was: 85, 75, 81, 79, 71, 95, 75, 77, 75, 90, 71, 75, 79, 95, 75, 77, 84, 75, 81, 75.

The mode or most frequently occurring value is 75. Mode is rarely used in medical studies. The advantages of mode are that it is easy to understand and is not affected by the extreme items. The disadvantage is that the exact location is often uncertain and often not clearly defined that is why it is not often used in medical statistics.

Out of the three measures of central tendency, mean is better and is utilized more often because it uses all the observations in the data and is further used in the test of significance.

MEASURES OF DISPERSION OR VARIABILITY

Measure of variability of observations helps to find how individual observation is dispersed around the mean of large series. There must be individual variation. If we examine the data of blood pressure or height or weight of a large group of individuals, we may find that the values may vary from person to person. Even within the same individual there may be variation from time. There are several measures of variation or dispersion of which the widely used are:

- **Range:** The range is the simplest measure of dispersion. It is defined as the difference between the highest and lowest figures in a given sample. For example, the range from the diastolic blood pressure of ten individuals can be calculated by subtracting the lowest reading from the highest one:

$$83, 75, 81, 79, 71, 90, 75, 95, 77, 94$$

In this series, the highest reading is 95 and the lowest one is 71.

$$\text{Range is } 95 - 71 = 24$$

The range is not of practical importance as it indicates the extreme value only and nothing about the dispersion of values between the two extreme values.

- **Mean or average deviation:** It is the average of the deviation from the arithmetic means. It is given by the formula.

$$MD = \sum \frac{(x - \bar{X})}{x}$$

Where x is the series of reading and $\bar{X}$ is the arithmetic means and $(x - \bar{X})$ is the deviation from mean. The mean deviation from the diastolic blood pressure of 10 individual is 83, 75, 81, 79, 71, 95, 75, 77, 84, 90.

$$\text{Arithmetic Mean} = \frac{83 + 75 + 81 + 79 + 71 + 95 + 75 + 77 + 84 + 90}{10} = 81$$

$$\bar{X} = 81$$

Systolic BP x	Arithmetic mean $\bar{X}$	Mean deviation Deviation from the mean $(x - \bar{X})$
83	81	2
75	81	−6
81	81	0
79	81	−2
71	81	−10
95	81	14
75	81	−6
77	81	−4
84	81	3
90	81	9
Total = 810		**Total = 56 (ignoring ± sign)**

$$\text{Arithmetic Mean} = \frac{810}{10} = 81$$

$$MD = \sum \frac{(x - \bar{X})}{x}$$

$$= (x - \bar{X}) = 56$$

$$MD = \frac{56}{10} = 5.6$$

- **Standard deviation:** It is defined as "root – means – square – deviation." It is denoted by the Greek letter sigma (σ) or by the initial SD. It is the most frequently used measure of deviation. Standard deviation is calculated from the formula.

$$\text{Standard deviation (SD)} = \sqrt{\sum \frac{(x - \bar{X})}{\eta}}$$

The above formula is used when the sample size is >30.

Example: The diastolic blood pressure of 10 individual is: 83, 75, 81, 79, 71, 95, 75, 77, 84, 90. Calculate SD.

Solution:

x	$\bar{X}$	$x - \bar{X}$	$(x - \bar{X})^2$
83	81	2	4
75	81	–6	36
81	81	0	0
79	81	–2	4
71	81	10	100
95	81	14	196
75	81	–6	36
77	81	4	16
84	81	3	9
90	81	9	81

$x = 81$, $\eta = 10$

$$\text{SD} = \sqrt{\sum \frac{(x - \bar{X})^2}{\eta - 1}} = \sqrt{\frac{482}{10 - 1}} = \sqrt{\frac{482}{9}} = \sqrt{53.55} = 7.31$$

$\eta = 10$

$\text{SD} = 7.31$

The basic significance of standard deviation is that it is an abstract number that it gives us an idea of the spread of dispersion. The larger the standard deviation the greater is the dispersion value about the means than 30. For smaller size this formula tends to underestimate the standard deviation and needs correction which is done by subtracting the denominator by 1 ($\eta - 1$) from η.

Therefore, standard deviation (SD) can be calculated by the formula:

$$\text{SD} = \sqrt{\sum \frac{(x - \bar{X})^2}{\eta - 1}}$$

The steps for calculating the standard deviation are:
1. First of all, take the deviation of each value from the arithmetic means
2. Square each deviation
3. Add up the squared deviation
4. Divide the result by number of observations η or $(\eta - 1)$ in case sample size is <30
5. Take the square root which gives the standard deviation

DESCRIPTIVE STATISTICS

Definition

Descriptive statistics is the study of the amount and distribution of the diseases or health status within a population by person place and time.

It usually includes the determinants of incidence, prevalence and mortality rates for diseases in large population group. This is according to the characteristics such as age, sex, race, social customs, habits, etc. The descriptive statistic also describes the occurrence of diseases in relation to person, place and time. It is the first step in epidemiological investigations and provides data about the distribution and frequency of diseases or health-related states of the population by identifying the characteristics with which the diseases in question seems to be associated. It provides answers to the following questions:
- When the disease is occurring? Time distribution.
- Where is it occurring? That is place distribution.
- Who is getting the diseases? That is person distribution.

The procedures involved in descriptive methods are:
- Defining the population to be studied
- Defining the diseases under study
- Describing the disease by time, place and person
- Measurement of diseases
- Comparing with known indices
- Formulation of an etiological hypothesis

Defining the Population to be Studied

The descriptive studies are carried out in population; therefore population should be defined in terms of total number, age, sex, occupation and sociocultural characteristics, etc. Population defined should be large or whole population in an area or just a representative sample may be taken.

Defining the Diseases Under Study

Once the population under study is defined or specified then the diseases or condition under study to be defined stating its signs and symptoms and how diseases will be measured. If the definition is not valid it would lead to errors in presentation and findings would not be comparable with other findings.

Describing the Diseases by Time, Place and Person

After defining diseases the epidemiologist describes the occurrence of disease or health related events or characteristics with in the population in terms of time, place, and person.

- **Time distribution:** Three types of time distribution occur, i.e.
  1. **Short-term fluctuation:** The best-known short-term fluctuation in the occurrence of a disease is an epidemic.
  2. **Periodic fluctuations:** This refers to the seasonal variation in occurrence of a disease, e.g., many communicable diseases, like measles upper respiratory infections, malaria, and measles occur usually in early spring, whereas respiratory infections show rising trend in winter month
  3. **Long-term fluctuations:** This refers to changes in the occurrence of diseases over a long period of time generally many years or decades. Secular trend implies a definite upward or downward movement in occurrence of some diseases. Diabetes mellitus, hypertension and coronary heart diseases are showing an upward trend, whereas typhoid, diphtheria and polio are showing a downward trend.
- **Person distribution:** The descriptive study describes the occurrence of a disease by person according to age, sex, occupation, marital status, habits, social class, ethnicity, behavior, stress, migration, etc.
  - **Age:** Age is related to diseases as shown here:
    Childhood—measles
    Middle age—cancer
    Old age—atherosclerosis
  - **Sex:** Sex is another host characteristic linked with diseases occurrence. Certain chronic diseases are more common in women than men, e.g., hyperthyroidism and obesity are more common in women than men, whereas lung cancer and coronary heart diseases are more common in men than women.
  - **Occupation:** Different occupations are related to different diseases such as a person working in coal mines have silicosis occurring commonly and farmers working in fields have farmers lung diseases.
  - **Ethnicity:** Tuberculosis, sickle cell anemia and cancer are found to be distributed in certain racial and ethnic origin groups.
  - **Social class:** Disease distribution also shows social class difference. The upper classes show higher prevalence of coronary heart diseases, hypertension and diabetes, whereas lower class shows nutritional deficiency diseases and lower life expectancy.
  - **Behavior:** Certain behavior factors such as cigarette smoking, alcoholism and over eating are associated with coronary artery disease and obesity.
  - **Stress:** Stress has been shown to be related to susceptibility to diseases and patient's compliance with medical regimen, etc.
- **Place distribution:** By studying the distribution of a disease in different population of the geographical area, we gain perspective on the fascinating difference in disease pattern not only between the countries but also within the countries. The environmental change, standard of living, diet and other etiological factors influence the disease pattern in different geographical areas. The difference may be classified as:

- **International difference:** Cancer of the oral cavity and uterine cervix are exceedingly common in India as compared to industrialized countries.
- **National difference:** Distribution of endemic goiter, leprosy, malaria and nutritional deficiency diseases has all shown variations in their distribution in India. Some parts of the country are more affected and others less affected or not affected at all. Such distribution exists in every country. Such information is needed to show areas which are affected with diseases for providing proper healthcare services.
- **Rural urban difference:** Diseases, like cardiovascular disease, mental illness and drug abuse is more common in urban areas whereas skin diseases and warm infestations are more common in rural area.
- **Local distribution:** Diseases distribution may vary within the inner part and the outer part of the city. Infected sources of water in a particular area of city may cause outbreak of cholera or other water-borne diseases.

The geographical differences in disease distribution are important as these provide information about the sources of diseases, mode of spread to make etiological hypothesis.

Characteristics to be assessed in descriptive epidemiology in relation to person place and time.	
Person	Age, sex, occupation, marital status, ethnic group and race, social class and family variables.
Place	Natural boundaries, political subdivisions, environmental factors, urban/rural differences, international comparisons.
Time	Secular trends, cyclic changes, seasonal.

Measurement of Diseases

The disease is measured in term of morbidity, mortality and disability. Measurement of mortality is straightforward. Morbidity has two aspects: Incidence rate and prevalence rate.

1. Incidence rate can be obtained from the longitudinal studies
2. Prevalence rate can be obtained from cross sectional studies.

Descriptive study may use longitudinal design or cross-sectional design to obtain estimates of magnitude of health and diseases problems in human population.

Cross-sectional studies: It is the simplest form of an observational study. It is based on a single examination of a cross section of population at one point in time. The results of which can be projected on the whole population, provided the sampling has been done correctly. Cross-sectional study is also known as prevalence study.

Longitudinal study: In longitudinal study the observations are repeated in the same population over a prolonged period of time longitudinal study is used:

- To study the natural history of the diseases and its further outcome
- For finding out the incidence rate—a rare occurrence of new cases in the community
- For identifying the risk factors of diseases, longitudinal studies provide valuable information which cross-sectional study may not provide.

Comparing with the Known Indices

Comparisons between different population and subgroups of the same population are made about disease incidence and prevalence rates. It helps to know the disease etiology and identify those groups of population which are at risk for some diseases.

Formulating an Etiological Hypothesis

By knowing the distribution of diseases, hypothesis can be made out about disease etiology.

Uses of descriptive epidemiology:

* Provides data regarding the magnitude of the diseases and types of disease problems in the community in terms of morbidity and mortality rate and ratio.
* It provides clue to disease epidemiology and help in the formulation of an etiological hypothesis.

RESPONSIBILITY OF COMMUNITY HEALTH NURSE IN VITAL STATISTIC

The medical and nursing personnel have got an important role in health information system. The community health nurse is responsible for health information and vital statistics in her area. Some important responsibilities of community health nurse are listed as under.

* Collection of information regarding vital statistics in her area.
* Observation of the information collected by the health personnel working under her and guiding them.
* Classification of the data collected from nursing and health workers of her area working under her.
* Presentation of the data through tables, bar diagrams maps, etc., according to the need.
* Forwarding the data collected to the concerned official/institutions.
* Analyzing the data, making community diagnosis and provide treatment.
* Spreading the importance of vital statistics in the community, creating awareness regarding registration of vital events.
* Keeping up to date knowledge of data collection and communication.
* Taking an active role in health surveys.
* Maintaining all registers in the health centers regarding inpatient, outpatients and disease registers, etc.

Summary

* Health information system may be defined as "a mechanism for the collection, processing, analysis and transmission of information required for organizing and operating health services and also for research and training" therefore health information system is a process whereby health data (input) are recorded, stored, retrieved and processed for decision making.
* The concept of health information system is to provide reliable, relevant, up to date, adequate, timely and reasonably complete information to the health agencies at all levels, i.e., central, state and district.
* Components of HIS are demography, vital statistics health statistics, i.e., mortality, morbidity, disability and quality of life, health resources and utilization of health services, indices of outcome of medical care and financial statistic.

Contd...

- Sources of HIS are census, registration of vital event, sample registration system, notification of diseases, hospital records, disease registers, record linkage, epidemiology, surveillance, health data, health manpower statistics, population survey and other routine statistics related to health and nonquantifiable information.
    - Vital statistic is concerned with the study of human population, i.e., numerical data regarding important incidents occurring in a community and the method of analysis of this data. The important incidence such as birth, marriage, diseases and death, etc.
    - Important rates and indicators include birth rate, death rate, specific death rate, infant mortality, rate, neonatal mortality rate, perinatal mortality rate, maternal mortality rate, etc.
    - Morbidity indicators are incidence rate, attack rate, prevalence rate disability rate, environmental indicators social and mental indicators and socioeconomic indicators, etc.
    - Vital health records include birth register, death registers fetal death registers marriage registers divorce registers, adoption registers MTP and abortion registers, morbidity registers MCH records and k sheet, etc.
    - Basic statistical methods include tabulation, charts, diagrams, graphs, pictures and special curves. The statistic averages are mean, median and mode. Measure of dispersion include range, mean or average deviation and standard deviation.
    - Descriptive statistics is the study of the amount and distribution of the disease or health status within a population by person, place and time. It includes the determination of incidence, prevalence and mortality rates for diseases in large population.
    - Measurement of diseases is morbidity, mortality and disability. Descriptive study may use longitudinal design or cross-sectional design.
- Descriptive epidemiology provides data regarding the magnitude of the diseases and types of disease problems in the community in term of morbidity and mortality, rates and ratios.
- Responsibilities of community health nurse in vital statistic are collection of information regarding vital statistics in her area; observing the information collected by the health worker, classification of the data collected; presentation of data through tables, charts, bar diagrams maps, etc. according to need and forwarding data collected to the concerned officials.

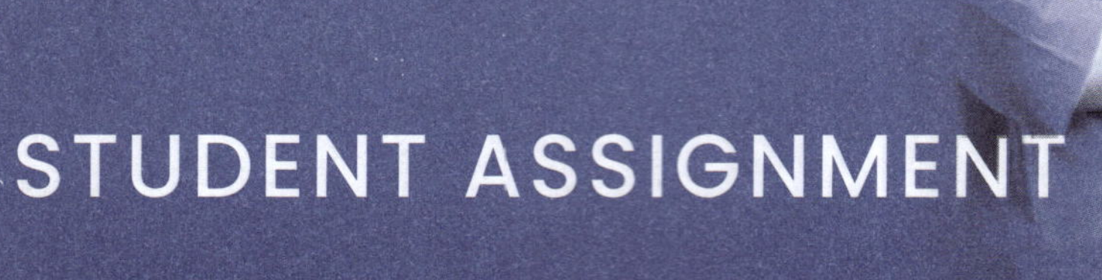

LONG ANSWER TYPE QUESTIONS

1. Describe the concept and components of health information system.
2. Explain the sources of health information system.
3. Describe the basic statistical methods.
4. Explain the mean, median and mode by giving examples.

SHORT ANSWER TYPE QUESTIONS

1. List the uses of health information system.
2. Define vital statistics. State the functions and purpose of vital statistic.
3. Write about the descriptive statistics.
4. Write short notes on the following:
   - a. Tabulation
   - b. Histogram
   - c. Frequency polygon
   - d. Pie chart
5. Define the following terms:
   - a. Birth rate
   - b. Death rate
   - c. Infant mortality rate
   - d. Neonatal mortality rate
   - e. Specific death rate
   - f. Maternal mortality rate

MULTIPLE CHOICE QUESTIONS

1. **Which is not correct about the primary data?**
   - a. Interviews
   - b. Observations
   - c. Hospital records
   - d. Questionnaire
2. **The scientific study of the human population is:**
   - a. Demography
   - b. Sex ratio
   - c. Family welfare
   - d. Urbanization
3. **Registration of birth should be done within:**
   - a. 7 days
   - b. 21 days
   - c. 10 days
   - d. 8 days
4. **The Central Birth and Death Registration Act came into force on:**
   - a. 1st April 1970
   - b. 14th Oct 1969
   - c. 1st January 1950
   - d. 1st Dec 1972
5. **To calculate vital statistic the population is taken as on:**
   - a. 1st January
   - b. 1st April
   - c. 1st July
   - d. 31st December

6. **Which of the following is incorrect about statistics?**
   a. It presents facts in definite form
   b. It converts data into information
   c. It is a tool of politicians
   d. It is used for comparison and help in prediction and planning effective strategy for future

7. **The study of collection and analysis of data regarding birth, death, fetal death, marriage, divorce and legal separation is:**
   a. Statistics
   b. Health statistics
   c. Biostatistics
   d. Vital statistics

8. **The sources of vital health statistic are:**
   a. Census
   b. Records of hospitals and health centers
   c. Journals publishing periodic events
   d. All of the above

9. **The basic statistical method are:**
   a. Tables and charts
   b. Diagrams and graphs
   c. Pictures and special curves
   d. All of these

10. **The statistical averages include:**
    a. Mean
    b. Median and mode
    c. Both (a) and (b)
    d. None of these

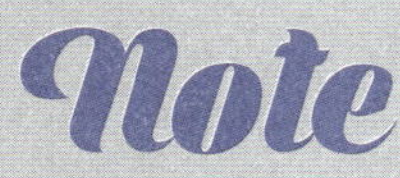

10

Health Agencies

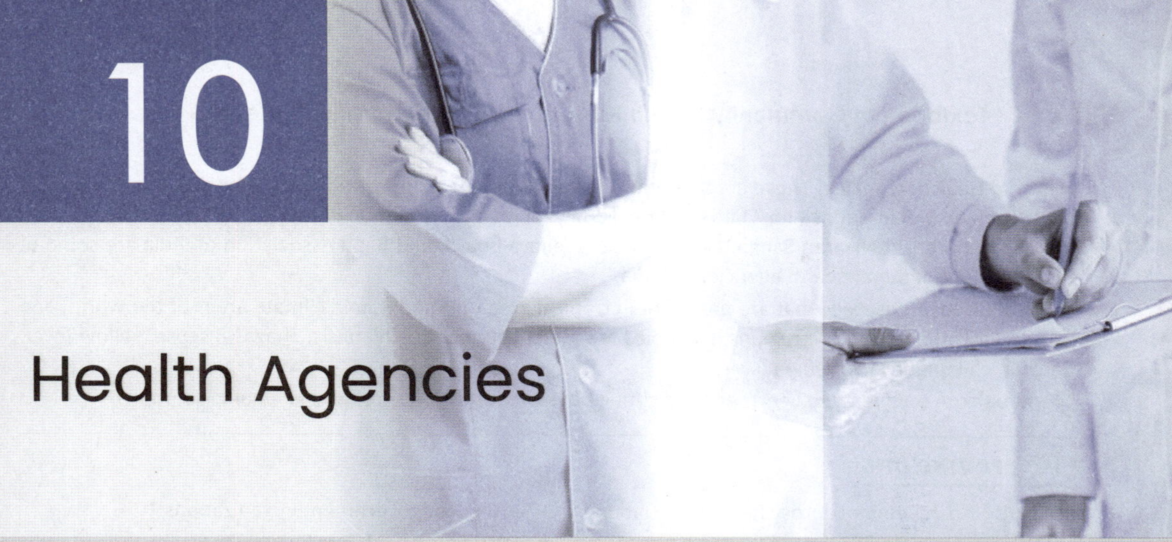

LEARNING OBJECTIVES

After the completion of the unit, the readers will be able to:
- Describe the national and international health agencies.
- Appreciate the role of various international health agencies toward the contribution of universal health.
- Explain the role of international health agencies in health development programs.
- Discuss the role of national health agencies.
- Quantify the contribution of national health agencies to uplift the living standard of the people.

UNIT OUTLINE

International Health Agencies
- World Health Organization
- United Nations Fund for Population Activities
- United Nations Development Program
- World Bank
- Food and Agriculture Organization
- United Nations International Children's Emergency Fund
- Danish International Development Agency
- European Commission
- International Red Cross
- United States Agency for International Development
- United Nations Educational, Scientific and Cultural Organization
- International Labor Organization
- Cooperation for Assistance and Relief Everywhere

National Voluntary Health Agencies of India
- Indian Red Cross Society
- Indian Council for Child Welfare
- Family Planning Association of India
- Tuberculosis Association of India
- Hind Kusht Nivaran Sangh
- Central Social Welfare Board
- All India Women's Conference
- All India Blind Relief Society
- Bharat Sevak Samaj
- Kasturba Memorial Fund

KEY TERMS

International Health Agencies: These are the nonpolitical, nonprofit voluntary organizations working to formulate policies for the health of global population with special focus on poor and underdeveloped population. They may engage in research related to communicable and noncommunicable diseases and to eradicate poverty and hunger. They may also provide financial assistance to tackle health-related issues and to start various projects for the development of nations. These agencies include WHO, UNICEF, UNFPA, FAO, World Bank, CARE, International Red Cross.

National Health Agencies: These are voluntary, nongovernment, nonprofit making agencies. The Indian Red Cross Society, Indian Council for Child Welfare, Family Planning Association of India, Tuberculosis Association of India, Hind Kusht Nivaran Sangh, Central Social Welfare Board, and Blind Association of India are some of the important national health agencies in India.

Tropical disease: Diseases that are prevalent in tropical area (hot and humid climate areas of the world) and less prevalent in temperate regions. Examples are malaria, lymphatic filariasis, chagas disease, yellow fever, dengue, chikungunya, dracunculiasis.

World bank: A unique global partnership fighting poverty worldwide through sustainable solutions.

Abbreviations

BELRA: British Empire Leprosy Relief Association

FFHC: Freedom from Hunger Campaign

IRCS: Indian Red Cross Society

MEDLARS: Medical Literature Analysis and Retrieval System

NGOs: Nongovernment Organizations

SEAR: South-East Asia Region

TCM: Technical Cooperative Mission

UBS: Urban Basic Services

INTERNATIONAL HEALTH AGENCIES

No single country can fulfil its health needs on its own resources. Every country needs help from other countries for the solution of its health problems. The role of international health agencies is vital with reference to this. There are a number of international health agencies who are extending help to India on regular basis. These are described in detail in this chapter.

WORLD HEALTH ORGANIZATION

World Health Organization (WHO) is a specialized, nonpolitical health agency of the United Nations with its headquarter at Geneva in Switzerland. It came into force on 7th April 1948 which is celebrated on 7th April every year as World Health Day. A World Health Day theme is chosen every year to focus attention on a specific aspect of public health.

Aims of WHO

- To provide access to fundamental and vital healthcare to each and every human being.
- Eradication of poverty and disease.

Objectives

- The main objective of WHO is the attainment of highest standard of health by all individual.
- Achievement of high standard of health without differentiating on the basis of caste, religion, politics and social status is the fundamental right of each individual.
- The current objective of WHO is the attainment by all the people of the world a level of health that will permit them to lead a socially and economically productive life, i.e., "Health for All" through primary healthcare.
- The WHO is unique among the UN specialized agencies; in that it has its own constitution, own governing bodies, own membership and own budget. It is a part of but not subordinate of United Nations. Two major policy developments have influenced the WHO. First the Alma-Ata

conference in 1978 on primary healthcare which provided both WHO and UNICEF with a common charter for health. The second is the global strategy for Health for All by 2000 AD and more recently the millennium development goals.

Membership

Any country of the world can become a member of WHO. It is open to all countries. Most of the countries are the members of WHO as well as UN. Every member country has to pay the budgetary contribution yearly and is entitled to the services and aid, the organization can provide. In 1948, the WHO had 56 members and now the WHO has 194-member states and two associate members. Territories which are not responsible for the conduct of their international relations may be admitted as associate members. Associate members participate without votes in the deliberations of the WHO.

Organization of WHO

World Health Organization (WHO) has three main wings:

1. *World Health Assembly*

This is the highest administrative wing, supreme governing body or Nation's "Health Parliament" of the organization.

Functions of World Health Assembly

* Formulation of international health policies and programs
* Review the previous year's activities
* Sanctioning the budget for the current year
* Elect members for the executive board

The world health assembly is constituted from representatives of each member country and its meeting is held once in a year.

2. *Executive Board*

This is constituted by experts from the field of health from member countries. The board has 31 members. Its meeting is held twice in a year. One-third of the members are renewed every year.

Functions of Executive Board

* To strengthen the decisions and policies passed and approved by the world health assembly
* The board has the power to take independent decisions during emergencies, epidemics, earthquakes, floods, etc.

3. *Secretariat*

This wing works under the director general who is the chief technical advisor and executive of the organization. The director general has five deputies and a staff of about 5000 persons. Under the secretariat, there are 14 departments, namely survey, communicable diseases, health education, environment, budget, finance, etc.

Functions of Secretariat

To make available technical and managerial help to the member countries in their national health development programs

Regional Organization

WHO organization has six regional organizations. These are:

1. South East Asia
2. Africa
3. America
4. Europe
5. Western Pacific
6. Eastern Mediterranean

India is a member of SEAR. Its headquarter is in New Delhi.

The other members of this region are Myanmar, Sri Lanka, Indonesia, Korea and Bhutan.

Budget of WHO

Each member state contributes a fixed amount to the WHO, depending upon its size and national health. This amount is the main financial basis of the organization.

Functions of WHO

- **Prevention and control of specific diseases:**
  - Almost all communicable diseases have been the subject of WHO activities. Eradication of smallpox is an outstanding example of international health cooperation and WHO now directing the global battle against poliomyelitis. Epidemiological surveillance of communicable diseases is an important activity of WHO.
  - It has also paid attention to the noncommunicable diseases, like cancer, cardiovascular diseases, genetic diseases, mental disorders, drug addiction and dental diseases.
  - WHO's activities have also branched out into the fields of vector biology and control, immunology, quality control of drugs and biological products, drug evaluation and monitoring and health laboratory technology.
  - Immunization against common diseases of childhood (expanded program on immunization) is now a priority program of WHO.
- **Development of comprehensive health services:**
  - The most important single function of WHO is to promote and support National Health Policy development and the development of comprehensive national health program
  - Appropriate technology for health (ATH) is another new program launched by the WHO to encourage self-sufficiency in solving health problems.
- **Family health:**
  - Family health is one of the major program activities of WHO since 1970.
  - Family health is again subdivided into maternal and child healthcare, human reproduction, nutrition and health education.
  - Chief concern is improvement of the quality of life of the family as a unit.
- **Environmental health:**
  - Environmental health is an important activity of WHO. WHO advises governments on national programs for provision of basic sanitary services.

- The activities are directed to the protection of air, water and food.
- Health conditions of work, radiation protection and early identification of new hazards originating from new technological developments.
- **Health statistics:**
  - Assistance is given to the countries in the improvement of their medical records, and in the planning and operating national health information system.
  - Dissemination of a variety of morbidity and mortality statistics relating to health problems and their publication.
  - In order that statistics from different countries may be comparable, WHO publishes international classification of diseases which is updated every 10th year.
- **Biomedical research:**
  - WHO stimulates and coordinates the research work.
  - It has established a world-wide network of WHO collaborating centers, besides awarding grants to research workers and research institutions for promoting research.
  - Six tropical diseases, i.e., malaria, schistosomiasis, trypanosomiasis, filariasis, leishmaniasis and leprosy are the target of WHO special program for research and training in tropical diseases to develop new tools, strengthen research institutions and training workers in the countries affected.
- **Health literature and information:**
  - The WHO literary is one of the satellite centers of the medical literature analysis and retrieval system (MEDLARS) of the US national library of medicine.
  - MEDLARS is fully computerized indexing system covering the whole of medicine on an international basis.
  - WHO also has a public information service both at headquarters and each of the regional offices.
- **Cooperation with other organization:**
  - WHO collaborates with the UN and with other specialized agencies and maintains various degrees of working relationship.
  - WHO has also established relations with a number of international governmental organizations.
  - The WHO has been active in nursing education and practice. It has offered guidance in setting up programs for nursing education and promoted training for auxiliary nursing personnel.
  - WHO promotes public health in many ways.

Activities of WHO

The activities of WHO in India and SEAR are as follows:

- Eradication of malaria
- Control of TB and communicable diseases
- Reproductive and child health
- Health laboratory services
- Health statistics
- Manufacture of vaccines
- Dental health
- Medical rehabilitation
- Public health administration
- Quality control of drugs
- Help in medical and nursing education

UNITED NATIONS FUND FOR POPULATION ACTIVITIES

United Nations Fund for Population Activities (UNFPA) is an international development agency that promotes the right of every woman, man and child to enjoy life of health and equal opportunity. UNFPA has been providing assistance to India since 1974. UNFPA supports countries in using population data for policies and programs to reduce poverty and to ensure that every pregnancy is wanted, every birth is safe, every young person is free of HIV and every girl and woman is treated with dignity and respect.

Areas of Focus

The main areas of focus are:
- Reproductive health
- Gender equality
- Population and development strategies
- Population dynamics including growth rates, age, structure, fertility and mortality, migration and more influence on every aspect of human, social and economic development
- Reproductive health and women's empowerment, powerfully affect the population trends.

Functions of UNFPA

- Family planning
- MCH services
- Treatment of infertility
- Prevention of abortion and management of its consequences
- Treatment of reproductive tract infections
- Prevention and treatment of sexually transmitted diseases including HIV infections
- Information, education and counseling on human sexuality and reproductive health
- Prevention of violence against woman, care of survivors of violence and other actions to eliminate traditional harmful practices
- Appropriate referral for further diagnosis and management.

Role of UNFPA in India

- UNFPA has assisted India in redirecting its population efforts away from family planning targets and quotas and instead focusing on providing high quality services within a comprehensive reproductive healthcare system.
- UNFPA is helping India in supporting the strategy endorsed by the 1994 International Conference on Population and Development which emphasized the inseparability of population and development and focused on meeting individual needs rather than demographic targets.
- The key to this new approach is empowering women and expanding access to education, health services and employment opportunities.

UNITED NATIONS DEVELOPMENT PROGRAM

The United Nations Development Program (UNDP) was established in 1966.

Objective of UNP

To help the poor countries in the development of human and natural resources.

UNDP is the main source of finance for technical cooperation. There are >170 countries and territories, UNDP offer global perspective and local insight to help empower lives and build strong nations. The projects of UNDP provide necessary help in economic and social fields like agriculture, industry, science, health, hospital administration, nursing services and training and social welfare.

Budget of UNDP

The contribution for the budget is made by the member countries of United Nations in their annual meeting.

Focus Area of UNDP

The UNDP is focused on four areas:
1. Poverty reduction and achieving the Sustainable Development Goals
2. Democratic governance
3. Crisis prevention and recovery
4. Environment and energy for sustainable development.

Functions of UNDP

- It is the global development network of UN, advocating for change and connecting countries to knowledge, experience and resources to help people in building a better life.
- UNDP works in 166 countries through a network of 135 country offices worldwide working with them on their solutions to global and national development challenges.
- UNDP advocates the millennium development goals, the concept of human development and the need to empower woman. Its series of global, regional and country-focused human development reports are powerful advocacy tool with a focus on people-centered, inclusive, equitable and sustainable growth.
- UNDP focuses on five inter-connected thematic areas, i.e., poverty reduction, democratic governance, crisis prevention and recovery, environment and energy and HIV/AIDS.

Role of UNDP in India

The UNDP is committed to help India in achieving the global millennium development goal as well as the national objectives articulated in consecutive Five-Year Plans. The goal of organization is to help, improve the lives of the poorest women, men and the marginalized people in India. UNDP works in the areas of democratic governance, poverty reduction, crisis prevention and recovery, environment and energy and HIV/AIDS.

WORLD BANK

The World Bank is a specialized agency of the United Nations. It was established in 1944. Its headquarter is in Washington. It has >10,000 employees in >100 offices worldwide.

Objectives

- To help in raising the standard of living of the underdeveloped countries who are comparatively poor.
- To fight poverty with compassion and professionalism for lasting results and to help people to be self-sufficient themselves with their environment by providing resources, knowledge, building capacity and partnership in the public and private sectors.

Functions

- The World Bank provides low interest loans, interest free credits and grants to developing countries.
- It also provides technical support for projects of economic development.
- World Bank provides financial assistance generally concerned with projects involving energy, transport, railways, industries, agriculture, education, family planning, health, environment, etc.
- WHO and World Bank jointly carry out many projects, like water supply, world food program, population control, AIDS control, etc.

Authority

The authority of World Bank is invested in Board of Governors.

World Bank in India

India is one of the oldest members of World Bank since its inception in 1944. The World Bank is one of the largest sources of funding. In India, the World Bank works in close partnership with the central and state governments. It also works with other development partners such as bilateral and multilateral donor organizations, nongovernmental organizations (NGOs), the private sector and the general public including academics, scientists, economists, journalists, teachers and local people involved in development projects.

FOOD AND AGRICULTURE ORGANIZATION

Food and Agriculture Organization (FAO) was established in 1945. Its headquarter is in Rome. This was the first organization of the United Nations. Organization specialized agency created to look after several areas of world cooperation.

Aims

- To help nations raise living standard of people.
- To improve nutrition of the people of all countries.
- To increase the output of agriculture, fisheries and forestry.
- To better the conditions of rural people and through all means, to widen the opportunity of all people for productive work.
- To increase food production in order to keep pace with the ever-growing world population.
- To combat malnutrition and disseminate information and education.

Functions

- Scientific, technological, social and economic research relating to nutrition, food and agriculture.
- Improvement of education and administration relating to nutrition, food and agriculture and the spread of public knowledge of nutritional and agricultural science and practice.
- Conservation of natural resources and the adoption of improved methods of agriculture production.
- Improvement of the processing, marketing and distribution of food and agricultural products.
- Adoption of policies on agricultural commodity arrangements.
- FAO also plays a major role in dealing with food and agricultural emergencies such as drought, famine, plant diseases and insect plagues.
- The most important aspect of FAO's work is toward ensuring that the food is consumed by the people who need it, in sufficient quantities and its right proportion and maintains a better state of nutrition throughout the world.
- FAO has organized a world freedom from hunger campaign (FFHC) in 1960. The main aim of the campaign is to control malnutrition and to disseminate information and education.
- FAO is also collaborating with other international agencies in the applied nutrition program.
- The joint WHO/FAO expert committees have provided the basis for many cooperative activities, like nutritional survey, training courses, seminars and the coordination of research programs on brucellosis and other zoonosis.

UNITED NATIONS INTERNATIONAL CHILDREN'S EMERGENCY FUND

The United Nations International Children's Emergency Fund (UNICEF) is one of the specialized agencies of the United Nations. It was established in 1946 by the United Nations General Assembly to rehabilitate the children in Post-war Europe. In 1950, the program was extended to provide long range benefits to children of all developing countries. In 1953, when the emergency functions were over, the General Assembly gave it a new name "UN Children's Fund" but retained the initial UNICEF. UNICEF is governed by 36 members' executive board. The headquarters of UNICEF is at United Nations, New York and has >200 offices in developing countries.

UNICEF's regional office is in New Delhi the region is known as the South Central Asian Region which covers Afghanistan, Sri Lanka, India, Maldives' Mongolia and Nepal. UNICEF works in close collaboration with WHO and the other specialized agencies of the United Nations, like UNDP, FAO and UNESCO. In the early years, UNICEF and WHO worked together on urgent problems such as malaria, tuberculosis and venereal diseases. Later, its assistance to countries covered the fields such as maternal and child health, nutrition environmental sanitation especially the provision of water supply to the rural community, health centers and health education, and programs which would directly or indirectly benefit child health.

Objectives

- The main objective is the improvement in the health of mothers and infants
- To look after children's welfare, especially in developing countries by providing people with low-cost community-based services in maternal and child health, nutrition and immunization, etc.
- UNICEF plays the main role in all programs which benefit the children's health directly or indirectly.

Functions

- **Child health:** UNICEF has provided substantial aid for the production of vaccines and sera in many countries:
    - UNICEF has also assisted environmental sanitation programs emphasizing safe and sufficient water for drinking and household use in rural areas for the purpose of improving the quality of life in villages.
    - Currently focusing attention on providing primary healthcare to mothers and children.
    - Emphasis is given on immunization, infant and young child care, family planning aspects of family health, safe water and adequate sanitation.
- **Child nutrition:** UNICEF gives high priority to improve child nutrition. It helped child nutrition first by supplementing child feed in the mid-1950s with the development of low-cost protein rich food mixtures. In collaboration with FAO, UNICEF began aiding "applied nutrition programs" through channels such as community development, agriculture extension, school and health services so as to motivate and help the rural population to grow and eat the foods it required for better child nutrition. UNICEF also supplied equipment for modern dairy plants in various parts of India.
- **Family and child welfare:** The purpose is to improve the care of children both within the home and outside their homes-through parent education, daycare centers, child welfare and youth agencies and woman's club. These services are carried out as a part of health, nutrition and education or home economics extension programs.
- **Education:** UNICEF in collaboration with UNESCO provides funds for training of the personnel including health and sanitation workers, teachers, nutritionists. Universal child immunization against preventable diseases in the 1990s was one of the leading goals of UNICEF.
- It provides technical supplies, equipment and other aids ranging from paper for textbooks to equipment and medicine to health clinics, and pipes and pumps for bringing clean water to villages.
- It assists government to plan, develop and extend community-based services in fields of maternal and child health, nutrition, clean water and sanitation.
- It provides help to mothers and children arising from natural calamities, civil strife and epidemics.
- It makes efforts to prevent diseases, like TB, malaria, eye diseases, skin diseases, etc.
- UNICEF performs various other functions on the behalf of children and upholds the convention on the rights of the children and works in its implementation.
- In short, activities cover programs assisting in child survival, protection and development, intervention, like immunization improved infant feeding practice, child growth monitoring, home-based diarrhea management, drinking water, environment, all sanitation, birth spacing, education of girls and income generating activities for women.

UNICEF Activities in India

- **Health**
    - **Immunization:** UNICEF has supported India's BCG vaccination program from its inception
    - It has donated two plants for the manufacture of triple vaccine and iodized salt
    - Donated DDT plant
    - Provided medical education and training
    - Helped in developing rural health services

- Provided aid to the primary health centers
- Helped in controlling communicable diseases.

- **Environment sanitation:** It has assisted environment and sanitation program emphasizing safe and sufficient water for drinking
  - Helping in digging well in rural areas
  - Promoting the use of ground water.
- **Nutrition:**
  - Applied nutrition program
  - Agricultural extension services
  - School health services
  - Helping dairy projects. UNICEF has supplied equipment for modern dairy plants in various parts of India, i.e., Maharashtra, Gujarat, Karnataka, Uttar Pradesh, West Bengal, Andhra Pradesh.

  Prevention of malnutrition:
  - Specific aid is given to nutritional deficiency diseases such as provision of large doses of vitamin A in areas where xerophthalmia is prevalent.
  - Enrichment of salt with iodine in goiter endemic areas.

  Provision of supplementary nutrition:
  - Provision of iron and folic acid supplements to combat anemia and enrichment of foods
  - Supply of milk powder, etc.
  - More recently FAO, UNICEF and WHO have been encouraging the development of national food and nutrition policies that make provision for child nutrition.
- **Education:**
  - Strengthening science laboratories
  - Arranging workshops
  - Supply of audio-visual aids
  - Providing books and other education material to nursing institutions.
- **Social welfare**
  - Reproductive and child health services
  - Contributing to primary healthcare
  - Promoting child safety and safe motherhood (CSSM)
  - Contribution for achievement of "Health For All"
  - Contribution of integrated management of neonatal and childhood illness (IMNCI)

Since 1976, UNICEF has been participating in urban basic services (UBS). The aim of UBS projects is to upgrade basic services of health, nutrition, water supply, sanitation and education, especially for children and women in selected cities and towns. The overall objective is to improve the degree and quality of survival and development of children of urban low-income families.

High Yield Point

The UNICEF is promoting a campaign known as GOBI campaign to encourage four strategies for a "Child Health Revolution".

- **G:** For growth charts to better monitor child development
- **O:** For oral rehydration to treat all mild and moderate dehydration
- **B:** For breastfeeding
- **I:** For immunization against measles, diphtheria, polio, pertussis, tetanus and tuberculosis

DANISH INTERNATIONAL DEVELOPMENT AGENCY

Danish International Development Agency (DANIDA) is the name of the government of Denmark's Development Cooperation. This is an area of activity under the Ministry of Foreign Affairs of Denmark. The term DANIDA appeared in 1963.

Focused Areas of Development

Denmark will concentrate on its development cooperation on four strategic priority areas which are interconnected and which enable Denmark to make its contribution toward combating poverty and promoting human rights. The strategies are:

- Human rights and democracy
- Green growth
- Social progress
- Stability and protections

Functions

- DANIDA's policy focuses on eradication of poverty and ensuring sustainable development.
- It works to select countries referred to as program countries and provides support to NGOs as well as government agencies.
- Other areas of development include social and economic development, human rights, democratization and good governance, stability, security and the fight against terrorism, refugees, humanitarian assistance and environment.
- It has also launched the "Strategy for Denmark's support" to the international fight against HIV/AIDS.
- The government of Denmark is providing assistance for the development of services under National Blindness Control Program since 1978.

EUROPEAN COMMISSION

The first commission was established in 1951 as the nine-member "High Authority" under president. The European Commission represents the interests of the European as a whole. It proposes new legislation to the European parliament and the council of European Union and it ensures that the European Union law is correctly applied by the member countries. The term "commission" refers to both the 28 commissioners and the wider institution itself.

Functions

- European commission proposes laws for adoption.
- European commission makes proposals to meet the obligations.
- Assessment of the potential economic, social and environmental impact of a given piece of legislation act is published along with the proposal list.
- The commission ensures that it is correctly applied by the EU member countries.

European Commission in India

The relationship between the European Commission and India has changed substantially from that of aid donor and recipient to one of the partnerships with opportunities for mutual benefit in recent years. India's current economic growth continues the demand for development assistance will go on decreasing. India is home to the largest number of poor with one-third of the world's 1.2 billion extreme poor living here. There are huge disparities in standard of living due to the unemployment. Minorities continue to suffer from disproportionate lack of basic services such as elementary education primary healthcare, safe drinking water, proper housing, etc. The EU-India strategy program (2007–2013) responds to two major challenges relating to millennium development goals by proposing two priority areas, i.e., health and education.

> **Recent Update**
>
> In 2023, the EU and Indian launched a trade and technology council focusing on digital transformation and green technologies.

INTERNATIONAL RED CROSS

International Red Cross is a nonpolitical, nonofficial international humanitarian organization devoted to the service of mankind in peace and war. It was founded by Henry Dunant, a young Swiss businessman, in 1864.

The first Geneva Convention took place in 1864, and a treaty was signed for the relief of the wounded and the sick of the armies in the field. Thus, the international committee of Red Cross came into existence an independent, neutral institution, the founder organization of Red Cross (ICRC). Since then, it has grown into branches all over the world symbolizing the spirit of compassion and universal brotherhood. In 1919, the league of the Red Cross Society was created with headquarter in Geneva to coordinate the work of the national societies which are now >90 in number. Later on, it was realized that natural calamities bring great human suffering, so the services of International Red Cross were extended to other programs which would prevent human suffering. These include services to the victims of disasters, sick and wounded soldiers of armies, services to war veterans, disaster service, first aid and nursing, health education and maternity and child welfare services.

Objectives

- To improve the health of people in countries that had suffered greatly during war.
- To strengthen and unite for health activities in already existing Red Cross societies.
- To promote the creation of new societies.
- To inspire, encourage, facilitate and promote at all times all forms of humanitarian endeavors.

Functions

- Provides services to the armed forces and take care of sick and wounded during war and peace.
- Carries out relief operations to assist victims of disasters and combine this with the development of work.
- Focuses on four core areas, i.e., promoting humanitarian values, disaster response, disaster preparedness and health, and community care.
- Provides unique network of national societies which cover almost every country in the world.

- Cooperation between national societies gives the International Federation of Red Cross (IFRC) greater potential to develop capacities and assist those most in need at a local level; the network enables the IFRC to reach individual communities.
- Coordinates and mobilizes relief assistance for international emergencies, promotes cooperation between national societies and represents these national societies in the international field.
- Assists and advises national societies with relief operations and development program, and also encourages regional cooperation.
- Assists in training in first Aid and home nursing, health education and MCH and child welfare services.

UNITED STATES AGENCY FOR INTERNATIONAL DEVELOPMENT

United States Agency for International Development (USAID) is a technical cooperation mission for international development. It was established on November 3, 1961 with spirit of program and innovation. November 3, 2011 marked USAID's 50th anniversary of providing US foreign development assistance from the American people. USAID is the leading US government agency that works to end extreme global poverty and enable resilient, democratic societies to realize their potential.

Objectives of USAID

USAID works in over 100 countries to:
- Promote broadly shared economic prosperity
- Strengthen democracy and good governance
- Protect human rights
- Improve global health
- Advance food security and agriculture
- Improve environmental sustainability
- Improve education
- Help societies to prevent and recover from conflicts
- Provide humanitarian assistance in the wake of natural and man-made disasters

Functions

USAID invests in ideas that help millions of men, women and children by:
- Extending help in investing in agriculture productivity so that countries can feed these people and become self-sufficient.
- Assisting to combat maternal and child mortality and deadly diseases, like HIV, malaria and tuberculosis.
- Rendering liesaving assistance in the wake of disaster.
- Promoting democracy, human rights and good governance around the world.
- Fostering private sector development and sustainable economic growth.
- Assisting communities to adapt to the changing environment.
- Raising the standard of women and girls throughout all work.

USAID in India

The US government presently extends aid to India through three agencies:
1. United States Agency in International Development (USAID)
2. Public law 480 (food for peace)
3. The US export – import – bank
   - USAID is in charge of activities previously administered by the Technical Cooperation Mission (TCM). USAID mission functions in New Delhi. Both grants and loans are extended by the agency.
   - USAID cooperates in India for the control and eradication of malaria and filaria.
   - Assistance in general nursing training.
   - Development of primary health centers.
   - Medical education and related institutes.
   - Different fields of health such as nutrition and control of communicable diseases.
   - Water supply and sanitation.
   - Presently USAID is also helping in agriculture and family planning programs.

UNITED NATIONS EDUCATIONAL, SCIENTIFIC AND CULTURAL ORGANIZATION

United Nations Educational, Scientific and Cultural Organization (UNESCO) is a specialized agency of the United Nations. A conference was held at London on November 16, 1945 for the established of an educational, scientific and cultural organization. This led to the establishment of UNESCO on 4th November 1946. The headquarters of UNESCO is in Paris. It has 93 member states and seven associate members. The organization is based in Paris with over 50 field offices and many institutes and centers throughout the world.

Objective

The main objective of UNESCO is to contribute to peace and security in the world by promoting collaboration among nations through education, science, culture and communication. This is undertaken to further respect for justice, for the rule of law and for the human rights for all human beings.

Functions

UNESCO pursues its objectives through five major programs, i.e., education, natural sciences, social and human sciences, cultural, communication and information.

Education

The largest sector of UNESCO is in the field of education.
- Removal of illiteracy by encouragement of adult education, distance education and the open school system.
- Emphasis on education of women and girls.

- Financial assistance for education of disabled children.
- Provision of grants and fellowship to teachers and scholars, organization of library system and promotion of international understanding through education.
- Organization of book fairs and festivals at international and national levels. Example: development of library system is an important component of continuing education. Delhi Public Library established in 1951 with financial assistance from UNESCO has developed into a big metropolitan public library system.
- Encouragement of science education by providing regional training centers.
- Promotion of education as an instrument for international understanding.

Scientific Activities

The scientific activities undertaken by UNESCO are:
- UNESCO organizes seminars and conferences of scientists of various countries and circulates information through journals, press and exhibitions. 'Courier' is the official monthly magazine of UNESCO.
- It promotes basic research in fields, like geology, mathematics, physics and oceanography. As a result, it finances engineering and technology schemes in a number of developing countries.
- It helps in correction of the imbalance in scientific and technological manpower that exists, because 90% of trained manpower is concentrated in the industrialized countries.
- It encourages the study of social sciences in order to focus attention on combating all forms of discrimination, improving the status of woman and helping the youth in solving their problems.

Communication

UNESCO develops communication for dissemination of information.
- It has set up regional networks, trained technologies and deals with both hardware and software aspects of informatics.
- It improves the quality of press, the films and video services.
- It assists developing countries to develop communications.
- It upholds countries to develop communications.
- It upholds the freedom of the press and independence of the media.

Preservation of Cultural Heritage

It encourages modernization without the loss of cultural identity and diversity:
- UNESCO provides technical advice and assistance, equipment and funds for the preservation of monuments and sites which are to be protected.
- It aims to protect the world inheritance of books, works of art and save manuscripts.
- It gives encouragement to artistic creations in literature and fine arts.
- It pays attention toward the cultural development through the medium of films.
- It sends cultural missions to different countries so that there would be development contracts which may promote peace and prosperity. In the past, it has provided travel grants to writers, artists under a project named "mutual appreciation of eastern and western cultural values". Under this scheme, India's talented exponents of classical music and dance traveled to Europe and America.

INTERNATIONAL LABOR ORGANIZATION

Soon after the World War, International Labor Organization (ILO) was recognized the problems of industry like—disease, working conditions and industrial hazards, etc. In 1919, ILO was established as an affiliate of the League of Nations to pursue a vision based on the promise that universal lasting peace can be established only if it is based on social justice and improve the working and living conditions of the working population all over the world. The ILO became the first specialized agency of UN in 1946. The headquarter of ILO is in Geneva, Switzerland.

Objectives

- To contribute to the establishment of lasting peace by promoting social justice.
- To promote rights at work, encourage descent employment opportunities, enhance social protection and strengthen dialogue on work-related issues.
- To improve through international action, labor conditions and living standards.
- To promote and realize standards and fundamental principles and rights at work.
- To create greater opportunities for women and men to descent employment and income.
- To enhance the coverage and effectiveness of social protection for all.
- To strengthen tripartism and social dialogue.
- To promote economic and social stability.

Functions

- Formulation of international policies and programs to promote basic human rights, improve working and living conditions and enhance employment opportunities.
- Creation of international labor standards backed by a unique system to supervise the application.
- An extensive program of international technical cooperation formulated and implemented in an active partnership with constituents, to help countries to put these policies into practice in an effective manner.
- Training, education and research activities to help in advance all of these efforts.
- ILO provides assistance to organizations interested in the betterment of living and employment standards.
- There is a close collaboration between ILO and WHO in the field of health and labor.

ILO in India

India has been a permanent member of the ILO governing body since 1922. The first ILO office in India was started in 1928. The decades of productive partnership between the ILO and its constituents has mutual trust and respect as underlying principles and is grounded in building sustained institutional capacities and strengthening capacities of partners. It has a two-directional focus for social-economic development, overall strategies and ground level approaches.

COOPERATION FOR ASSISTANCE AND RELIEF EVERYWHERE

Cooperative for Assistance and Relief Everywhere (CARE) was established in 1945 in North America in the wake of the Second World War. It is a major international humanitarian agency delivering broad spectrum emergency relief and long-term international development projects.

CARE is independent, nonsectarian, nonprofit, impartial and nongovernmental organization. It is one of the largest and oldest humanitarian aid organizations focused on fighting global poverty. CARE began its operation in India in 1950 till the end of the 1980s. The primary objective of CARE-India was to provide food for children in the age group of 6–11 years. From the mid-1980s CARE-India focused its food support in the ICDS program and in development of programs in the areas of health and income supplementation.

Objectives

- To serve individuals and families in the poorest communities in the world
- To draw strength from our global diversity, resources and experience
- To promote innovative solutions and advocate for global responsibility
- To strengthen capacity for self-help
- To provide economic opportunity
- To deliver relief services in emergencies
- To influence policy decisions at all levels
- To address discrimination in all its forms
- To meet international standards of quality and accountability.

Functions

CARE works on the following projects:
- Emergency response
- Food security
- Economic development
- Education
- Maternal health
- Water sanitation and hygiene
- Focus on improving women and girls health
- HIV/AIDS
- Climate change
- Advocacy

CARE in India

CARE is helping India in the following projects:
- Integrated nutrition and health project
- Anemia control project
- Improving women's health project
- Improved healthcare for adolescent girls project
- Child survival project
- Improving women's reproductive health and family spacing project
- Konkan integrated development project, etc.

CARE-India works in partnership with the Government of India, state governments, NGOs, etc. Currently it has projects in Andhra Pradesh, Bihar, Madhya Pradesh, Maharashtra, Odisha, Rajasthan, Uttar Pradesh and West Bengal.

NATIONAL VOLUNTARY HEALTH AGENCIES OF INDIA

Voluntary health agencies or organizations is a group of individuals who enters into an agreement as volunteer to form a body to accomplish a purpose. This is called voluntary sector and is the sphere of social activity undertaken by the organization. These organizations are nongovernmental, nonprofit making, nonpolitical agencies providing voluntary help to improve the health of the population and raise their living standard.

The national voluntary health agencies in India are as follows:

INDIAN RED CROSS SOCIETY

Indian Red Cross Society (IRCS) was established in 1920 under the Indian Red Cross Society Act. It is a voluntary humanitarian organization with >400 branches which are spread throughout the states, districts and subdivisions of the country. Indian Red Cross works in the direction of reducing human sufferings. The national headquarters of Indian Red Cross is in Delhi.

Objectives

- To make Red Cross societies and communities more aware of the risks they face, how to reduce their vulnerability and how to cope when disaster strikes.
- To influence the behavior of all the people.
- To enable communities to reduce their vulnerability to disease and prepare for and respond to public health crisis.

Programs and Activities

The main core areas of the Indian Red Cross programs:

- **Armed force:** The care of the sick and wounded among the members of the forces is one of the primary obligations of the Red Cross society. It runs a well-equipped hospital "the Red Cross home" in Bengaluru the only one of its kind in India.
- **Red Cross promotes the humanitarian values:** IRCS encourage respect for other human beings and a willingness to work together to find solutions to problems.
- **Disaster response:** Disaster response continues to represent the largest portion of IRCS work, with assistance to millions of people annually ranging from refugees to victims of natural disasters.
- **Disaster preparedness activities:** The sharp increase in the number of natural disasters countrywide has prompted the Red Cross to devote more attention to disaster preparedness activities.
- **Health and care in the community:** Health and community care has become a cornerstone of humanitarian assistance and accounts for a large part of Red Cross spending.
- **Major activities of Indian Red Cross:**
  - Immediate relief to victims of natural calamities, like floods, cyclones, earthquakes, drought, epidemics, etc.
  - Workshops for workers on disaster management
  - Blood bank and promotion of voluntary blood donation

- Milk and medicine supplies
- HIV/AIDS programs and care of the persons with HIV/AIDS
- Home for disabled ex-servicemen—society runs a well-equipped hospital for the disabled ex-servicemen "the Red Cross Home" in Bengaluru the only one of its kind in India and the Far East.
- Vocational training centers, St John Ambulance Association in India which is part of Red Cross, have trained lakhs of men and women in first aid and home nursing and allied subjects.
- Hospital services and caring of the sick and wounded during war
- Maternal and child health and family welfare services
- Community services
- Ambulance services, nursing services and junior Red Cross activities
- Preparedness and prevention of communicable and infectious diseases
- Relief operations in fire, railway and other accidents and events.

The commendable services provided by IRCS are:

- During cyclones in Odisha
- Kargil War
- Floods of 2008
- Gujarat Earthquakes

The priorities and focus of Red Cross services are on strengthening activities in following areas:

- Such as disaster management
- Disaster preparedness
- Healthcare
- Organizational development
- Humanitarian values

INDIAN COUNCIL FOR CHILD WELFARE

Indian Council for Child Welfare (ICCW) was formed in 1952. This is connected with international children's welfare council. It is a voluntary organization engaged in promoting development services for children. It has 32 State/Union Territory Councils all over the country, which in turn have district councils. The state council for child welfare is constituted of elected representatives from life members of the organization. In some states the governor of the state is head of the state council. ICCW serves to secure Indian children those "opportunities and facilities by law and other means" which are necessary to enable them to develop physically, mentally, socially and spiritually in healthy and normal manner and in conditions of freedom and dignity.

Objectives

- To promote the opportunity and facility for the development of the children.
- To ensure the promotion of physical, social and mental health of children through legal or any other means.

Activities

- **Crutches/Daycare center:** These centers provide services to small children (0–3 years) by providing them with food, care and protection. The scheme has been found very fruitful and essential for working mothers.

- **Preschool:** These centers cater to children aging between 3 and 6 years. Nonformal education is implemented and nutrition is also given to them.
- **Orphanages:** The department provides grant-in-aid to voluntary organizations properly registered under Society Registration Act and who are engaged in the welfare of orphans.
- **Recreational center cum children's library:** Recreational center cum children's library has been opened at different places to enable the children to spend their leisure time in a beneficial manner and to guide them in their future lives. Selected books and materials have been supplied to these centers for this purpose.
- **State council for child welfare:** It was constituted to provide services to the children in need of care and protection and to promote child development in line with the aims and objectives of the Indian Council of Child Welfare.

FAMILY PLANNING ASSOCIATION OF INDIA

Family Planning Association of India (FPAI) was founded in 1949 with its headquarters in Mumbai. It has been recognized as India's leading and largest reproduction and sexual health organization. It has got 38 branches and special projects spread across the country assisted by national and international funding. The association has trained several hundreds of doctors, health visitors and social workers. Its branches are running family planning clinics with grants-in-aid from the government. One of the activities of the headquarters is to answer enquiries on family planning by correspondence or by personal interviews.

Mission

Family Planning Association of India (FPAI) envisions health, particularly sexual and reproductive Health for All, especially marginalized and young people.

FPAI strengthens a voluntary and nongovernment commitment to promote sexual and reproductive health and rights including family planning. It supports the rights of individuals to reproductive choices including legal and safe abortion, works toward reducing the spread and the impact of STIs/HIV/AIDS and increasing access to gender sensitive information, education and services to all, especially the young and marginalized and eliminating violence, discrimination and abuse.

Services Provided by FPAI

It runs clinics for the following terms:
- Maternal and child healthcare
- Treating infertility
- Adolescent sexual and reproductive health
- Providing contraceptives including emergency contraceptives
- Facilities for abortion
- Diagnosis and treatment of reproductive tract infections and sexually-transmitted infections
- Prevention and management of HIV/AIDS
- Counseling services
- Pathological/diagnosis facilities.

TUBERCULOSIS ASSOCIATION OF INDIA

The Tuberculosis Association of India was formed in 23 February, 1939 with its headquarters at Delhi. It is a voluntary organization and is a registered society. It has branches in all the states of the country. The Association providing training to the doctors, health visitors and other health workers in antituberculosis program and health education. Some of the institutions run by the association are:

- Lady Linlithgow Tuberculosis Sanatorium, Kasauli
- King Edward VII Sanatorium at Dharampur
- Tuberculosis Hospital at Mehrauli
- New Delhi Tuberculosis Center

Objectives

- To work toward prevention, control, treatment and relief from tuberculosis
- To encourage and assist in the establishment throughout India
- To affiliate or control and render assistance to any institution
- To undertake the research work and investigation on subjects concerning tuberculosis and allied chest diseases

Activities

- Organizing TB seal campaign every year to raise funds
- Publication of the prestigious Indian Journals of tuberculosis quarterly since 1953 and this is the only journal of India devoted exclusively to the cause of tuberculosis and chest diseases
- Providing up to date quality diagnostic and treatment services
- Supplementary revised National Tuberculosis Control Program and Directly Observed Therapy Shortcourse (DOTS) services of Government of India
- Increasing public awareness about the disease
- Involvement of community leaders in the control efforts
- Enlisting cooperation of patients and their families in seeking proper diagnosis and to complete treatment

HIND KUSHT NIVARAN SANGH

Hind Kusht Nivaran Sangh (HKNS) was established on 27th January 1925. Its precursor was the Indian Council of the British Empire Leprosy Relief Association (BELRA). It was renamed as LEPRA in 1950 after the independence. The headquarters of Hind Kusht Nivaran Sangh is at New Delhi. It was registered in 1950 under the registration of Societies Act 1860 as Hind Kusht Nivaran Sangh (Indian Leprosy Association). It is an old and prestigious body of people committed toward treatment, rehabilitation of leprosy patients and elimination of leprosy from India, Sangh has branches throughout India which are active in leprosy eradication program with the help of voluntary and government agencies.

Objectives

- To carry out research on various aspects of leprosy.

- To provide short courses of training and treatment of leprosy.
- To carry out propaganda.

Activities

- Production and dissemination of health education activities and publicity material on leprosy
- Publication of quarterly Indian journal of leprosy and bimonthly news bulletin Kusht vinashak for leprosy workers and the general public.
- Production and distribution of leprosy seals to create awareness about leprosy and help other organizations in raising funds for their work through the sale of these seals.
- Antileprosy day is observed on 30th January every year to create mass awareness about leprosy.
- Conducting training courses on nine months duration for physiotherapy technicians through leprosy training centers, i.e., Naini in Allahabad, Uttar Pradesh and Purulia in West-Bengal.
- Organizing the all India Leprosy Workers Conference and regional Leprosy Workers conferences in collaboration with the state branches and other voluntary organizations providing assistance to voluntary organizations and leprosy patients.
- Maintaining a house called "Shanti Illam" at Vellore (Tamil Nadu) where leprosy patients who come for surgical treatment at the Christian Medical College and Hospital, Vellore are provided free boarding and lodging facilities
- Running of two mobile leprosy treatment units in two districts of Delhi (Northeast and West) with funds provided by the Government of India
- Organizing exhibitions on leprosy in Delhi.

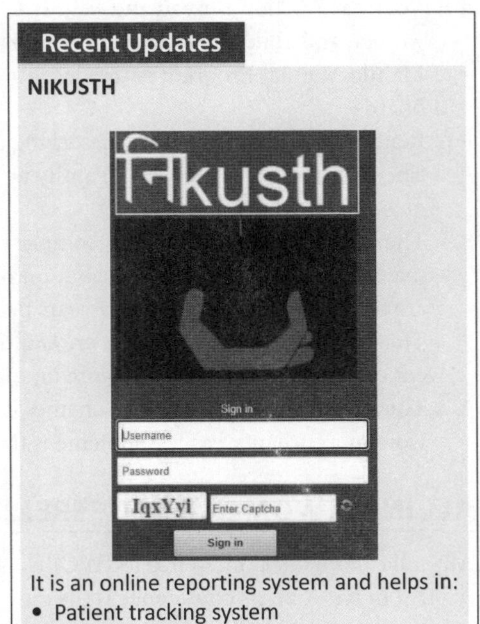

It is an online reporting system and helps in:
- Patient tracking system
- Early data analysis
- Prompt action

CENTRAL SOCIAL WELFARE BOARD

The Central Social Welfare Board (CSWB) is an autonomous, organization under the general administrative control of the ministry of education. It is an apex national body set up by the Government of India as an initiative of Pt Jawaharlal Nehru on 13th August 1953. It is also known as Kendriya Samaj Kalyan Board.

Objectives

- To bring a positive transformation in women's empowerment and economic development by reinforcing the spirit of voluntarism
- To recommend gender-specific policy initiatives to meet the new challenges for women and children in emerging areas.

- To strengthen voluntary organizations and expand coverage of 'engendered' schemes in areas where they have not reached.

Functions

- Surveying the needs and requirements of voluntary welfare organizations in the country.
- Promoting and setting up of social welfare organizations on a voluntary basis.
- Condensed courses of education and vocational training (CCE & VT).
- Awareness generation program for rural and poor women.
- The provision of support services to woman in the major thrust area of CSWB.
- Voluntary Action Bureau and Family Counseling Center is to provide rehabilitative services to women and children who are victims of family maladjustments and atrocities.
- Mahila Mandal Program is the decentralized program of the board and being run by the state boards.
- Rendering of financial aid to deserving existing organizations and institutions.
- The board initiated in 1968, "Family and Child Welfare Services" in rural areas for the welfare of women and children.
- The activities of the project comprise teaching of craft, social education, literary classes, maternity aid for women, distribution of milk, supplementary foods, and recreational facilities are provided to children of 3–5 years belonging to low income families.
- The welfare extension projects are multiprojects which extend services such as primary school education, craft activities for woman, maternity services and recreation facilities in rural areas.
- The board has also started a scheme of industrial cooperatives to help the lower-middle class woman in urban areas to supplement their family income by doing paid work.

ALL INDIA WOMEN'S CONFERENCE

All India Women's Conference (AIWC) is a nongovernmental organization based in Delhi.

All India women's conference is the only women's voluntary welfare organization in the country. It was formed in 1927 to function as an organization dedicated to upliftment and betterment of woman and children. It was registered in 1930 under the Societies Act XXI of 1850. It has >1,56,000 members in >500 branches of AIWC across the country. It is recognized as premier organization working for women's development and empowerment.

Objectives

- To work for a society based on the principle of social justice, personal integrity and equal rights and opportunities for all.
- To secure recognition of the inherent right of every human being to work and to achieve the essentials of life, by planned social distribution.
- To support the claim of every citizen to the right to enjoy basic civil liberties.
- To stand against all separatist tendencies and to promote greater national integration and unity.
- To work actively for the general program and welfare of women and children and to help women utilize fundamental right conferred on them by the constitution of India.
- To work for permanent international unity and world peace.

Functions

- Most of the branches of AIWC are running MCH clinics, health centers, adult education centers, milk centers and family planning clinics
- Organizes health and family welfare and population education program
- Organizes literary campaign and educational program
- Organizes socioeconomic activities
- Micro credit program to eradicate poverty among women
- Rural programs
- Establishes computer training centers
- Provides institutional care
- Integrated skill development and literacy program
- Scholarship program for women
- Legislation legal awareness
- Nonconventional and renewable energy
- Start textile printing units
- Research studies.

ALL INDIA BLIND RELIEF SOCIETY

All India Blind Relief Society (AIBRS) was established in 1946, in Mumbai with a view to coordinate different institutions working for the blind. It is India's largest voluntary organization working for the welfare of visually impaired people through a network of 65 regional branches and 24 state branches.

Vision

Empowered and well-informed visually challenged population of the country, thus enabling them to lead a life of dignity and productivity.

Mission

- Prevention of preventable and care of curable visual impairment
- Socioeconomic, rehabilitation of the visually challenged in main stream, through education, training and employment
- To take up advocacy against all types of individuals and structural discrimination and ensure full legal capacity
- Assure accessibility to the world of information

Functions

- Prevention of blindness
- Organizing eye relief camps
- Education
- Providing Audio books
- Vocational training
- Rehabilitation
- Research library and information
- Advocacy
- Recreation
- Community-based rehabilitation
- Women welfare

BHARAT SEVAK SAMAJ

Bharat Sevak Samaj (BSS) was formed in 1952. It is a nonpolitical, nongovernment, voluntary organization. It has branches in all states and in nearly all the districts.

Objectives

The main objective of BSS is to help people to achieve health by their own actions and efforts.

Activities

The main activities of the organization are:
- Improvement in the environmental sanitation in the rural areas.
- Education on environmental health.

KASTURBA MEMORIAL FUND

Kasturba Memorial Fund was created in commemoration of Kasturba Gandhi after her death in 1944. This fund was raised for the improvement of women's status.

Objectives

The main objective of this fund is to raise the standard of Indian women.

Activities

This fund is utilized for the programs and activities which benefit the women, especially in the villages through Gram Sevikas.

Summary

- The National and International Health Agencies play a vital role in the healthcare system.
- The standards, guidelines, laws and regulations, financial and technical aid, training of manpower, research in health and environment, assistance and support in implementing health related and other developmental programs in developing and developed countries are supported by the International Health Agencies.
- Since India is a member of the International Health Agencies, it is privileged to receive all types of aid in any kind.
- The main objective of WHO is the attainment of highest standard of health by all individuals without differentiating on the basis of cast, religion, politics; and social status is the fundamental right of each individual.
- UNFPA is an International Development Agency that promotes the right of every woman, man and child to enjoy life of health and equal opportunities.
- UNDP was established in 1966. Objective of UNDP is to help the poor countries in the development of human and natural resources.

Contd...

- World Bank provides low interest loans, interest free credits and grants to developing countries, provides financial assistance concerned with projects involving energy, transport, railway, industries, agriculture, education, family planning and health services.
- FAO helps nations in raising the living standard of people, improving nutrition, and growth of agriculture, fisheries and forestry, combating malnutrition and disseminating information and education.
- UNICEF was established to improve the health of mothers, infants and children's welfare.
- DANIDA works to select countries referred to as program countries and provides support to NGOs as well as government agencies, eradication of poverty and ensuring sustainable development.
- European Commission represents the interest of Europe as a whole, proposes new legislation to the European Parliament and Council of European Union and ensures European Union Law is correctly applied by the member countries.
- International Red Cross helps to improve the health of people of the countries who suffered during war, to strengthen and unite for health activities in already existing Red Cross Societies to promote the creation of new societies and to inspire, encourage, facilitate and promote at all times all form of humanitarianism.
- USAID's objectives are to promote economic prosperity, strengthen democracy, protect human rights, improve global health, advance food security and agriculture, improve environmental sanitation, education, help societies prevent and recover from conflicts.
- UNESCO's objective is to contribute to peace and securities in the world by promoting collaboration among nations through education, science, culture and communication.
- The objectives of ILO are to contribute to the establishment of social justice, lasting peace, to promote right at work, descent employment, enhance social protection and improve through international action the condition and living standard of labors.
- CARE was established in 1945. It is a major International Humanitarian Agency delivering broad spectrum emergency relief and long-term international development projects.
- The National Health Agencies are voluntary, nongovernmental, nonprofit making, nonpolitical agencies providing voluntary help to improve the health of the population and raise their living standard such as Indian Red Cross Society, Indian Council For Child Welfare, Family Planning Association of India, Tuberculosis Association of India, All India Blind Relief Society, etc.

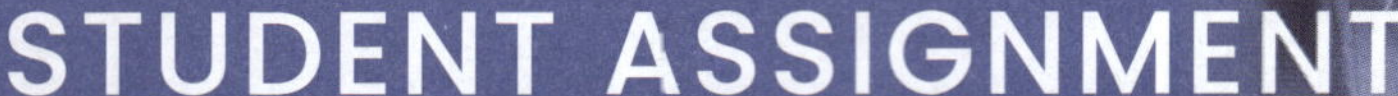

STUDENT ASSIGNMENT

LONG ANSWER TYPE QUESTIONS

1. Describe the functions of WHO.
2. Explain the activities of UNFPA and its role in India.
3. What is the objective of UNDP? How is UNDP financed? Describe its main functions.
4. State the aims of FAO and describe its functions.
5. What are the objectives of UNICEF? Explain its functions and its activities in India.
6. Who was the founder of International Red Cross? State its objectives and explain the main functions.
7. Describe briefly the functions of UNESCO.
8. List the objectives of CARE and explain its functions.

SHORT ANSWER TYPE QUESTIONS

1. Write about the structure of WHO.
2. What is the role of World Bank?
3. Write about the European Commission.
4. Write the functions of ILO.
5. State the functions of IRCS.
6. What are the activities of Tuberculosis Association of India?
7. Write the functions of Hind Kusht Nivaran Sangh.

MULTIPLE CHOICE QUESTIONS

1. **WHO was established in the year:**
   - a. 1946
   - b. 1948
   - c. 1951
   - d. 1960

2. **The principal organ of WHO:**
   - a. The world health assembly
   - b. The executive board
   - c. The secretarial
   - d. All of the above

3. **The main objective of WHO is:**
   - a. Achievement of highest standard of health by all individuals without differentiating on the basis of caste, religion, politics and social status
   - b. To provide monetary grants to countries
   - c. To extend technical help
   - d. None of the above

4. **The main areas of focus of UNFPA are:**
   a. Reproductive health
   b. Gender equality
   c. Population and development strategies
   d. All of the above

5. **UNDP was established in the year:**
   a. 1946
   c. 1950
   b. 1949
   d. 1966

6. **The focused area of UNDP is:**
   a. Supporting strategic planning for successful justice and security reforms through developing guidance on assessing needs and capacities and measuring impact
   b. Legal empowerment through supporting legal assistance and legal awareness
   c. Strengthening the position of women in different legal areas
   d. All of the above

7. **The World Bank was established in the year:**
   a. 1946
   c. 1947
   b. 1944
   d. 1950

8. **UNICEF was founded in the year:**
   a. 1945
   c. 1959
   b. 1946
   d. 1960

9. **The activities of UNICEF in India are:**
   a. Health and environment sanitation
   c. Education and social welfare
   b. Nutrition
   d. All of these

10. **European Commission was established in the year:**
    a. 1951
    c. 1958
    b. 1947
    d. 1960

11. **International Red Cross was founded in the year:**
    a. 1864
    c. 1929
    b. 1919
    d. 1944

12. **The focused areas of International Red Cross are:**
    a. Promoting humanitarian values
    b. Disaster response and disaster preparedness
    c. Health and community care
    d. All of the above

13. **The US government extends aid to India through:**
    a. United States Agency for International Development
    b. Public law 480 (food for peace)
    c. The US export-import bank
    d. All of the above

14. **The headquarters of UNESCO is in:**
    a. Colombo
    c. Paris
    b. Geneva
    d. Washington

15. **ILO was established in the year:**
   a. 1919
   b. 1922
   c. 1943
   d. 1948

16. **CARE was formed in the year:**
   a. 1920
   b. 1945
   c. 1948
   d. 1950

17. **The objectives of the Indian Red Cross society are:**
   a. To make Red Cross Societies and Communities more aware of the risks they face, how to reduce their vulnerability and how to cope when disaster strikes
   b. To influence the behavior of all the people
   c. To enable communities to reduce their vulnerability to disease and prepare for and respond to public health crisis
   d. All of the above

18. **The main objectives of Indian Council for Child Welfare are:**
   a. To promote the opportunity and facility for the development of the children
   b. To ensure the promotion of physical, social and mental health of children
   c. All of the above
   d. None of the above

19. **The headquarters of Family Planning Association of India is at:**
   a. New Delhi
   b. Mumbai
   c. Bengaluru
   d. Kolkata

20. **The Tuberculosis Association of India was formed in the year:**
   a. 1939
   b. 1949
   c. 1953
   d. 1954

21. **The objectives of Hind Kusht Nivaran Sangh are:**
   a. To carry out research on various aspects of leprosy
   b. To provide short courses of training and treatment of leprosy
   c. To carry out propaganda
   d. All of the above

22. **The Central Social Welfare Board was constituted in the year:**
   a. 1953
   b. 1959
   c. 1962
   d. 1964

23 **All India Women's Conference was established in the year:**
   a. 1926
   b. 1929
   c. 1940
   d. 1943

24 **The main functions of All India Blind Society are:**
   a. Prevention of preventable and care of curable visual impairment
   b. Socioeconomic rehabilitation of visually handicapped
   c. Education and vocational training
   d. All of the above

ANSWER KEY

1. b.	**2.** d.	**3.** a.	**4.** d.	**5.** d.	**6.** d.	**7.** b.	**8.** b.
9. d.	**10.** a.	**11.** a.	**12.** d.	**13.** d.	**14.** c.	**15.** a.	**16.** b.
17. d.	**18.** c.	**19.** b.	**20.** a.	**21.** d.	**22.** a.	**23.** a.	**24.** d.

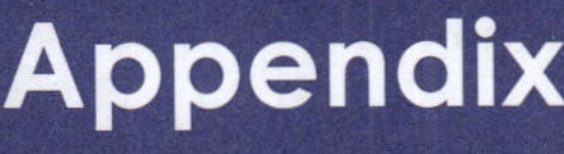

Management of Biomedical Waste

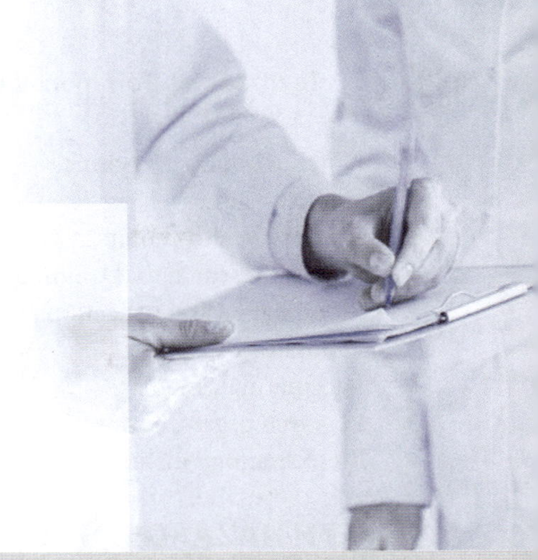

The waste produced in the course of healthcare activities carries higher risk of infection than any other type of waste. Inadequate and inappropriate handling of healthcare waste may have serious public health hazards and significant impact on environmental health. Therefore, it is essential to have safe methods of handling and disposal of healthcare waste.

The Biomedical Waste (Management and Handling) Rules, 1998 were notified under the Environment Protection Act, 1986 (29 of 1986) by the Ministry of Environment and Forest, Government of India on 20th July, 1998. The Act is now superseded by Biomedical Waste Management Rule-2016, which came into force from 28th March 2016. Guidelines have been prepared to enable each hospital to implement the said rules, by developing comprehensive plan to hospital waste management, in term of segregation, collection, treatment, transportation and disposal of the healthcare waste.

POLICY ON HEALTHCARE WASTE MANAGEMENT

The policy statement aims to provide a system for management of all potentially infections and hazardous waste in accordance with the Biomedical Waste (Management and Handling) Rules, 2016.

DEFINITION OF BIOMEDICAL WASTE

According to Biomedical Waste (Management and Handling) Rules, 1998 of India, "Biomedical waste means any waste, which is generated during the diagnosis, treatment or immunization of human beings or animals, or in research activities pertaining thereto or in the production or biological testings.

Between 75% and 90% of the waste produced by the healthcare providers is nonrisky or general. It comes from administrative and housekeeping functions of healthcare establishments, and may also include waste generated during maintenance of healthcare premises. The remaining 10–25% of healthcare waste is regarded as hazardous and may create a variety of health risk.

SOURCES OF HEALTHCARE WASTE

The institutions that generate healthcare waste are:
- Hospitals and dispensaries

- Nursing homes and clinics
- Dentist's clinics
- Primary health centers
- Medical research and training establishments
- Blood banks and collection centers
- Laboratories
- Vaccinating centers
- Research organizations
- Biotechnology institutions

HEALTH HAZARDS OF HEALTHCARE WASTE

The healthcare waste contains:
- Infectious agents
- Toxic or hazardous chemicals or pharmaceuticals
- Broken glass pieces of ampoules or vials
- Sharp needles, blades, etc.
- Healthcare waste may contain genotoxic and radioactive materials.

The healthcare workers who are at risk are:
- Doctors, nurses and paramedical staff
- Hospital maintenance personnel
- Patients in healthcare establishment
- Visitors to healthcare establishment
- Workers in support service allied to healthcare establishment such as laundries, waste handling and transportation.
- Workers in waste disposal facilities such as land-fills or incinerators including scavengers.

The hazards include:
- **Hazards from infectious waste:** The pathogens present in the waste may enter the human body through a puncture or abrasions on the skin or by inhalation, HIV, Hepatitis B and C have strong evidence of transmission via healthcare waste.
- **Hazardous from chemicals and pharmaceuticals:** These substances are toxic, genotoxic, corrosive, flammable, reactive, explosive or shock sensitive. The acute or chronic exposure to these chemicals and pharmaceuticals can cause injuries and burns, etc.
- **Hazardous from genotoxic waste:** The exposure to these genotoxic waste may occur during preparation of or treatment with particular drug. These chemicals enter the body either through inhalation of dust or aerosol. It may be absorbed through the skin.
- **Hazards from radioactive waste:** The type of disease caused by radioactive waste depends upon the type and extent of exposure. It may range from headache, dizziness, vomiting or it may affect genetic material.
- **Public sensitivity:** Apart from health hazards, the general public is very sensitive to visual impact of healthcare waste particularly the animal waste.

CATEGORIES OF BIOMEDICAL WASTE AND THEIR COLLECTION

The hazardous and toxic biomedical waste has been categorized for the purpose of safe transportation to a specific site for specific treatment. Certain categories of infectious waste require specific treatment (disinfection, decontamination) before transportation to disposal. These categories of biowaste for collection of color code container, their treatment and disposal option has been listed in Table 1.

TABLE 1: Categories of biomedical waste for collection of color code bags with their treatment and disposal option

Category	Type of waste	Type of bag to be used	Treatment and disposal option
Yellow	**Human anatomical waste:** Human tissues, organs, body parts and fetus below the viability period	Yellow-colored nonchlorinated plastic bags	Incineration or plasma pyrolysis or deep burial
	Animal anatomical waste: Experimental animals carcasses, body parts, organs, tissues including the waste generated from animals used in experiment or testing in veterinary hospitals or college or animal houses	do	Incineration or plasma pyrolysis a deep burial
	Soiled waste: Items contaminated with blood body fluids like dressing plaster casts, cotton swabs and bags containing residual or discarded blood and blood components	do	Incineration or plasma pyrolysis or deep burial. In the absence of above facilities, autoclaving or microwaving/hydroclaving followed by shredding or mutilation or combination of sterilization and shredding. Treated waste to be sent to energy recovery
	Expired or discarded medicines: Pharmaceutical waste like antibiotics, cytotoxic drugs including all items contaminated with cytotoxic drugs along with glass or plastic ampoules, vials, etc.	do	Expired cytotoxic drugs and items contaminated with cytotoxic drugs to be returned back to manufacturer or supplier for incineration at temperature >1200°C or to a common biomedical waste treatment facility hazardous waste treatment, storage and disposal facility for incineration >1200°C.
	Chemical waste: Chemicals used in production of biological and used or discarded disinfections	Yellow-colored nonchlorinated plastic bags	Disposed by incineration or plasma pyrolysis

Contd…

Category	Type of waste	Type of bag to be used	Treatment and disposal option
	Chemical liquid waste: Liquid waste generated due to use of chemicals and used or discarded disinfectants, silver X-ray films developing liquid, discarded formalin, infected secretions aspirated body fluids, liquid from laboratories and floor washing, cleaning, housekeeping and disinfectant activities, etc.	Separate collection system leading to effluent treatment system	After resource recovery, line chemical liquid waste shall be pretreated before mixing with other waste water. The combined discharge shall conform to the discharge norms given in Schedule III
	Discarded linen, mattresses beddings contaminated with blood or body fluid	Nonchlorinated yellow plastic bags or suitable packing material	Nonchlorinated chemical disinfection is followed by incineration or plasma pyrolysis or for energy recovery in the absence of above facilities, shredding or mutilation or combination of sterilization and shredding treated waste to be sent for energy recovery or incineration or plasma pyrolysis.
	Microbiology, biotechnology and other chemical laboratory waste – Blood bags, laboratory cultures, stocks or specimens of microorganism, live or attenuated vaccines, human and animal cell culture, used in research, industrial laboratories, production of biological residual toxins, dishes and devices used for culture	Autoclave safe plastic bags or container	Pretreat to sterilize with nonchlorinated chemicals on site as per National AIDS control organization or world health organization guidelines thereafter for incineration.
Red	**Contaminated waste (Recyclable):** Waste generated from disposable items such as tubings, bottles, Intravenous tubes and sets, catheters, urine bags, syringes (without needles and fixed needle syringes) and vacutainers (with their needles cut) and gloves	Red-colored nonchlorinated plastic bag of container	Autoclaving or microwaving/hydroclaving followed by shredding or mutilation or combination of sterilization and shredding, treated waste to be sent to registered or authorized recyclers or for energy recovery or plastic to diesel or fuel oil or for road making, whichever is possible. Plastic waste should not be sent to landfill site

Contd...

Category	Type of waste	Type of bag to be used	Treatment and disposal option
White translucent	**Waste sharp including metals:** Needles, syringes with fixed needles, needles from needle tip cutter or burner scalpel, blades or any other contaminated sharp object that may cause puncture and cuts. This includes both used, discarded and contaminated metal sharps	Puncture proof, leak proof tamper proof container	Autoclaving or dry heat sterilization followed by shredding or mutilation or encapsulation in metal container or cement concrete; combination of shredding cum autoclaving; and sent for final disposal to iron foundries (having consent to operate from the State Pollution Control Board of Pollution Control Committee) or sanitary landfill or designated concrete waste sharp pit
Blue (a)	**Glassware:** Broken or discarded and contaminated glass including medicine vials and ampoules except those contaminated with cytotoxic wastes	Cardboard boxes with blue-colored marking	Disinfection (By soaking the washed glass waste after cleaning with detergent and sodium hypochlorite treatment) or through autoclaving or microwaving or hydroclaving and then sent for recycling
Blue (b)	Metallic body implants	Cardboard boxes with blue-colored marking	

SEGREGATION OF BIOMEDICAL WASTE

It should be done at the site of generation of biomedical waste. This includes all patients care activity areas, diagnostic service areas, operation theaters, labor rooms, treatment rooms, dressing rooms, etc. The responsibility of segregation should be with the generation of biomedical waste, i.e., doctors, nurses, technicians, etc. The biomedical waste should be segregated as per the color coding plastic containers with symbols of biohazard and cytotoxic hazard.

The yellow plastic container (Fig. 1) with biohazard symbol is meant for receiving human tissues, organs, body parts, experimental animal carcasses, body parts, organs, tissues including their waste generated from animals, soiled dressing, linens, plaster casts, cotton swabs, bags containing residual blood and blood components.

The yellow container with symbol of cytotoxic hazard (Fig. 2) is meant to receive pharmaceutical waste, like cytotoxic drugs including all items contaminated with cytotoxic drugs along with glass or plastic ampoules, vials, all expired or discarded medicines, antibiotics, etc.

Contaminated Waste (Recyclable)

The waste generated from disposable items such as tubing, bottles, intravenous tubes and sets, catheters, urine bags, syringes (without needles and fixed needle syringes) and vacutainers (with their needles cut) and gloves should be received in red plastic containers.

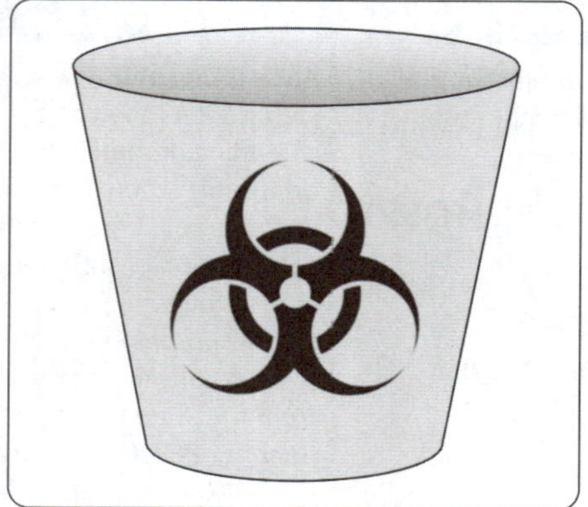

Figure 1: Container with biohazard symbol

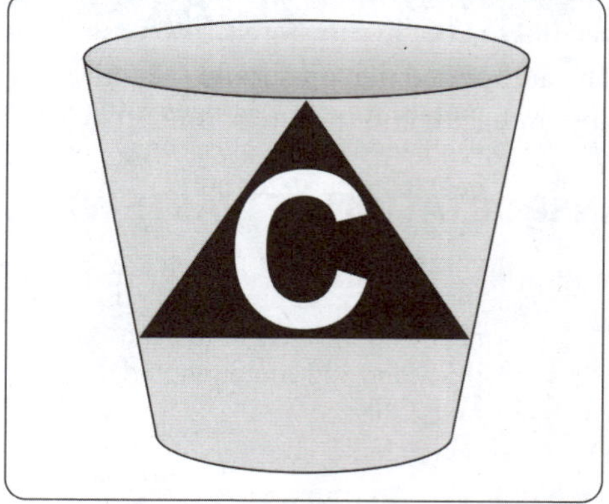

Figure 2: Bag with cytotoxic hazard symbol

Glassware

Broken or discarded and contaminated glass including medicine vials and ampoules except those contaminated with cytotoxic drugs.

Waste Sharp Including Metals

Needles, syringes with fixed needles, needles from needle tip cutter or burner, scalpels, blades or any other contaminated sharp object that may cause puncture and cuts. This includes both used, discarded and contaminated mental sharps.

General Waste

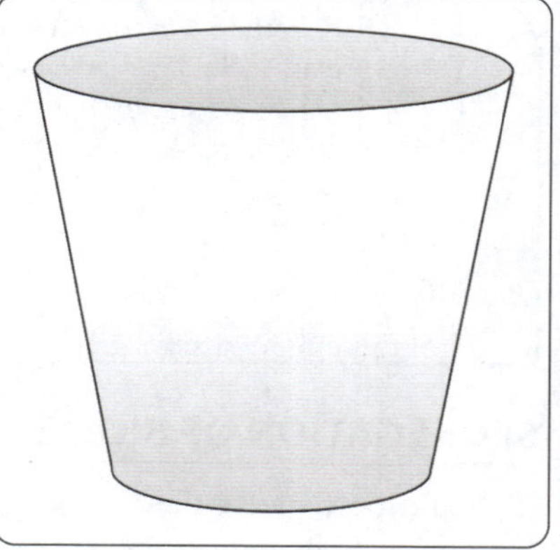

Figure 3: White container (translucent)

A separate container or bag of any color other than above mentioned color code, should be placed at every point of generation for general waste to be disposed of through municipal activity (Fig. 3).

COLLECTION OF BIOMEDICAL WASTE

The collection bags and the containers should be labeled as per guidelines of Schedule III, i.e. symbols for biohazards and cytotoxic hazards. A separate container shall be placed at every point of generation for general waste to be disposed of through municipal authority. The trolleys which can be used to collect hospital waste should be designed in such a way that there should be no leakage or spillage of biomedical waste while transporting to designated site.

STORAGE OF WASTE

Storage implies to the holding of biomedical waste for a certain period of time for treatment and final disposed.

- No untreated biomedical waste shall be kept stored beyond a period of 48 hours.

- The authorized person must take the permission of the prescribed authority, if for any reason it becomes necessary to store the waste beyond 48 hours.
- The authorized person should take measures to ensure that the waste does not adversely affect human health and the environment, in case it is kept beyond the prescribed time.

TRANSPORTATION OF WASTE WITHIN THE HOSPITAL

- Within the hospital, routes for the disposal of waste must be designated to avoid the passage of waste through patient care areas as far as possible.
- Separate time schedule should be prepared for the disposal of general waste and biomedical waste to reduce the chances of their mixing up.
- Dedicated wheeled containers, trolleys or carts with proper label (as per Schedule IV of Rule b) should be used to transport the waste from the site of storage to the site of treatment.
- Trolleys or carts should be thoroughly cleaned and disinfected in the event of any spillage.
- The wheeled containers should be designed in such a manner that the waste can be easily loaded, could remain secured during transportation, does not have any sharp edges and easy to clean and disinfect.

TRANSPORTATION OF WASTE FOR DISPOSAL OUTSIDE THE HOSPITAL

- Not withstanding anything contained in the Motor Vehicle Act, 1988 or rules thereunder, biomedical waste shall be transported only in such vehicles as may be authorized for the purpose by the competent authority.
- The containers for transportation must be labeled as given in Schedule III and IV of BMW 1998.

Safety Measures

The personnel handling the biomedical waste should wear disposable gloves, latex surgical gloves, heavy-duty rubber gloves (up to elbows) for the cleaners, simple and cheap mask to prevent healthcare workers against aerosols, splashes and dust protective glasses, plastic aprons, special footwear, etc.

- Immunization against hepatitis B and tetanus should be given to all hospital staff.
- Adopt universal precautions and appropriate safety measures while doing therapeutic and diagnostic activities and also while handling the biomedical waste.
- All the sanitation workers engaged in the handling and transporting should be made aware of the risks involved in handling the biomedical waste.
- Any worker reporting with an accident injury due to handling of biomedical waste should be given prompt first aid. Necessary investigations and follow-up actions as per requirement may be carried out.

TRAINING IN HANDLING BIOMEDICAL WASTE

- Each hospital should have well-planned awareness and training program for all categories of personnel including administrators to make them aware about safe hospital waste management practices.

- Training should be conducted category wise and emphasis should be given in training modules per category of personnel.
- Training should be conducted in appropriate language/medium and in an acceptable manner.
- Wherever possible audio-visual aids should be used and experienced trainers should be appointed for the training.
- Training about color coded bags, categorization and chemical disinfectant, can be given to the concerned employees.
- Training should include demonstration of lessons, behavioral science approach should be adopted with emphasis on established proper practices. Training is a continuous process and require constant reinforcement.

WASTE MANAGEMENT IN SUBCENTERS

Infection management and environment plan, "guidelines for healthcare workers for waste management and infection control in subcenters" of Ministry of Health and Family Welfare, Government of India are to be followed:

- A 2 m-deep pit or trench should be dug. It should be half filled with waste, then covered with lime within 50 cm of the surface before filling the rest of the pit with soil.
- It must be ensured that animals do not have any access to burial sites. Covers of galvanized iron/ wire meshes may be used.
- On each occasion, when wastes are added to the pit, a layer of 10 cm of soil shall be added to cover the wastes.
- Burial must be performed under close and dedicated supervision.
- The deep burial site should be relatively impermeable and no shallow well should be close to the site.
- The pits should be at a distant from habitation and sited so as to ensure that no contamination occurs of any surface water or ground water. The area should not be prone to flooding and erosion.
- The location of deep burial site will be authorized by the prescribed authority.
- The institution must maintain a record of all pits for deep burial.

Must Know

COVID-19 had serious impact on all aspects of our society including waste management. The biomedical waste during COVID-19 had increased amount of potentially infected waste which required additional careful handling and treatment process to safeguard the health of workers associated with such health care facilities. To safeguard the healthcare personnel and the community, following measures must be taken:

- Foot operated lids in color coded bins must be introduced to avoid contact.
- General solid waste should not be contaminated by patients' secretions and body fluids.
- All the waste handlers must follow the preventive measures such as hand washing, using gloves, wearing mask. In addition, gown should be worn while handling the biomedical waste of acute, highly infections life-threatening cases as happened during COVID-19 epidemic.

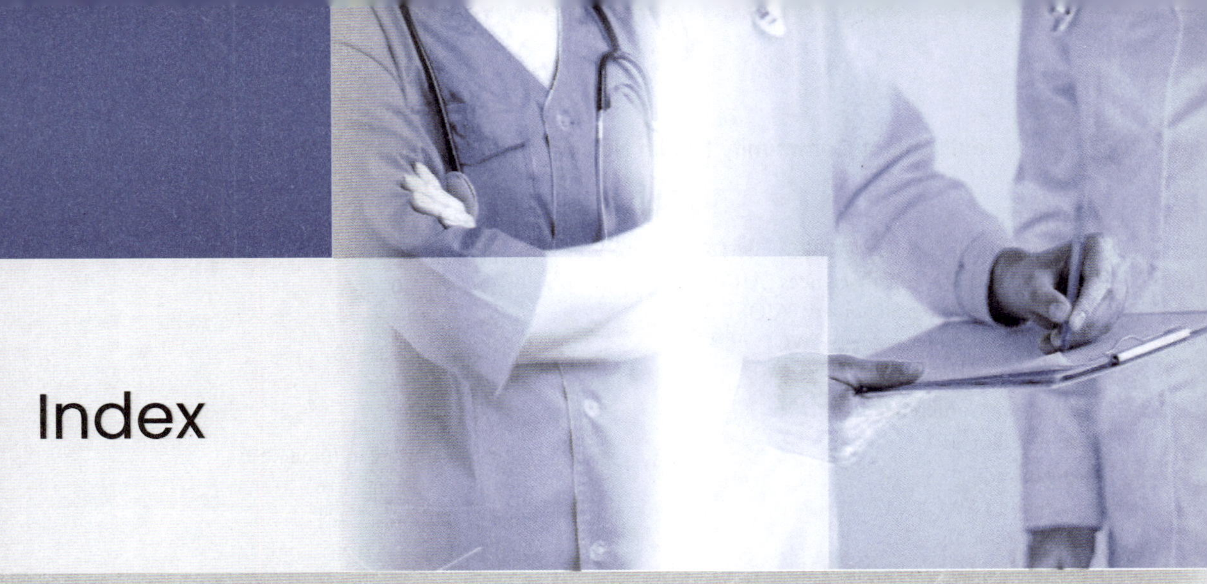

Index

Refer 'f' for figure and 't' for table respectively.

A

Abiotic factors 147
Abortion 313
   rate 290, 377
   ratio 290
Accelerated Rural Water Supply Program (ARWSP) 232
Accelerating
   toward leprosy free world 209
Accredited Social Health Activist (ASHA) 36, 340
Achievements of
   RNTCP 196
   the program 199
Acquired Immunodeficiency Syndrome
   (AIDS) 213, 285, 302
Active
   neglect 148
   surveillance 200
Activities
   of
      ASHA 207
      National Malaria Eradication Program 199
      NMHP 251
      team members 165
      the program 243
   under NACP 215
   undertaken for malaria control 198
Acute
   encephalitis syndrome 41, 358

flaccid paralysis (AFP) 239
respiratory
   diseases 175
   infection 29
      control program 187
Administrative units 247
Adolescent
   friendly health clinics (AFHC) 254
   health 39
      program 253
   Reproductive and Sexual Health
      Program 254
   services (ARSH) 253
Advantages
   and disadvantages of
      Cu-T 309t
      oral pills 310, 310t
   of
      planned small family 296
      single dose mass therapy 203
Aerosol-space spray 201
Age-specific
   fertility rate (ASFR) 288, 375
   marital fertility rate (ASMFR) 289, 377
Aims
   and objectives of family welfare 301
   of
      Family Welfare Program 325
      participation 259

All India
  Blind Relief Society (AIBRS) 59, 423
  Institute of Medical Sciences (AIIMS) 52
  Ophthalmological Society (AIOS) 221
  Women's Conference (AIWC) 59, 422
Allergic reaction 231
Alma-Ata Conference 1978 19
Amoxicillin 191
Anganwadi
  center (AWC) 247
  workers 35
Animal anatomical waste 431
Antiretroviral therapy (ART) 216
Anxiety 151
Applied Nutrition Program 133
Aspects of
  family welfare 301
  school health services 130
Ayurveda 54
Ayushman Bharat 33
  Program 236

B

Bag with cytotoxic hazard symbol 434*f*
Bajaj Committee (1986) 94
Ban on TB serology 197
Bar chart 383, 383*f*
Barrier/s
  methods 305
  of small family norms 297
Basal body temperature method 316
Basic
  health services 19, 24
  human needs 294
  principle/s
    for the single dose of DEC 203
    of the family welfare program 324
  statistical methods 381, 395
Benefits of
  DOTS 191
  fertility regulation 287
Bharat Sevak Samaj (BSS) 58, 424
Bhore Committee (1946) 89
Biological
  agents 135

hazards 137
Biomedical
  research 403
  waste 429, 436
Biostatistics 365, 373
Biotic factors 147
Birth
  and death rate in India 291
  control vaccine 316
Block health nurse 361
Body mass index (BMI) 255
Branches of rehabilitation 64
British Empire Leprosy Relief Association
  (BELRA) 420
Budget of
  UNDP 405
  WHO 402

C

Cancer 177
  services under the NCCP 242
Capreomycin 191
Cardiovascular
  disorders 177
  system 146
Cataract 179
Categories of
  biomedical waste 431, 431*t*
  mental retardation 162
Causes of
  blindness 160, 220*t*
  increase in elderly population 144
  infertility 293
  mental retardation 162
  population explosion 282
  speech impairment 158
Census 265, 369
Central
  auditory disorder 157
  Birth and Death Registration Act 1969 380
  Council of Health and Family Welfare 10
  Government Health Scheme (CGHS) 51, 127
  health education bureau 10
  Social Welfare Board (CSWB) 58, 421

Cervical mucus method 316
Chadha Committee (1963) 90
Characteristics of
    effective health team 346
    health
        information system 367, 368*f*
        team 341
    ideal contraceptive 304
Charaka Samhita 54
Chemical
    hazards 137
    liquid waste 432
    methods 306
    waste 431
Chief Executive Officer (CEO) 13
Child
    development officer 247
    health 37
        components 112
    mortality rate 256
    survival and safe motherhood (CSSM) 223, 327
Chittaranjan National Cancer Institute (CNCI) 241
Cholera 356
Chronic
    lung disease 178
    obstructive pulmonary disease (COPD) 148
Classification of
    disability 156
    hearing loss 157
    speech disorders 158
Clofazimine 191, 206
Coitus interruptus 315
Cold chain 224
College counseling services 252
Combined
    injectable contraception 312
    pills 310
Common problems of school children 130
Communicable diseases 174, 353, 356, 359
Community 1, 3
    -based
        MLOP 221
        nursing 5
        rehabilitation 166
        testing (CBT) 218
    Development Program 50

diagnosis 28
health 1, 4
    center (CHC) 16
    nurse 395
    nursing 1, 5
        team 341
    nursing centers 217
Complications of
    abortion 315
Components of
    DOTS 194
        treatment 191
    EMCP 200
    health information system 368, 369*f*
    minimum needs program 235*f*
    NMHP 251, 251*f*
Composition of health team at
    community health center 343, 343*t*
    primary health center 342, 342*t*
Compound bar chart 384
Comprehensive
    healthcare 19, 23
    primary healthcare (CPHC) 33, 122
Concept/s of
    family welfare 298, 299*f*
    fertility and infertility 285
    health team 340
    healthcare 20
    of health information system 394
Conductive hearing loss 157
Congenital 293
    disorder 160
Container with biohazard symbol 434*f*
Contaminated waste 432, 433
Contraception 288
Contraceptive
    methods 304, 305*t*
    services under NFWP 328
Contraindication of
    mifepristone and misoprostol 313
Copper T 308, 308*t*
Crude
    birth rate 292*f*
    rate 375
Cycle of planning 69*f*

D

Daily out patients (OPD) 252

Dais training 356

Dapsone 206

Data 365

Death rate 291, 375

Decline in fertility rate 278*t*

Deforestation 284

Delirium 150

Dementia 150

Demographic
- cycle 267
- goals 303
- processes 268
- profile of tribal population 255
- studies 267
- trends in
  - India 271
  - the world 268

Demography 265, 266

Dengue and chikungunya 41

Density of population 276
- in India 277*t*

Dental health 133

Depot medroxyprogesterone acetate (DMPA) 311

Designated microscopy center (DMC) 190

Detection of
- deafness 157
- speech disability 158

Diabetes mellitus 177

Diaphragm 306

Diarrheal
- disease/s 29, 175
  - control 107

Diastolic blood pressure 382*t*

Differences between
- district hospital and district health center 50*t*

Digestive system 145

Directly Observed Treatment Short-course (DOTS) 190

Directorate General of Health Services (DGHS) 8

Disability 154

Diseases
- due to
  - biological agents 138

chemical agents 138*t*
physical agents 138*t*
- of psychological origin 138

Distinction between
- data and information 366

Distribution of estimated population 274*t*

District
- Blindness Control Society (DBCS) 221
- health officer (DHO) 346
- mental health program 252
- Public Health Nursing Officer (DPHNO) 346

DOTS strategy 194

E

Early
- detection of diseases 129
- diagnosis and intervention 157

Education 295
- of handicapped children 134

Electronic Vaccine Intelligence Network (eVIN) 224

Emergency obstetric care 103, 108, 109

Empaneled healthcare providers (EHCPs) 237

Employees State Insurance
- Act, 1948 125
- Scheme (ESI) 51

Empowered action group 103, 108

Endocrine
- factors 293
- system 147

Enhanced Malaria Control Project (EMCP) 200

Eradication strategies 204

Ergonomics 103, 142

Esophagus 146

Essential
- newborn care 107
- obstetric care 106, 108

Ethambutol 191

Ethionamide 191

Eugenic 314

European
- Commission in India 410
- union law 425

Expanded program of immunization 186, 223

Eye
- Bank Association of India (EBAI) 221
- diseases 160

F

Facility-based
  counseling services 254
  newborn care (FBNC) 117
Factors affecting
  health planning 69
  national health planning 70
Family
  and child welfare services 422
  health awareness campaign 216
  life education 134
  Planning 38, 286, 302
    Association of India (FPAI) 59, 419
    counseling 320
    Insurance Scheme 128
  Welfare 298
    Program 300*f*
Features of
  CBR 166
Female
  health worker (FHW) 348
  infertility 293
  sterilization 318
Fertility 265
  regulating methods 304
Fever treatment depots (FTDs) 357
Fields of health information system 368
Filariasis 29, 176
First line regimen for drug sensitive TB 191
Food and Agriculture Organization (FAO) 283, 406
Freedom from hunger campaign (FFHC) 407
Frequency
  distribution table 382*t*
  polygon 365, 385, 385*f*
Function of
  IRLs 190
  vital statistics 374
Functional household tap connection (FHTC) 233
Functionaries of
  NFWP at center level 327
Functions of
  executive board 401
  health team 344
  NIHFW 328
  nursing personnel in occupational health 143

  primary health center 46*f*
  school health nurse 135
  secretariat 402
  state health directorate 12*f*
  the central organization 203
  UNDP 405
  UNFPA 404
  WHO 402
  World Health Assembly 401

G

General
  fertility rate (GFR) 288, 377
  functions of Directorate General of Health
    Services 9*f*
  marital fertility rate (GMFR) 288, 375
  marriage rate (GMR) 290, 377
  principle of tabulation 381
Genitourinary system 146
Geriatric nursing 144
Gerontological nursing 103
Gerontology 103
Glassware 433, 434
Global
  leprosy strategy 209
  scenario 204
  warming 284
Goal of
  NLEP 205
Gonadotrophic suppression 293
Gonadotropin-releasing hormone (GnRH) 293
Government Health Insurance Schemes 124, 168
Gram
  Panchayat 1, 15
  Sabha 1, 15
Gross reproductive rate (GRR) 289, 378
Growth rate 265, 271, 272, 292
Guinea Worm Eradication Program in India 204

H

Hazards
  from
    infectious waste 430
    radioactive waste 430

of
immunization 231
unplanned large family 295
Health 2, 295
aspects 301, 304
under occupational health services 139
assessment 153
checkup 248
committees and reports 88
education 133
and counseling 140
finance 99
hazards of healthcare waste 430
information system (HIS) 365, 366, 367, 394
insurance 124
schemes 125
intelligence 10
management information 99
system 366
manpower statistics 371
organization at the
central level 6, 6f
district level 12
state level 10
planning 69
problems in India 174, 174f
sector planning 72
statistics 365
system 1, 16
performance 98
strengthening 99
team 339
Healthcare 19, 340, 361
agencies 50
model 27
services 20
system 21
in public sector 32f
Hearing 145
and speech disability 156
Hereditary factors 147
High
birth rate 282, 290
-dose isoniazid 191
Hind Kusht Nivaran Sangh (HKNS) 57, 420
Histogram 365, 384, 384f
Historical development of
family welfare program 326

Home-based newborn care 115
Homeopathy system of medicine 55
Hormonal 311
device LNG-20 309
Hormone releasing IUDS 309
Hospital-based MLOP 221
Human
anatomical waste 431
chorionic gonadotropin (hCG) 316
health resource 258
resources 210
Hypertension 150, 176, 257
Hypospadias 293

I

Immunization 37, 107, 247
Impact of
population explosion 283, 283f
Importance of
family welfare 300
Inactivated poliovirus vaccine (IPV) 240
Incidence
of infertility 293
rate 378
Income tax exemption 153
India Newborn Action Plan (INAP) 327
Indian
council for child welfare (ICCW) 58, 418
leprosy association 420
medical association (IMA) 221
Penal Code (IPC) 314
Red Cross Society (IRCS) 57, 417, 425
System of Medicine (ISM) 285, 323
Indigenous system of medicine (ISM) 53
Individual family planning counseling 321
Infant mortality 255
rate 376
Infertility 266
Information
education and communication (IEC) 217
system 219, 365, 366
Ingestion 137
Inhalation 137
Injectable
contraceptive 311
inactivated poliovirus vaccine 240

Institutional-based rehabilitation 166
Integrated
    Child Development Scheme (ICDS) 35, 246
        program 246
    counseling and testing center (ICTC) 217, 254
    management of neonatal and childhood illness
        (IMNCI) 114, 117, 409
    set-up at the district level 14*f*
    vector control program 358
Integumentary system 146
Intelligent quotient 103
Intensified Malaria Control Project 200
Intermediate reference laboratories (IRLs) 190
Internal sterilization 318
International
    Classification of Impairment, Disabilities and
        Handicaps (ICIDH) 154
    conference on population development
        (ICPD) 324
    development agency 424
    Federation of
        Antileprosy Association (ILEP) 209
        Red Cross (IFRC) 412
    health
        agencies 399, 400
        relations and quarantine 9
    Labor Organization (ILO) 415
    Red Cross 411, 425
Intraocular lens 173
Intrauterine device (IUD) 351
Iodine deficiency 186
    disorder/s 180
        control program 222
Isoniazid 191

J

Jal Jeevan Mission (JJM) 233
Janani
    Shishu Suraksha Karyakram (JSSK) 121, 122
    Suraksha Yojana (JSY) 110, 121
Japanese encephalitis 41, 353, 358
Jungalwalla Committee (1967) 92
Juvenile mass treatment 243

K

Kala-azar 353, 358
    elimination 41
        plan 122
Kanamycin 191
Kartar Singh Committee (1973) 92
Kasturba Memorial Fund 58, 424
Kendriya Samaj Kalyan Board 421

L

Lady health visitor (LHV) 348, 350
Laparoscopic sterilization 319
Leprosy 29, 175, 256, 354
    in India 57
Level/s
    of
        healthcare system 21
        urbanization in the country 278*f*
Life expectancy 255, 266, 281
Linezolid 191
Lippes loop 308, 308*f*
Literacy rate in India 279*f*
Liver 146
Long-
    acting pills 310
    time measure 89
Low
    birthweight babies 180
    stationary 267
Lymphatic filariasis 41, 353

M

Mahila Mandal Program 422
Major
    health problems in India 186
    initiatives 206
        under NHRM 120
    interventions under RCH-1 106
Malaria 29, 174, 353, 357
    action plan (MAP) 199
    and other vector-borne diseases 257

Male
    health worker (MHW) 348
    infertility 293
    sterilization 317
Malnutrition 150, 160
Management
    of
        infertility 294
        locomotors 155
        mentally handicapped 163
        stress 152
        visually handicapped 161
    protocol of MDR-TB and pregnancy 193*f*
Manual vacuum aspiration (MVA) 110
    technique 315
Mass
    drug administration (MDA) 173, 353
    media 324
Maternal
    and child health (MCH) 11, 244, 297, 349
        wings 122
    health 37
    mortality 255
        rate 376
Mean 365, 387
Measles 188
Measure of variability 388
Median 365, 388
    of diastolic blood pressure 388*t*
Medical
    and nonmedical health team 340
    care problems 30, 181
    education 9
    literature analysis and retrieval system
        (MEDLARS) 403
    method of abortions 110
    officer (MO) 242, 351
    rehabilitation 166
    research 9
    store depots 9
    team dealing emergency ambulance services 124
    Termination of Pregnancy 118, 297, 351, 354
        Act 1971 314
Mehta Committee (1983) 94
Menstrual
    hygiene 254
    induction 313
    regulations (MR) 312

Mental
    disorders 178
    Health 133
        and addiction 257
        Policy 250
    retardation and mentally handicapped 161
Method/s
    of family planning 304
    to regulate fertility 288
Midday Meal 132
    Program 248
    Scheme 249
Millennium development goals (MDG) 324
Mini pills 310
Minilap operation 319
Minimum Needs Program (MNP) 47, 235
Ministry of Health and Family Welfare 118
Mirena 309
Mixed hearing loss 157
MMR
    and chicken pox vaccines 188
Mode 365, 388
    of action of oral pills 310
Model of
    healthcare
        delivery system 28*f*
        system in India 31*f*
    primary level of healthcare 22*f*
    referral system 23*f*
    secondary level of healthcare 22*f*
Morbidity 378
    indicators 395
    management and disability prevention
        (MMDP) 202
Moxifloxacin 191
Mudaliar Committee 90
Mukherjee Committee 91
Multidrug therapy 186
Multiload-375 309
Multiple bar charts 384
Municipal
    board 13
    corporation 13
Municipality 13
Musculoskeletal system 146

N

National
AIDS
control
organization (NACO) 214
program 213
Prevention and Control Policy (NAPCP) 214
ambulance service 121
and International Health Agencies 424
Antimalaria Program 198
blindness control programs 358
Cancer Control Program 241
Council of AIDS (NCA) 214
development council 74
diabetes control program 238
drinking water mission (NDWM) 232
Family
Planning Insurance Scheme (NFPIS) 328
welfare policy 322
welfare program 231, 323
Filaria Control Program (NFCP) 201
Guinea Worm Eradication Program 204
health
agencies 400
mission 103, 117
planning 70
policy 94
programs 60, 187
protection scheme 237
immunization
day (NID) 239
schedule for infants 225*t*
Institute of
Communicable Diseases (NICD) 243
Family Planning (NIFP) 328
health
administration and education
(NIHAE) 328
and Family Welfare (NIHFW) 327, 328
mental health and neuroscience 52
Iodine Deficiency Disorders Control Program
(NIDDCP) 41, 222
iron-plus 122
Leprosy Eradication Program (NLEP) 40, 204,
358
Malaria Control Program 40
medical library 10
Mental Health Program (NMHP) 250
mobile medical unit 121
Nutritional Anemia Prophylaxis Program
(NNAPP) 244
pediatric AIDS initiative 216
Program for
Control of Blindness (NPCB) 219
and Visual Impairment (NPCBVI) 257
Healthcare for Elderly (NPHCE) 152
reference laboratories (NRLs) 190
Rural
Drinking Water Program (NRDWP) 233
health mission 119
sanitation program 233
socio-demographic goals 323
STD control program 218
strategic plan for TB elimination 196
Tuberculosis Elimination Program 39
Urban Health Mission (NUHM) 118
Vector-Borne Disease Control Program
(NVBDCP) 40, 357
voluntary health agencies of India 417
Water Supply and Sanitation Program 232
Natural family planning methods 316
Naturopathy system 56
Navjaat Shishu Suraksha Karyakram (NSSK) 115, 117
Neonatal mortality rate 376
Nervous system 145
Net reproduction rate (NRR) 289, 378
Nikshay 197
Nirmal Bharat Abhiyan (NBA) 234
NITI Aayog 67, 72, 88
Nodal organization 214
Noncommunicable
disease/s 176, 257, 354, 359
problems 29
Nongovernmental Organizations (NGOs) 406
Norethisterone enanthate (NET-EN) 311
No-scalpel vasectomy (NSV) 288, 317
Nursing management of
neurological and psychological problems 150
physiological problems 150
Nutrition 39, 134, 286
Nutritional
anemia 180
health education 247

problems 29, 179
rehabilitation centers (NRCs) 112
Nyaya panchayat 1, 15

O

Objectives
of
NAPCP 214
national health planning 71
NNPP 284
RNTCP 189
Occupational
cancers 138
dermatosis 138
diseases 138
environment 135
eye health services 221
hazards 136, 136*f*
health
nursing 141, 142
services 139
healthcare team 141
Oral
abortifacient 313
cavity 145
healthcare 179
pills 310
polio vaccine (OPV) 239, 240
Organization of
Directorate General of Health Services 8*f*
health system in India 6, 6*f*
National Family Welfare Program 327
Revised National Tuberculosis Control Program
(RNTCP) 189, 189*f*
at state level 198
State Ministry of Health 11*f*
Union Ministry of Health and Family Welfare 7*f*
Osteoporosis 150
Other backward classes (OBC) 301
Outpatient health facility 115

P

Pancha Mahabhutas 54
Panchayat Samiti 1
at the block level 15

Panchayati Raj
at village level 15
institutions (PRIs) 232
system 14
Para-aminosalicylic acid 191
Perinatal mortality rate 376
Period prevalence 379
Periodical health check-up 139
Permanent disablement benefit 126
Phases of
National AIDS Control Program 215, 215*f*
Pictogram/s 366, 386
Pie
charts 385
diagram 386*f*
Plague 356
Planning 67, 68
Commission 71
for responsible parenthood 300, 302
Pneumococcal
conjugate vaccine (PCV) 226
vaccines 188
Polio eradication—pulse polio program 239
Poliomyelitis 356
Population
-based nursing 5
density 266
explosion 28, 282, 298
of India 271*t*, 382*t*
in different years 382*t*
per physician in different countries 387*f*
problems 30, 182
Postcoital contraception 311
Postconceptional methods 312
Postgraduate Institute (PGI) 52
Postpartum sterilization 318
Poverty 283
line 298
Pradhan Mantri Jan Arogya Yojana (PMJAY) 237
Pregnancy
rate (PR) 289, 377
with MDR-TB 193
Premature retinopathy 160
Prevalence
of disease 205
rate 379
states present in the country 213

Prevention
  and control of
    anemia 107
    respiratory diseases 188
    vitamin A deficiency in children 107
  of
    communicable diseases 131
    malnutrition 409
    mental retardation 162
Primary
  care concept 161
  eye care 160, 220
  health center (PHC) 16, 45, 348, 351
  healthcare 19, 24, 219
    in India 32
  infertility 293
Principles of
  fertility regulation 287
  hospital-based management 113
  IMNCI guidelines 114
  Swajaldhara 233
Problem implementation plans (PIPs) 328
Progestogen-only
  injectable 311
  pills (POP) 310
Program/s
  implementation plan 208
  integrated to NRHM 120
  leadership 210
  management 243
  strategy 208
Proportional mortality rate (PMR) 378
Protein-energy
  malnutrition (PEM) 29
  undernutrition (PEU) 180
Prothionamide 191
Provision of
  TB health visitors 256
  welfare facilities 140
Psychological
  rehabilitation 166
  hazards 138
Public
  health 3
    engineering departments (PHED) 232
    nurse (PHN) 339, 348, 361
    sector 31
  -private partnership (PPP) 52

Pulse polio
  immunization program 224
  initiative (PPI) 239
Pyrazinamide 191

R

Radiations 137
Rajiv Gandhi
  National Drinking Water Mission
    (RGNDWM) 232
  Shramik Kalyan Yojana 127
Ramalingaswami Committee (1992) 94
Rashtriya
  Bal Swasthya Karyakram (RBSK) 121
  Kishor Swasthya Karyakram (RKSK) 121
  Swasthya Bima Yojana (RSBY) 237
Red cross
  services 418
  societies 425
Referrals health facility 115
Regional
  cancer center scheme 241
  certification commission (RCC) 240
  Institute of Ophthalmology (RIO) 220
Rehabilitation 155, 158
  allowance 127
  medicine 63
  nursing 163
  phase 113
  services
    for visually handicapped 161
    in India 167
  team 165
Reproductive
  and Child Health (RCH)
    Program 104
    services 103
    tract infections (RTI) 285, 323
Respiratory system 146
Revised
  midday meal scheme 250
  National
    Cancer Control Program 241
    Tuberculosis Control Program
      (RNTCP) 189, 359
Rifampicin 191, 206
Rogi Kalyan Samiti (RKS) 120, 329

Role of
a nurse in National Health Programs 258
district public health nursing officer 346, 346f
geriatric nurse in management of geriatric
people 149
health
assistant 352
worker 354
nurses in healthcare services 60f
public health nurse 349
school health nurse 134
UNDP in India 405
UNFPA in India 404
Rural
administration 14
hospitals 50
Sanitation Program 233

S

Sample registration system (SRS) 370
Schedule tribal component (STC) 258
School
AIDS education program 216
eye health services 220
health
administration 134
committee 134
records 134, 135
services 128
mental health services 252
Secondary
infection 219
infertility 293
prevention 155, 162
Secretariat 401
Sector diagram 385
Selective mass treatment 243
Sensitive TB pediatric cases 192t
Sensory neural hearing loss 157
Sex ratio 255, 274
at birth 275
Sexually transmitted infection (STI) 323
Shanti illam 421
Short
course chemotherapy 186
-term measure 89

Siddha medicine system 54
Social
rehabilitation 166
welfare measures 219
Socio-economic caste census (SECC) 237
Soiled waste 431
Sources of
demography 268
health information system 369
Sparsh 210
leprosy awareness campaign 208
Specific
death rate 376
rate 375
Sperm granules 318
Spontaneous recanalization 318
Srivastava Committee (1974–1975) 93
Stabilization phase 113
Stages of
demographic transition 267f
Standard deviation 390
State
cancer institute (SCI) 242
health directorate 11
Institute of Health and Family Welfare
(SIHFW) 328
Ministry of Health 11
-wise literacy rate in India 280t
Statista 373
Statistic/s 366, 373
maps 386
Statistical data 381
Steps of
health planning 73
planning 68
in health sector 73f
problem solving 346f
Sterilization 288
Stomach 146
Strategic
implementation of RNTCP 194
pillars and roadmap for leprosy 210
plan for vision 2020 221
Strategies
of
family welfare program 324

intervention 253
    NUHM 118
    RNTCP, India (2019) 196
    the program 220, 243
  to control STDs 219
  for leprosy eradication till 2027 211*f*
Stress 151
Stroke/s 150, 179
Structure of Panchayati Raj institution at village
  level 15*f*
Suicide prevention services 253
Survey education and treatment (SET) 208
Sustainable development goals (SDGs) 33
Swachh Bharat Mission–
  Gramin (SBM–G) 234
  Urban (SBM–U) 234
Swajaldhara 233
Systemic diseases 160

T

Technical Cooperation Mission (TCM) 413
Temporary disablement benefit (TDB) 126
Total
  dependency ratio 276
  fertility rate (TFR) 284, 289, 377
  marital fertility rate (TMFR) 289, 378
  mass treatment 243
Town area committee 13
Traditional tubectomy 318
Transfusion transmissible infection (TTIs) 216
Translucent 434*f*
Treatment
  of TB under RNTCP 190
  plan for drug sensitive TB adults 191
Triage 113
Tribal
  health 255
  sub plan (TSP) 258
Tropical disease 400
Tubectomy 318*f*
Tuberculin reaction 385*t*
Tuberculosis (TB) 29, 175, 256, 302, 354
  Association of India (TAI) 58, 420

Type/s
  of
    averages 387
    bar charts 384
    contraceptives 305
    copper T available 309*t*
    health services 60
    IUDs currently in use 307*f*
    rehabilitation 166, 166*f*
    surveys 372

U

Ultraviolet (UV) radiation 137
Unani system of medicine 55
Union
  Ministry of Health and Family Welfare 7
  territory councils 418
United
  Nations
    Development Program (UNDP) 404
    Educational, Scientific and Cultural
      Organization (UNESCO) 413
    Fund for Population Activities (UNFPA) 271,
      404
    International Children's Emergency Fund
      (UNICEF) 407
  States Agency for International Development
    (USAID) 329, 412
Universal
  health coverage (UHC) 33, 122
  Immunization Program (UIP) 223, 354, 356
  NCDs screening 41
Urban
  administration 13
  basic services (UBS) 409
  community health center 119
  local bodies (ULBs) 235
  Malaria Scheme (UMS) 200
  primary health center 119
  Sanitation Program 233
Urinary incontinence 150
Uses of
  health information system 368
  vital health records 381

V

Vaginal
   rings 312
   sponge 306
Vande Mataram Scheme 111
Vasectomy 317, 317*f*
Village Health
   Guide (VHG) 328
   Sanitation and Nutrition Committee
      (VHSNC) 121
Vision 145
Vital
   health record 380
   statistics 366, 372
Vitamin A prophylaxis 221
Vocational rehabilitation 166
Voluntary
   Action Bureau and Family Counseling
      Center 422
   counseling and testing centers (VCTC) 217
   health services 57

W

White container 434*f*
Widowhood 147
Workplace stress management 252
World 159
   Bank 400, 405
      in India 406
   Health
      Assembly 401
      Organization (WHO) 367, 400
   Leprosy Day (WLD) 210

X

Xerophthalmia 180

Y

Yaws Eradication Program 242
Yoga 56

Z

Zila Parishad 16

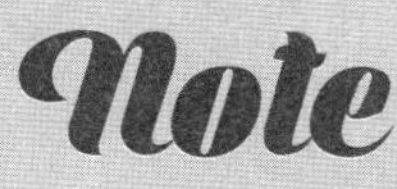

Note

Note